Dentine Hypersensitivity

David G. Gillam
Editor

Dentine Hypersensitivity

Advances in Diagnosis, Management, and Treatment

Second Edition

Springer

Editor
David G. Gillam
Centre for Oral Bioengineering,
Institute of Dentistry
Barts and the London School
of Medicine and Dentistry
Queen Mary University of London
London, UK

ISBN 978-3-031-74323-8 ISBN 978-3-031-74321-4 (eBook)
https://doi.org/10.1007/978-3-031-74321-4

This Springer imprint is published by the registered company Springer Nature Switzerland AG
The registered company address is: Gewerbestrasse 11, 6330 Cham, Switzerland

I would like to extend my sincere gratitude to my friends and colleagues, who are established individuals in their respective fields of research and clinical practice, for their generosity in sharing their time and energy to contribute to this book. I would also like to extend my appreciation to Dr. Alison Wolf (Springer), who initially discussed with me the possibility of editing a book to provide an overview on dentine hypersensitivity to both educate and update readers on the latest advances in research and the practical implications for everyday clinical practice. My appreciation is also extended to Professor Gottfried Schmalz, who kindly provided the foreword for this book, and to Dr. Ken Markowitz for the helpful comments during the proofreading of the book chapters. I would also like to extend my gratitude to the staff at Springer for their support and encouragement throughout the preparation and publication of this book. Finally, I would like to express my appreciation to my family, particularly my wife Joyce, for her understanding, constant support, and patience throughout my professional career.

Foreword

Dentine hypersensitivity has gained increasing interest in recent years due to several reasons. For example, the success of caries prevention programs and improved periodontal treatment modalities are factors considered to be responsible for an increased number of patients of all ages having more natural teeth than in the past. Consequently, these patients apparently suffer more frequently from what they call "sensitive teeth" (dentine hypersensitivity), mainly after exposure to cold and sweet drinks/food or to tactile stimuli. The quality of life of these patients is markedly compromised, and they may ask the clinician for pain relief. This is a challenge for both the dental clinician and the dental scientific community. It is reflected, for example, in a constantly increasing number of publications in the scientific literature, scientific workshops, and continuing education courses over the past two decades on the topic. It is known that patients with dentine hypersensitivity also exhibit gingival recession, sometimes as a sequel of periodontal treatment. They also experience the loss of enamel, e.g., due to increased consumption of erosive drinks and other acidic food products, extensive tooth brushing with abrasives in the toothpaste, or other factors. This may lead to exposed dentine surfaces, which are a prerequisite for dentine hypersensitivity. However, it should be noted that not all exposed dentine surfaces lead to dentine hypersensitivity. Further light on the topic was provided by the introduction of the hydrodynamic theory, as first proposed by Gysi around 1900 and then further elaborated by Martin Brännström in the middle of the last century. The open dentine tubules on the exposed dentine surface have been considered essential for the fluid shifts in the dentine tubules following thermal, osmotic, or other stimulation, subsequently activating mechanoreceptors at the nerve endings associated with the odontoblast processes close to the pulp. However, not all phenomena can be satisfactorily explained by this theory. For instance, the role of pulp inflammation, tertiary dentine formation, nerve transduction, occlusal stress responsible for cervical abfractions, and periodontal involvement is still being discussed in this context. Thus, further research on dentine hypersensitivity needs a multidisciplinary approach, involving the classical discipline of operative dentistry but also periodontology, endodontics, including pulp biology, immunology, occlusal stress, and the essential aspects of prevention of the condition.

Manufacturers of cosmetics (e.g., toothpaste and mouth rinse products) and dental materials (e.g., dentine adhesives and desensitizing products) have rapidly responded to the needs of both patients and dental professionals by introducing a wide range of products into the consumer market for the treatment of dentine hypersensitivity. Different approaches to reduce dentine hypersensitivity have been developed; most of these products are based on the concept of covering or obturating the tubule openings on the exposed dentine surface. Both the potential effectiveness and clinical efficacy have often been demonstrated by in vitro studies and mainly short-term clinical trials, respectively. Again, several problems have arisen, for example, the clinical relevance of the in vitro tests used in this context, the mainly limited efficacy of these treatments, with the need for constant application, the lack of pain relief in certain cases, or the question of possible pulp damage induced by certain therapies. Dentine hypersensitivity is a challenge, and this book addresses the challenge posed by this condition. Here, all aspects of dentine hypersensitivity are comprehensively covered and updated. The array of topics ranges from basic research on etiology to treatment modalities and finally to preventive aspects, including patient communication, motivation, and compliance. A group of well-known authors from both clinical and laboratory research, under the wise guidance of David Gillam, have not only provided a compilation of the relevant evidence from the published literature but also critically pinpointed the weaknesses of the presently available information and the missing gaps in our understanding of dentine hypersensitivity. Finally, interesting ideas for the formulation of new products and an innovative design for future studies are presented. Reading this book is certainly a gain not only for researchers but also for the clinician.

Chairman ISO TC 106 Dentistry
Poliklinik für Zahnerhaltung und Parodontologie/
Department for Conservative Dentistry
and Periodontology
Regensburg, Germany
gottfried.schmalz@ukr.de

Prof. Dr. Dr. h.c.mult.
Gottfried Schultz

Acknowledgements

The authors would like to acknowledge the contributions of our colleagues in the development and evaluation of the novel products currently being developed at QMUL, namely: Professor Graham Davis, Professor Mangala Patel, Professor Delia Brauer, Dr. Natalia Karpukhina, Professor Padhraig Fleming, Dr. Saroash Shahid, Dr. Melissa Tiskaya, as well as the numerous undergraduate and postgraduate students who have been invaluable in these formative studies.

Disclosure Statement

The authors have one or more patents on the bioactive glass formulations and other oral care products and are currently directors of BioMin Technology Ltd, UK.

Contents

Introduction and Overview: Statement of the Problem

1

Martin Addy and David G. Gillam

1.1 Aim and Objective

It is more than four decades since dentine hypersensitivity (DH) was described as "an enigma being frequently encountered but ill-understood" (Johnson et al. 1982). Since this time, the "three R's" of research, writing and review have, considerably but not completely, improved the understanding of DH. This said surveys, in several countries, suggest that DH remains ill-understood by a considerable proportion of dental healthcare professionals (Canadian Advisory Board on Dentine Hypersensitivity 2003; Rao et al. 2010). With respect, it would not seem unreasonable or derogatory to suggest that the topic of DH has received limited attention in dental undergraduate and postgraduate curricula. Also, it would appear the plethora of literature on the subject which has grown enormously over relatively recent years has been read by a minority of dental professionals. The overall aim of this book must be therefore to address this imbalance in the understanding of the problem. Specifically using question-based, section headings, the aim of this first chapter is to provide a brief overview of DH, including current concepts of the condition and possible future innovations in diagnosis, management and treatment. The hoped-for objective is to provide a basis for subsequent chapters and authors to detail specific aspects of the diagnosis, management and treatment of DH.

1.2 How Common Is Dentine Hypersensitivity?

There have been several surveys on the prevalence and distribution of DH in a variety of subject groups (for reviews, see Addy 2000, 2002; West 2006) (Chap. 2), but whether any used selection protocols for classical population based epidemiological studies is open to question. Indeed, some were only from patients attending dental practices or hospitals, or question and answer only based studies and several predated the now agreed definition of the condition and may have included subjects that would be excluded by the said definition: one frequently quoted study was published only as an abstract (Graf and Galasse 1977). This all said, averaging across studies spanning nearly 35 years, that used a dental inspection, suggests that 15% of adults suffer from DH from one or more teeth at any one time, although much lower, 3%, and much higher, >50%, prevalence figures have been published (for review, see West 2006). A recent review on

M. Addy
School of Oral and Dental Science, University of Bristol, Bristol, UK
e-mail: Martin.Addy@bristol.ac.uk

D. G. Gillam (✉)
Centre for Oral Bioengineering, Institute of Dentistry, Barts and the London School of Medicine and Dentistry, Queen Mary University of London, London, UK
e-mail: d.g.gillam@qmul.ac.uk

D. G. Gillam (ed.), *Dentine Hypersensitivity*, https://doi.org/10.1007/978-3-031-74321-4_1

the burden of DH by Cuhn-Cruz and Wataha (2014) from the published studies would appear to suggest that the best estimate of the prevalence of DH is 10% with an average of 33% across the studies. Even though DH can be diagnosed in persons at the extremes of age, teenagers to octogenarians, most commonly it appears to afflict young people between 20 and 40 years. Females have been reported to be more commonly affected than males and at a younger mean age but not all data reached statistical significance. Available distribution data mostly indicate four features of DH: canines and first premolars, then incisors and second premolars and finally molars is the order of teeth most affected; left-sided teeth are more frequently afflicted than their right-sided, contra-lateral counterparts; the site of predilection by far is buccal cervical; lesions show little or no plaque (Addy et al. 1987; Fischer et al. 1992).

What is largely missing from the prevalence and distribution data is numbers of teeth affected and range of pain scores experienced per individual. This lack of information makes difficult an accurate judgement of how DH impacts on the quality of life of sufferers (see Chap. 3). Thus, although DH is stated to be a common painful condition of the teeth, do 15% of all populations in developed countries visit the dentist at anyone time to report suffering from the condition? Unlikely! Indeed, do 15% of adults who regularly attend the dentist report voluntarily, as suffering from DH? Also, most unlikely! Furthermore, over many years authors have reported DH to be cyclical, which suggests lesions "self-heal" through tubule occlusion and then restart by tubule exposure: is this really the case? Possibly, but other explanations are available, including seasonal variation in aetiological factors and stimuli, stimuli avoidance tactics by sufferers and periodic self-medication with home use desensitising products: all of these would preclude the need for professional intervention. At this early stage of this chapter, it is apparent that there are important gaps in our knowledge of DH. In summary, prevalence and distribution data associates DH more commonly with younger adults, specific teeth, tooth sides and sites, good oral hygiene, and possibly females. Such information must beg the question: are these associations indicative even supportive of present-day thoughts on the aetiology of DH? Probably!

1.3 Awareness of Dentine Hypersensitivity by Dental Professionals

As previously indicated, DH remains ill-understood by a considerable proportion of dental healthcare professionals (Canadian Advisory Board on Dentine Hypersensitivity 2003; Rao et al. 2010), which can have an impact in the awareness and treatment of the condition in practice. Recent surveys have indicated that DH is poorly understood by clinicians, possibly due to lack of education on the topic at both dental undergraduate and postgraduate schools, although it is evident that this may be changing in some areas of the world. Nevertheless, most surveys still indicate that there is confusion with the underlying mechanism of DH, its prevalence, diagnosis and management (see Chap. 2). Despite the plethora of literature on the subject which has continued to grow enormously over relatively recent years, it is apparent that only a minority of dental professionals show an interest in the topic as most clinicians consider DH to have a limited impact on the QoL of their patients (Chap. 2). Is there still a need for further education on? Definitely?

1.4 Definition and Terminology: Hypersensitivity or Sensitivity?

At an international meeting, DH was defined as: short sharp pain arising from exposed dentine in response to stimuli, typically thermal, evaporative, tactile, osmotic or chemical, and which cannot be ascribed to any other form of dental defect or pathology (Holland et al. 1997). Essentially, the definition is a clinical descriptor of DH as a specific dental condition which needs to be distinguished from other causes of dentinal pain and calls out for a diagnosis of DH by exclusion (for reviews, see West 2006; Addy and Smith 2010). Moreover, the definition is recommending the continued use of the term DH, perhaps if only because of long time common usage. This, however, does not end the long running debate over the accuracy of the term and the conclusion of many authors that the exposed dentine is merely sensitive and therefore lesions should be termed dentine sensitivity. Whilst for many years being sympathetic even supportive of this view, the authors, clearly playing with the semantics of the definition, would like to put forward a counter argument in favour of the term DH. Available evidence indicates that lesions of DH have many more and wider dentinal tubules open at the dentine surface and patent to the pulp than non-sensitive dentine (Ishikawa 1969; Absi et al. 1987). According to Poiseuille's law, the potential for fluid flow is therefore increased exponentially in DH lesions (see Chap. 5). Thus, the affected tooth may be "sensitive", but the exposed dentine is hyper-reactive to appropriate stimuli and thereby "hyper-sensitive". One condition, within the spectrum of those causing dentine pain, that should be discussed separately, is root sensitivity (RS), not least because, until publication of the definition of DH, it was the same as DH. The European Federation of Periodontology recommended the term RS to describe short sharp pain from exposed dentine of periodontally involved teeth or following periodontal treatments (Sanz and Addy 2002). Three points need to be made in support of the term: periodontally involved teeth do not fit the definition of DH; available figures put the prevalence of RS very much higher than DH (Chabanski et al. 1996); deep bacterial invasion of dentinal tubules has been reported in periodontally involved teeth (Adriaens et al. 1988) and thus far not in true DH. Further confusion regarding the terminology of DH and its definition of exclusion has also emerged when investigators are linking with DH with other dental conditions that normally would be excluded by the original definition of DH. For example, when describing, post-operative sensitivity (including bleaching related sensitivity, cracked tooth syndrome), molar incisor hypomineralisation, or other types of facial pain such as atypical odontalgia (persistent dentoalveolar pain) (Markowitz 2010; Sharav 2013; Gillam and Chatzopoulou 2019; Gupta et al. 2022; Santos et al. 2024). It is, however, clear when comparing clinical features of these other conditions, there are distinct differences in their development and subsequent pain history. In the light of this and its potential confusion in terms of differential diagnosis and subsequent management that the terminology used to distinguish these conditions should be reassessed.

1.5 Mechanism of Dentine Sensitivity: Does It Apply to Dentine Hypersensitivity?

Three hypotheses have been proposed to explain the sensitivity of dentine: nerves extending to the outer end of dentinal tubules; odontoblast transducer mechanism; hydrodynamic mechanism. Significant evidence against the first two hypotheses is available but will not be propounded upon further (for reviews, see Pashley 1990; Addy and Smith 2010) (see Chap. 5). Based upon knowledge that fluid flows outward from the pulp along dentine tubules, Gysi 1900 proposed the hypothesis of a hydrodynamic mechanism explaining dentine sensitivity. Unfortunately, there was a wait of more than 60 years before the eloquent experiments of Brannstrom and co-workers provided evidence to turn hypothesis into theory (for reviews, see Brannstrom 1963, 1966). Essentially, the hydrodynamic theory of dentine sensitivity postulated that stimuli applied to exposed dentine, such as those listed in the definition of DH, caused an increase in fluid flow in the dentine tubules: the resulting pressure change triggering a mechano-receptor response in A-beta and A-delta nerve fibres in and around the pulp dentine border. All stimuli applied to dentine were reported to cause an increased outward flow of fluid except heat where there was inward flow. Interestingly, when fluid flow in tubes is increased, a pressure-related streaming potential is triggered suggesting that stimulation of pulp nerves could also be electrical (Anderson and

Matthews 1967; Griffiths et al. 1993). For the hydrodynamic theory to apply to DH, lesions would have to exhibit open tubules at the dentine surface and patent to the pulp. Evidence, alluded to already, indeed, supports that this is the case. Furthermore, the extensive work of Pashley and co-workers into dentine permeability, including the development and use of the dentine fluid flow cell, provided strong support for a hydrodynamic mechanism explaining the pain mechanism in DH (for reviews, see Pashley 1990, 1992) (Chap. 5). Of note and over the last two-three decades, the flow cell model demonstrated some DH treatments reduced fluid flow across dentine (Greenhill and Pashley 1981). More recently, albeit indirectly, treatments known to block dentinal tubules in vitro and in situ have been proven to be effective in DH (for review, see Addy and West 2013) (Chaps. 6 and 8).

1.6 Aetiology of Dentine Hypersensitivity: Are Lesion Localisation and Initiation Tooth (and Gingival) Wear Phenomena?

The preceding sections indicate that for DH to occur, at any site on a tooth, dentine has to be exposed (lesion localisation) and the tubule system opened (lesion initiation). Evidence concerning the aetiology of these two distinct, but interrelated processes unfortunately has been drawn at best from studies in vitro and in situ and epidemiological derived associations and at worst case reports and clinical anecdote. As no classical randomised controlled trials (RCTs) exist, proving cause and effect, available data are circumstantial albeit quite compelling. Chapter 4 will consider aetiology in detail and a list of relevant reviews can be found in Addy and Smith (2010), so here only the salient points will be discussed.

Lesion localisation through dentine exposure can occur by loss of enamel and/or gingival recession (with loss of cementum). Loss of enamel, outside acute trauma, is a tooth wear process involving attrition, abrasion and erosion alone or more usually in combinations. Abfraction (cervical tensile stress) has been hypothesised to predispose cervical enamel to abrasion and/or erosion, but opinion is divided (for review, see Grippo 1991). Numerous publications, including a conference report (Addy et al. 2000) and a monograph (Lussi 2006), have considered these wear processes and in particular the combination of abrasion and erosion acting at buccal cervical tooth surfaces (for review, see Addy and Shellis 2006). There seems little doubt that erosion is a major factor in enamel loss, causing dissolution and demineralisation (softening) of this tissue: the more common source of the acid being extrinsic and dietary rather than intrinsic, gastric acid. Extensive data, drawn from developed nations also, "implicate" toothbrushing with toothpaste as the main abrasive cause of enamel loss, particularly at buccal cervical areas. Given the resistance of enamel to toothbrushing abrasion, it is further theorised that enamel loss from toothbrushing arises from abrasion of enamel softened by erosion: data suggest additive, even synergistic effects of the two wear processes.

Exposure of dentine by gingival recession can be usefully classified as "unhealthy" or "healthy". The aetiology of the former is quite well understood, whereas the latter is poorly explained and as with DH has been described as an enigma (Smith 1997). As dentine exposure, through unhealthy gingival recession, falls outside the definition of DH and is more relevant to RS, it will not be considered further. Reviews on healthy gingival recession using clinical anecdotes, case reports and epidemiological data cite chronic trauma, particularly toothbrushing, as the major aetiological factor (Watson 1984; Smith 1997; Addy and Hunter 2003) (see Chap. 4). RCTs of toothbrushing and "gingival recession" have been conducted but have concentrated only on recording gingival damage (lacerations or excoriations) by different toothbrush characteristics and have been of insufficient duration to measure recession. Interestingly, even surprisingly, the role of toothpaste in gingival damage or recession has rarely been discussed, particularly since toothpaste rather than toothbrushes produces most wear to dentine. It is probable that exposure of dentine at the buccal cervical area of teeth more commonly occurs through gingival recession than enamel loss but has not been studied; indeed, differentiating between the two processes could prove difficult.

Lesion initiation to open the dentine tubule system has mainly been investigated by studies in vitro and in situ. Scanning electron microscopic examination of extracted teeth or replicas reveals that non-sensitive dentine has few if any open tubules on the dentine surface whereas and alluded to already, sensitive dentine has large numbers of open tubules on the dentine surface (Absi et al. 1987). Assuming, with some degree of caution, that tubules in non-sensitive dentine are covered by a "smear layer" made up of collagen and hydroxyapatite (Pashley 1984), to initiate DH such a layer has to be removed. Available topographical studies reveal that artificially induced smear layers are very acid labile, thereby implicating again erosion as a major aetiological factor in DH (Absi et al. 1992). Abrasion of dentine as an initiating factor in DH, mainly but not exclusively, has been concerned with the effects of toothbrushes and toothpaste on dentine. Toothbrushes alone are very slow to remove a smear layer and therefore have been discounted as initiating factors; nevertheless brushes, used after an acid challenge, readily open tubules (Absi et al. 1992). Toothbrushing with toothpaste, considered the most common oral hygiene practice in developed countries (Frandsen 1986), has been studied extensively for abrasive effects on dentine, including the propensity to open dentinal tubules. The findings are not consistent but appear to depend on the toothpaste formulation. Most toothpaste appears to remove the smear layer and body dentine by an interaction of their abrasive and detergent systems (Moore and Addy 2005). With some toothpaste, however, the loss of smear layer is followed by tubule occlusion with abrasive particles and/or specific ingredients formulated for such a purpose: Chaps. 6 and 8 will discuss such effects under treatment options for DH. As with toothbrushes, erosion alone appears to promote abrasive effects of toothpaste and also can detach or dissolve some tubule occluding compounds. In conclusion, is DH a tooth and gingival wear phenomenon? Almost certainly, yes (for review, see Addy 2005)!

1.7 Management Strategies for Dentine Hypersensitivity: Logical or Biological?

For decades, it has been appreciated that in the condition known as DH, dentine is exposed, usually at the buccal cervical area of teeth. For more than 40 years, it also has been known that tubules are open at such sites. Such pieces of knowledge led to a management strategy that was almost entirely treatment orientated: formulations being developed to cover the exposed dentine and/or block the tubules. This approach is clearly logical but hardly biological as it does not consider the aetiology of DH: not unlike the past approach to the management of caries. Two main issues arise with this logical management approach: first, the lack of primary, and more particularly, secondary prevention for the condition, and second and related, the development of treatments to withstand aetiological impacts. The present-day knowledge of the aetiology of DH, outlined in the previous section, strongly implies that management should have a biological basis with prevention at the core (for review, see Addy and West 2013) (see Chap. 9).

Primary prevention of DH would of course be ideal but at this time is a utopian goal. Removal or limitation of erosive and abrasive factors to prevent exposure of dentine and dentine tubules is made difficult by the fact that this would impact particularly on common if not recommended dietary and oral hygiene practices. Also, to date, no agent has been discovered which provides significant protection against erosion of enamel and more particularly dentine and could be used as a dental public health measure (for review, see Ganss et al. 2013). Modification of the erosive potential of beverages has been achieved, but such products are not widely available (for review, see Lussi and Jaeggi 2006). Nevertheless, dental professionals should continue to advise moderation to limit erosive/abrasive loss of enamel and abrasive gingival recession and should be on the lookout for early signs of these conditions. The nature of such professional advice and recommendation has been reviewed (West 2006; Addy and West 2013) and will be considered in Chaps. 4 and 8. In essence, such advice appears sensible rather than scientific as it has yet to be subjected to the rigours of RCTs. In particular, bar anecdotal reports, no information is available to indicate whether such advice motivates a change in behaviour to limit aetiological impacts. Nevertheless, such recommendations are also relevant to the secondary prevention of DH and dovetail well with the treatment planning approach recommended for the condition which can be found in several reviews (Orchardson 2000; West 2006; Addy and Smith 2010; Addy and West 2013) and Chap. 8. In particular, the treatment plan must include a diagnosis based on the definition, the exclusion and/or management of other causes of dentine pain and the identification of aetiological and predisposing factors (see Chap. 4).

1.8 Treatments for Dentine Hypersensitivity: Are They Proven, and Do They Resist Aetiological Insults?

On the one hand, as already alluded to, the logical approach to manage DH is to treat the dentine with an agent that coats the surface and blocks the tubules, thereby stopping the hydrodynamic mechanism; quod erat demonstrandum! The biological approach, outlined in the above reviews and Chaps. 6 and 8, on the other hand, is to first put in place a recommended secondary preventive-based treatment plan to avoid recurrence, where treatment is the last item in the plan (see Chap. 8). Over the past decades, numerous agents and formulations have been used in the treatment of DH. Indeed, the number, range and diversity in apparently effective treatments put DH on a par with treatments for haemorrhoids: one early review suggesting that some DH clinical studies "belonged in the realms of testimonials" (Addy and Dowell 1983) (see Chap. 8). Of course, it is only in recent decades, as in most if not all branches of medicine and dentistry, that treatments for DH have been tested in RCTs, which conform to the principles of good clinical practice (GCP): large subject areas with texts (Holland et al. 1997; International Conference on the Harmonisation for Good Clinical Practice 2021; see also EMA 2018 report).

At this juncture, however, it is worth raising several issues in respect of "proving" efficacy of treatments for DH. First and foremost, must be the need for caution in extrapolating data drawn from studies in vitro and in situ to outcome in vivo: a problem appreciated many years ago for chemical plaque control agents (for review, see Addy and Moran 2007). Thus, DH studies in vitro and in situ can be supportive, even explanatory for results of RCTs, but cannot standalone. Second, the question must be asked, how close to real life are the testing methods or stimuli used in DH RCTs? It is evident, however, that some of these stimuli do not relate to those experienced in daily life, for example, electrical stimulators based on electrical pulp testers relying on voltage are more relevant in evaluating the status of the pulp in endodontic diagnosis rather than evaluating DH. It should also be acknowledged that even the established assessment tools such as dental probes and cold air syringes (airblast) have their own drawbacks. This probably explains why at least two different types of stimuli were recommended for use in DH RCTs (Holland et al. 1997; Gillam et al. 2000). Third, study outcomes are based almost entirely on statistically significant improvement of the test formulation over control and rarely if ever on numbers of subjects with complete pain relief: raising the difficult question of statistical versus clinical significance. Finally, one pertinent point, relevant to RCTs in DH specifically and painful conditions in general, is the confounding influence of regression to the mode and the placebo response creating considerable improvement in symptoms in the control group: reductions of 40% having been cited (for reviews, see Curro et al. 2000; West 2006; Addy and West 2013, Curro and Gillam 2015).

Other chapters will consider treatments for DH and only a brief overview will be given here (see Chaps. 8 and 10). Essentially, treatments can be classified by mode of delivery and action. Thus, delivery can be "professional or in office" or "over the counter or home use", whereas action is either "interruption of pulp nerve response" or "tubule occlusion". There is some overlap in the classifications, as the majority of professionally delivered treatments aim to occlude tubules, whereas most formulations to interrupt pulp nerves are home use products. Of course, professional interruption of pulp nerve response can be achieved through endodontic or extraction procedures, but except in the rare variant of DH where irreversible pulp inflammation is present (Dachi 1965), these approaches are not considered as valid treatment options.

Tubule occlusion using many in office treatments has been "proven" to occur by clinical observation and studies in vitro and in situ (for reviews, see Orchardson and Gillam 2006, Pashley 2000; West 2006). Unfortunately, the resistance of the deposited material to aetiological agents, notably abrasion and/or erosion, is rarely tested and certainly some deposits are very acid labile. Also, given the number of very varied in office treatments, relatively few have been tested in RCTs. Perhaps, with the exception of in office treatments which deposit a coating visible to the naked eye, such as adhesive restorative materials, this lack of information makes difficult recommendations for their use in the management programme for DH. Certainly, there is a great deal of professional anecdote and opinion on their use, including efficacy, when to use in the overall treatment plan and frequency of reapplication.

Home use treatments typically use toothpaste as the vehicle, although some mouth rinse formulations are available: here only toothpaste will be discussed. The "actives" in such products either interrupt pulp nerve response or occlude tubules. Various potassium salts have been incorporated into toothpaste to interrupt pulp nerve response and many products exist, but few manufacturers have subjected their formulations to RCT and "generic" products appear to "piggyback" claims of efficacy. This said, there are conflicting scientific opinions and data for the efficacy of potassium toothpaste in DH, which has been reviewed and summarised under "for" and "against" headings and a conclusion of "unproven with the caveat of this not translating to ineffective" (for review see Addy and West 2013). One rather compelling physiological argument revolves around whether the very water labile potassium ion can actually pass through dentinal fluid in vivo when delivered over the relatively short period of toothbrushing times. If indeed, however, potassium is an effective treatment, one hypothesis propounded by Addy and West (2013) is absorption of potassium into the body of dentine eventually forming a depot at the pulp dentine border: such would fit with the apparent delayed therapeutic time scale (see Chap. 6).

Toothpaste formulated to occlude tubules has contained a considerable array of agents and compounds. Here only those for which there are compelling data from RCTs, often supported by studies in vitro and or in situ will be elaborated upon (for review, see Addy and West 2013) (see also Chap. 7).

Strontium chloride, and later acetate, containing toothpastes have been available for decades and the product name was perhaps the most well-known to dental professionals and lay public. That the strontium ion actually occludes tubules has been questioned, since drawing proof from an auto-radiographic study (Kun 1976) is of course flawed and scanning electron microscopy failed to show occlusion (Addy and Dowell 1986). Nevertheless, for those products which formulated the strontium salt with artificial silica abrasive and non-ionic detergent systems tubule occlusion was seen in vitro and in situ, the deposit was largely silica and insoluble in water and dietary acid. Clinical studies have been largely supportive and certainly not negative for efficacy against controls. Interestingly, for many years based on studies in vitro, one of the authors (MA) has recommended not only brushing with these Sr/Si products but topical application with a finger: a regimen recently re-invented by the same manufacturer and others for tubule occluding toothpaste technologies.

Arginine/calcium carbonate toothpaste has been shown effective in DH, producing a tubule occluding deposit made up largely of calcium and phosphate. This deposit as would be expected is soluble in dietary acid; however, given the recommended twice daily (and topical) use may not be a factor as any dissolved deposit would be replaced.

Stannous fluoride (chloride) solutions, gels and toothpaste have all been shown to occlude tubules with a stannous containing deposit which is relatively acid resistant. Clinical studies have shown that this effect translates into efficacy.

Calcium sodium phosphosilicate anhydrous toothpaste has been shown effective in treatment of DH. As with the previous agents in toothpaste, studies in vitro show tubule occlusion by calcium, phosphate and silica, together with titanium when the formulation includes titanium dioxide: the deposit appears water and acid resistant (see Chaps. 7 and 9).

The available data on all products that claim to block the dentine tubules is quite compelling even though recent systematic reviews have reported a lack of homogeneity in some of the published clinical studies (Karim and Gillam 2013; Talioti et al. 2014). Nevertheless, this gives the profession a choice in recommending several toothpaste products as first-line treatments for this common painful condition. All contain a fluoride source and therefore users are not disadvantaged in the preventive properties of this ion. Moreover, the promotional material of the manufacturers has provided the profession, even the public, with additional useful education on DH.

1.9 What Is Missing in Our Knowledge and Understanding of Dentine Hypersensitivity: A Personal Wish List?

It is probably not unreasonable at this time to promote DH from an enigmatic to a moderately well-understood condition, particularly in respect of aetiology. This said, however, if erosion/abrasion action is involved in loss of enamel and opening of tubules, future epidemiological studies usefully could include dietary, toothbrushing and plaque data. Such data could also be drawn from subjects, with and without DH, matched for age, gender and dentine exposure. Protocols for RCTs involving modification of diet and/or oral hygiene practices to cause or reduce sensitivity could be devised but are likely to be lengthy and some may skirt close to ethical boundaries.

A wish list, for future research to help further understanding of DH, would include:

1. "Healthy" Gingival Recession: This very common condition, most frequently seen at buccal cervical surfaces of teeth, is for many people an aesthetic problem, and potentially the associated exposed dentine can become sensitive. Indeed, several "plastic surgical, periodontal procedures" have been developed to deal with the problem (see Chaps. 7 and 9). Yet so little is known about the aetiology and pathogenesis of the condition, and it remains the "poor relation" in respect of dental research. Epidemiological associations are already referred to implicate toothbrushing as a major causal factor. Perhaps now is the time to try and turn an association into cause and effect, using RCTs. Unfortunately, it should be recognised that the time scale and difficulties of such clinical studies would be quite different from those, which, for example, turned the strong association of plaque to gingivitis (Ash et al. 1964) into proof of causation (Loe et al. 1965): protocols for such studies would be gratefully received!
2. Tooth Wear: The research interest in this subject area recently has been large and continues to be so. Reviews have identified the historical switch in main dietary aetiological interactions from formally abrasion/attrition to more recently abrasion/erosion (for review, see Addy and Shellis 2006). A previous monograph, entitled *Dental Erosion* (Lussi 2006), suggests a good understanding of tooth wear processes and their interactions and management of the worn dentition, but primary prevention at a public health level appears a needed but distant goal. More recently, Lussi et al. (2011) provided a very clear understanding on the chemical and histopathological

aspects of erosion and the Royal College of Surgeons (England 2021) have published clinical guidelines for dental erosion (see also Chap. 4).

3. Treatment Effects: Whilst studies in vitro and in situ can show the morphological changes that occur when treatments are applied to dentine with open tubules, it is not necessarily safe to assume the same happens in vivo: further discussion occurs in the final section of this chapter (see also Chaps. 7 and 9).
4. Management Strategies: As alluded to earlier, management strategies for DH have been proposed and are based on biological rather than logical principles but have not been subjected to scientific testing: such evaluation would be perfect!

The above wish list for future research includes the use of RCTs to a greater or lesser degree. Such trials in DH are notoriously difficult with many potential problems. A short second wish list for methods that might overcome some of the problems is:

1. Visualise the Dentine Surface and Tubules: This would aid with diagnosis, treatment effects and possibly even grading severity (tubule numbers and diameters). To some degree, this wish has been granted by using studies in situ and replicas. The former thus far has not modelled for fluid flow in tubules and the latter, from experience is exacting, clinically difficult and, with respect to those who have tried, clinician sensitive: both methods are also very time consuming and need SEM facilities. Clinical magnification instruments would be ideal but need to visualise structures of less than 1 μm: could SEM be used in the clinic?
2. Objective Criteria for Clinical Trials: Two main changes can occur when DH treated by tubule occlusion agents: a reduction in fluid flow in tubules and subjective pain scores. To date neither change has so far been measured objectively. Theoretically, change in fluid flow could be indirectly assessed by measuring the capacitance or impedance of dentine from the exposed surface. Similarly, and hypothetically, pain caused by stimuli applied to sensitive dentine could be measured as a central response in the brain using, for example, an electroencephalogram. Also, what about lie-detector equipment?

Are these wish lists achievable or just science fiction, even fairy tales? Only time will tell!

References

Absi EG, Addy M, Adams D. Dentine hypersensitivity: a study of the patency of dentinal tubules in sensitive and non-sensitive cervical dentine. J Clin Periodontol. 1987;14:280–4.

Absi EG, Addy M, Adams D. Dentine hypersensitivity. The effects of toothbrushing and dietary compounds on dentine *in vitro*: a SEM study. J Oral Rehab. 1992;19:101–10.

Addy M. Dentine hypersensitivity: definition, prevalence, distribution and aetiology. In: Addy M, Embery G, Edgar WM, Orchardson R, editors. Tooth wear and sensitivity. London: Martin Dunitz; 2000. p. 239–48.

Addy M. Dentine hypersensitivity: new perspectives on an old problem. Int Dent J. 2002;52(Suppl 5/02):367–75.

Addy M. Tooth brushing, tooth wear and dentine hypersensitivity—are they associated? Int J Dent. 2005;55(Suppl 4):261–7.

Addy M, Dowell P. Dentine hypersensitivity—a review: clinical and *in vitro* evaluation of treatment agents. J Clin Periodontol. 1983;10:351–63.

Addy M, Dowell P. Dentine hypersensitivity—effect of interactions between metal salts, fluoride and chlorhexidine on the uptake by dentine. J Oral Rehab. 1986;13:599–605.

Addy M, Hunter ML. Can toothbrushing damage your health? Effects on oral and dental tissues. Int Dent J. 2003;53(Suppl 3):177–86.

Addy M, Moran J. Chapter 36: Chemical supragingival plaque control. In: Lindhe J, editor. Clinical periodontology and implantology. London: Backwell Munkgaard; 2007. p. 734–65.

Addy M, Shellis RP. Interaction between attrition, abrasion and erosion in tooth wear. In: Lussi A, editor. Dental erosion. From diagnosis to therapy: Monographs in oral science 20. Basel: Karger; 2006. p. 17–31.

Addy M, Smith SR. Dentin hypersensitivity: an overview on which to base tubule occlusion as a management concept. J Clin Dent. 2010;21:25–30.

Addy M, West NX. The role of toothpaste in the aetiology and treatment of Dentine Hypersensitivity. In: Van Loveren C, editor. Toothpastes. Monographs in oral science 31, vol. 23. Basel: Karger; 2013. p. 75–87.

Addy M, Mostafa P, Newcombe R. Dentine hypersensitivity: the distribution of recession, sensitivity and plaque. J Dent. 1987;15:242–8.

Addy M, Embery G, Edgar WM, Orchardson R. Tooth wear and sensitivity: clinical advances in restorative dentistry. London: Martin Dunitz; 2000. p. 1–400.

Adriaens PA, DeBoever JA, Loesche W. Bacterial invasion in root, cementum and radicular dentine of periodontally diseased teeth in humans—a reservoir of periodontopathic bacteria. J Periodontol. 1988;59:222–30.

Anderson DJ, Matthews B. Osmotic stimulation of human dentine and the distribution of pain thresholds. Arch Oral Biol. 1967;12:417–26.

Ash MM, Gitlin BN, Smith WA. Correlation between plaque and gingivitis. J Periodontol. 1964;35:424–9.

Brannstrom M. A hydrodynamic mechanism in the transmission of pain-produced stimuli through the dentine. In: Anderson DJ, editor. Sensory mechanisms in dentine. London: Pergamon Press; 1963. p. 73–9.

Brannstrom M. The sensitivity of dentine. Oral Surg Oral Med Oral Path. 1966;21:517–26.

Canadian Advisory Board on Dentine Hypersensitivity. Consensus-based recommendations for the diagnosis and management of dentine hypersensitivity. J Canad Dent Assoc. 2003;69:221–8.

Chabanski MB, Gillam DG, Bulman JS, Newman HN. Prevalence of cervical dentine sensitivity in a population of patients referred to a specialist periodontology department. J Clin Periodontol. 1996;23:989–92.

Cuhn-Cruz J, Wataha JC. The burden of dentine hypersensitivity. In: Robinson PG, editor. Dentine hypersensitivity: developing a person-centred approach to oral health. New York: Academic Press; 2014. p. 34–44.

Curro FA, Gillam DG. Chapter 7: Challenging the traditional approach to the conduct of dentine hypersensitivity studies: person-centric studies connecting the patient with their practitioner to optimize the clinical outcome. In: Gillam DG, editor. Dentine hypersensitivity: advances in diagnosis, management, and treatment. Cham: Springer International Publishing; 2015. p. 85–99. https://doi.org/10.1007/978-3-319-14577-8.

Curro FA, Friedman M, Leight RS. Design and conduct of clinical trials on dentine hypersensitivity. In: Addy M, Embery G, Edgar WM, Orchardson R, editors. Tooth wear and sensitivity. London: Martin Dunitz; 2000. p. 299–314.

Dachi SF. The relationship of pulpitis and hyperaemia to thermal sensitivity. Oral Surg Oral Med Oral Path. 1965;19:776–85. https://doi.org/10.1016/0030-4220(65)90350-6.

European Medicines Agency, 2018. ICH harmonised guideline integrated addendum to ICH E6(R1): guideline for good clinical practice ICH E6(R2) International Conference on Harmonisation of technical requirements for registration of pharmaceuticals for human use. https://ichgcp.net/. Accessed 21 May 2024.

Fischer C, Fischer RG, Wennberg A. Prevalence and distribution of cervical dentine hypersensitivity in a population in Rio de Janeiro, Brazil. J Dent. 1992;20:72–276.

Frandsen A. Mechanical oral hygiene practices. In: Loe H, VKleinman D, editors. Dental plaque control measures and Oral hygiene practices. Oxford: IRL Press; 1986. p. 93–116.

Ganss C, Schulze K, Schlueter N. In: van Loveren C, editor. Toothpastes. Monographs in oral science. Basel: Karger; 2013. p. 89–99.

Gillam DG, Chatzopoulou D. Post-operative pain following non-surgical and surgical periodontal procedures. In: Manakil J, editor. Periodontology and dental implantology. Rijeka: IntechOpen; 2019. https://doi.org/10.5772/intechopen.78728. Available from: https://www.intechopen.com/chapters/62139.

Gillam DG, Orchardson R, Narhi MVO, Kontturi-Narhi V. Present and future methods for the evaluation of pain associated with dentine hypersensitivity. In: Addy M, Embery G, Edgar WM, Orchardson R, editors. Tooth wear and sensitivity. London: Martin Dunitz; 2000. p. 283–98.

Graf H, Galasse R. Morbidity, prevalence and intraoral distribution of hypersensitive teeth. J Dent Res. 1977;56(Special issue A):162.

Greenhill D, Pashley DH. Effects of desensitizing agents on the hydraulic conductance of human dentine in vitr*o*. J Dent. 1981;60:686–98.

Griffiths H, Morgan G, Williams K, Addy M. The measurement in vitro of streaming potentials with fluids flow across dentine and hydroxyapatite. J Periodontal Res. 1993;28:59–65.

Grippo JO. Abfractions: a new classification of hard tissue lesions of teeth. J Esthetic Dent. 1991;3:14–9.

Gupta R, Patel A, Nikhade P, Chandak M, Rajnekar R, Dugar M. Comparative evaluation of postoperative sensitivity using three different tooth-colored restorative materials in non-carious cervical lesions: a split-mouth design in vivo study. Cureus. 2022;14(8):e27861. https://doi.org/10.7759/cureus.27861.

Gysi A. An attempt to explain the sensitiveness of dentine. Brit J Dent Sci. 1900;43:865–8.

Holland GR, Nahri MN, Addy M, Gangarosa L, Orchardson R. Guidelines for the design and conduct of clinical trials on dentine hypersensitivity. J Clin Periodontol. 1997;24:808–13.

International Conference on the Harmonisation for Good Clinical Practice. 2021. FDA-2018-D-2173-0030_content.pdf downloads.regulations.gov › FDA-2018-D-2173-0030.

Ishikawa S. A clinico-histological study on the hypersensitivity of dentine. J Japan Stomatol Soc. 1969;36:68–88.

Johnson RH, Zulgar-Nairn BJ, Kovall JJ. The effectiveness of an electro-ionising toothbrush in the control of dentinal hypersensitivity. J Periodontol. 1982;53:353–9.

Karim BF, Gillam DG. The efficacy of strontium and potassium toothpastes in treating dentine hypersensitivity: a systematic review. Int J Dent. 2013;2013:573258. https://doi.org/10.1155/2013/573258. Epub 2013 Apr 8.

Kun L. Etude biophysique des modifications des tissues dentaires prevoquees par l'application totale de strontium. Schweiz Monatschr Zahnheilk. 1976;86:661–76.

Loe H, Theilade E, Jensen SB. Experimental gingivitis in man. J Periodont. 1965;36:177–87.

Lussi A. Dental erosion from diagnosis to therapy. In: Lussi A, editor. Monographs in oral science, vol. 20. Basel: Karger AG; 2006. p. 1–219.

Lussi A, Jaeggi T. Chemical factors. In: Lussi A, editor. Monographs in oral science, vol. 20. Basel: Karger AG; 2006. p. 77–87. Chapter 7.1.1.

Lussi A, Schlueter N, Rakhmatullina E, Ganss C. Dental erosion—an overview with emphasis on chemical and histopathological aspects. Caries Res. 2011;45(Suppl 1):2–12. https://doi.org/10.1159/000325915. Epub 2011 May 31. PMID: 21625128.

Markowitz K. Pretty painful: why does tooth bleaching hurt? Med Hypotheses. 2010;74(5):835–40. https://doi.org/10.1016/j.mehy.2009.11.044. Epub 2009 Dec 31. PMID: 20045265.

Moore C, Addy M. Wear of dentine in vitro by toothpaste abrasive and detergents alone and combined. J Clin Periodontol. 2005;32:1242–6.

Orchardson R. Strategies for the management of dentine hypersensitivity. In: Addy M, Embery G, Edgar WM, Orchardson R, editors. Tooth wear and sensitivity. London: Martin Dunitz; 2000. p. 315–26.

Orchardson R, Gillam DG. Managing dentin hypersensitivity. J Am Dent Assoc. 2006;137(7):990–8; quiz 1028–9

Pashley DH. Smear layer: physiological considerations. Oper Dent Suppl. 1984;9(Suppl 3):13–29.

Pashley DH. Mechanisms of dentine sensitivity. Dent Clinics North Am. 1990;34:449–74.

Pashley DH. Dentin permeability and dentin sensitivity. Proc Finn Dent Soc. 1992;88(Suppl 1):215–4.

Pashley DH. Potential treatment modalities for dentine hypersensitivity: in-office products. In: Addy M, Embery G, Edgar WM, Orchardson R, editors. Tooth wear and sensitivity. London: Martin Dunitz; 2000. p. 351–66.

Rao CB, Kohli A, Addy M. Dentine hypersensitivity: information document for Indian dental professionals. Dental Council of India; Google Scholar. 2010.

Santos PS, Vitali FC, Fonseca-Souza G, Maia LC, Cardoso M, Feltrin-Souza J, Fraiz FC. Dentin hypersensitivity and toothache among patients diagnosed with molar-incisor hypomineralization: a systematic review and meta-analysis. J Dent. 2024;145:104981. https://doi.org/10.1016/j.jdent.2024.104981. Epub 2024 Apr 4. PMID: 38582436.

Sanz M, Addy M. Group D summary. J Clin Periodontol. 2002;29(Suppl 3):195–6.

Sharav Y. Atypical odontalgia. In: Gebhart GF, Schmidt RF, editors. Encyclopedia of pain. Berlin/Heidelberg: Springer; 2013. https://doi.org/10.1007/978-3-642-28753-4_322.

Smith RG. Gingival recession. Reappraisal of an enigmatic condition and a new index for monitoring. J Clin Periodontol. 1997;24:201–5.

Talioti E, Hill R, Gillam DG. The efficacy of selected desensitizing OTC products: a systematic review. ISRN Dent. 2014;2014:865761. https://doi.org/10.1155/2014/865761. eCollection 2014. Review.

Watson PJC. Gingival recession. J Dent. 1984;12:29–35.

West NX. Dentine hypersensitivity. In: Lussi A, editor. Dental erosion. Monographs in oral science 20. Basel: Kager; 2006. p. 173–89.

The Prevalence of Dentine Hypersensitivity

2

Sahar Taha and David G. Gillam

In this chapter, the various methods of studying the prevalence of DH together with the different contributing and confounding factors are discussed. In addition, a review of papers assessing the awareness and understanding of DH by dental professionals will be discussed. A review of the prevalence and awareness of DH data with summary tables will also be provided. Finally, suggestions for future research on the topic are presented.

2.1 Methods of Reporting DH Prevalence

Two main methods were reported in the published literature for studying the prevalence of DH, namely: self-reported questionnaires and clinical examination. Higher prevalence values were reported in studies that relied primarily on self-reported questionnaires rather than studies which were combined with clinical examination (Table 2.1). In the self-reported questionnaires, the prevalence values are generally considered to be overestimated due to the complexity of the other diseases or conditions that may present with pain, for example, caries, cracks, and fractures (Scaramucci et al. 2014; Rees and Addy 2002, 2004) (see Chap. 4). In addition, patients may not always understand what is required of them by the clinician and may therefore be too embarrassed, or not sufficiently concerned, to ask for clarification (Clayton et al. 2002).

Moreover, the nature of the questions in the survey may also influence the reported prevalence values. Nonspecific questions that identify pain or sensitivity, relying on the participant's own pain threshold as a trigger for identifying a positive result, will exclude patients who do not perceive their DH to be a problem that requires attention (Cunha-Cruz et al. 2013).

There are relatively few studies that interviewed the subjects and asked them questions related to pain or discomfort before a clinical exam was performed (Costa et al. 2014; Dhaliwal et al. 2012; Kehua et al. 2009; Que et al. 2013). However, this method may also have an interviewer bias effect on the reporting of the condition (Clayton et al. 2002).

The clinical examination for DH generally has focused on two main methods: thermal by air blast or tactile by probing (Chap. 5). Greater numbers of teeth testing positive to the stimulus were usually achieved using the thermal/evaporative technique than other available techniques, e.g., tactile stimulation (Liu et al. 1998). The proposed reason behind the lower values achieved

S. Taha
Brentwood Smiles Dentistry and Orthodontics, Brentwood, CA, USA

D. G. Gillam (✉)
Centre for Oral Bioengineering, Institute of Dentistry, Barts and the London School of Medicine and Dentistry, Queen Mary University of London, London, UK
e-mail: d.g.gillam@qmul.ac.uk

D. G. Gillam (ed.), *Dentine Hypersensitivity*, https://doi.org/10.1007/978-3-031-74321-4_2

Table 2.1 Summary of selected prevalence studies on DH

Study	Country	*n*	Study type	Method of clinical assessment	Setting	Prevalence (%)	Peak of age	M:F ratio	Commonly affected teeth	% with GR[a]
Clayton et al. (2002)	UK	250	Q[b]	NA[j]	GDP[f]	50%	Third decade	1:1	Mand right sextant	NA
Gillam et al. (2001)	UK and Korea	557	Q	NA	GDP	52–55.4%	Third to fourth decades	NA	NA	NA
Gillam et al. (1999)	UK	277	Q	NA	GDP	52%	Third decade	1:1.4	NA	NA
Colak et al. (2012a)	Turkey	1463	Q	NA	University students	8.4%	NA	1:1.2	NA	NA
Rane et al. (2013)	India	960	Q + CE	AB	Dental hospital	42.5%	Fourth decade	1.6:1	Lower anterior teeth	NA
Bamise et al. (2007)	Nigeria	2165	Q + CE[c]	AB[d]/Probing	University	1.34%	Fourth decade	1.4:1	Molars	12.8%
Rees and Addy (2004)	UK	5477	Q + CE	AB/PDA[e]	GDP	2.8%	Fourth decade	1:1.5	Max[g] first molars	93%
Taani and Awartani (2001)	Saudi Arabia	259	Q + CE	AB/PDA	GDP	42.4%	Fourth decade	GDP 1:4	Max molars and mand anteriors	5%
Fischer et al. (1992)	Brazil	635	Q + CE	AB/ Probing	Marine dental clinic	17%	M: sixth, F: third decade	1:1	Incisors and premolars	NA
Flynn et al. (1985)	Scotland	369	Q + CE	CWMR[k]/ Probing	University	8.7%	Fourth decade	1:1	Premolars	NA
Liu et al. (1998)	Taiwan	780	Q + CE	AB/Probing	University	32%	NA	1:1	Premolars and molars	23%
Amarasena et al. (2011)	Australia	12,692	Q + CE	NA	GDP	9.1%	Fourth to fifth decades	1:1.5	Max premolars and molars	39%
Chrysanthakopoulos (2011)	Greece	1450	Q + CE	AB	GDP	18.2%	Fifth in males Seventh in females	1:1.25	Premolars	85.9%
Ye et al. (2012)	China	2120	Q + CE	AB	GDP	34.1%	Fifth decade	1:1.5	Premolars	84.3%
Tengrungsun et al. (2012)	Thailand	420	Q + CE	AB	University	30.7%	Fourth decade	1:2.4	First molar	NA
Bahsi et al. (2012)	Turkey	1368	Q + CE	AB/Probing	GDP	5.3%	Fifth decade	1:2	Max premolars	88.4%

Colak et al. (2012b)	Turkey	1169	Q + CE	AB	University	7.6%	Fifth decade	1:1.5	Max premolars	95.7%
Dhaliwal et al. (2012)	Punjab, India	650	Q + CE	AB	Screening participants in villages	25%	Sixth decade	1:1.6	Mand incisors	NA
Cunha-Cruz et al. (2013)	USA	787	Q + CE	AB	GDP	12.3%	18–44	1:2.6	Premolars and molars	85.6%
Que et al. (2013)	China	1023	Structure interview+ CE	AB	General population	27.1%	Seventh decade	1.06:1	Premolars	15.5% for the age group (60–69)
West et al. (2013)	Europe (seven countries)	3187	Q + CE	AB (Schiff air score)	Population-based cross-sectional study	41.9% (CE) 26.8% (Q)	18–35	1420 M (44.6%): 1767 (55.4%) F	All teeth excluding second/third molars	Significant association between DH and EW and GR $P < 0.0001$
Scaramucci et al. (2014)	Brazil	300	Q + CE	AB/Probing	University	46%	NA	1:2.56	NA	NA
Al-Khafaji (2013)	UAE	204	Q + CE	AB	GDP	27%	Third decade	1.3:1	Lower anterior	15%
Vijaya et al. (2013)	India	655	Q + CE	A/Cold water confirmation (cotton pledget)	Dental college	**55%**	Second decade	360/295 Male	Upper and lower posteriors	N/A
Haneet & Vandana (2016)	India	2000	Q + CE	AB (Schiff air score)	Dental hospital/ satellite centres	**22.4%**	Second to fourth decade	More males sensitive than females	Evaluated by quadrants	Not recorded although gingival recession was noted as a cause of DH in 7.4%
Naidu et al. (2014)	India	212	Q + CE	Probe (VAS)/ AB/water	Dental school (rural)	32%	35–54 years	94/118	Premolars/ molars	28%
Pereira et al. (2018)	India	548 4200	Q + CE	Probe (VAS)/ AB	Dental college	13% (Q) 8.2% (CE)	30–39 years	1:1	Mandibular central incisors and first molars	N/A

(continued)

Table 2.1 (continued)

Study	Country	*n*	Study type	Method of clinical assessment	Setting	Prevalence (%)	Peak of age	M:F ratio	Commonly affected teeth	% with GR[a]
Ramlogan et al. (2017)	Trinidad and Tobago	130	Q + CE	AB	Dental school	73.1%	18–78 years	41% M; 59% F	Full mouth	Both the percentage of sensitive teeth and DS patients increased with increasing recession severity categories (NB cross-sectional study of periodontal patients)
Seong et al. (2018)	UK	350	Q + CE	AB (Schiff air score)	15 sites across Southwest of England		18–35 years	128 M (36.7%); 221 F (63.3%)	All teeth excluding second/third molars	349 participated (1 incomplete data was excluded) Secondary analysis from West et al. (2013) Every participant exhibited at least one tooth with recession. Not all participants exhibited DH despite the prevalent recession and severe erosive tooth wear
Savage et al. (2019)	Nigeria	1349	Q + CE	AB patient pain rating (yes/no) Schiff ordinal scale (0–3)	Rural and urban dental clinics in six geopolitical zones (seven states)	32.8% (CE) 32.9% (Schiff scale ≥1) 41.2% (Q)	18–35 years	592 M (44.5%); 737 F (55.5%) 20 not recorded?	. All eligible teeth excluding the second and third molars	Significant associations between elicited DH and erosive tooth wear ($p < 0.001$) were noted Identified risk factors should be considered in prevention and management

Demirci et al. (2022)	Turkey	1210	Q + CE	Probe/AB	Dental clinics (hospital)	10.2% (Q) 29.4%	18–70 years	32 M (25.8%); 92 F (74.2%)	Full mouth (excl: third molars)	Buccal surfaces (40.9%) of sensitive teeth showed a higher prevalence of gingival recession compared to the lingual surfaces (15.7%). The prevalence of sensitivity associated with loss of attachment (81.5%) was higher than teeth with gingival recession (36.8%)

[a]gingival recession (GR)
[b]questionnaire
[c]clinical examination
[d]sensitivity to air blast
[e]periodontal disease assessment
[f]general dental practice
[g]maxillary
[h]periodontal specialty clinic
[i]mandibular
[j]not applicable
[k]cold water mouth rinse
[i]erosive wear

with probing techniques (tactile) was probably due in part to the fact that only a small area of the exposed dentine was sensitive, and if the probe did not touch this area, the subject will not probably respond (Scaramucci et al. 2014).

Other investigators, for example, Flynn et al. (1985), used a cold water mouth rinse to diagnose DH. However, this method does not necessarily provide an accurate response from the teeth affected by this condition as pain arising from other dental conditions may also respond during the rinsing process.

2.2 Contributing and Confounding Factors to the Prevalence of DH

2.2.1 Non-carious Cervical Lesions

In a Chinese population, 1010 teeth diagnosed with DH, 644 (63.8%) were also diagnosed to have non-carious cervical lesions (NCCL) (Que et al. 2013). Erosion was also recognized as a predisposing factor for DH in an Australian population (Amarasena et al. 2011) (see Chap. 4). In the same study, abfraction was the least associated predisposing factor. Similarly, Bamise et al. (2007) reported a 10.9% prevalence for attrition with DH, 7.4% abrasion, 3.5% erosion, and 2.7% abfraction. Abrasion was reported to have the highest prevalence in Emirati patients with DH (27%), whereas abfraction was the least associated with only a 5% occurrence in DH patients (Al-Khafaji 2013). The lack of consistency in relating the different NCCL and DH factors may also attribute to the difficulty in diagnosing these lesions. For example, Cunha-Cruz et al. (2013) in a cohort of 787 American reported that there was no association with NCCLs whereas other studies such as Que et al. (2013) and Teixeira et al. (2018) did report an association between NCCLs and DH (see also Chap. 4 for further discussion on NCCLs).

2.2.2 Periodontal Disease

Gingival recession has been widely associated with DH (Amarasena et al. 2011). Loss of attachment was a major associative factor leading to an increased incidence of DH in younger age groups (Que et al. 2013). The percentage of DH patients who have gingival recession may be as high as 95.7% (Colak et al. 2012b). West et al. (2013) also reported that there were significant associations between clinically elicited DH and erosive tooth wear and gingival recession in adults aged between 18 and 35 years; Seong et al. (2018) in a secondary analysis of young UK from the West et al. study reported that despite the prevalence of both gingival recession and severe erosive wear present in subjects it was evident that not all teeth with associated gingival recession exhibited DH.

The incidence of DH increases following periodontal treatment (Lin and Gillam 2012; Splieth and Tachou 2013). Al-Sabbagh et al. also reported that the incidence increased from 30% preoperatively to 79% after 1 week of open-flap periodontal debridement (Al-Sabbagh et al. 2010). Furthermore, Fischer et al. (1992) reported that supragingival and subgingival scaling procedures may also cause a transient occurrence of DH. Lin and Gillam (2012), in their systematic review, reported that the prevalence for DH following nonsurgical therapy was between 62.5% and 90% 1 day following treatment, decreasing to approximately 52.6–55% after 1 week. The prevalence of DH following surgical therapy was between 76.8% and 80.4% 1 day after treatment, subsequently decreasing over time to 36.8% after 1 week, 33.4% after 2 weeks, 29.6% after 4 weeks, and 21.7% after 8 weeks. It was suggested that DH may be relatively mild/moderate in nature and transient in duration following periodontal therapy and as such reassurance and monitoring of the symptoms should be sufficient.

2.2.3 Sample Selection

Studies conducted at hospitals or specialty practices tend to report higher prevalence values (Chabanski et al. 1996, 1997), presumably this may be due to the greater risk of root exposure because of periodontal attachment loss and gingival recession following periodontal treatment.

However, a clear pattern for prevalence values according to the sample selected is still lacking (Table 2.1).

2.2.4 Teeth Location and Surfaces

Various intraoral locations may be affected with DH. The sites of predilection in descending order for DH are canines and first premolars, incisors and second premolars, and molars (Dababneh et al. 1999). However, the literature has not been consistent in reporting the intraoral distribution of the condition (Bamise et al. 2007). The buccal surface appears to be the most affected, followed by labial, occlusal, distal, and lingual surfaces with the incisal and palatal surfaces which were the least affected (Amarasena et al. 2010; Splieth and Tachou 2013). Interestingly, the occlusal surface was reported to have the highest sensitivity by 56%, while the buccal surface sensitivity was about 28% (Bamise et al. 2007) but this may be due to differences in the study populations.

2.2.5 Gender

Several studies have reported an association between DH and gender. Relatively few studies have reported that females were more affected with the condition (Scaramucci et al. 2014; Rees and Addy 2004; Taani and Awartani 2001; Amarasena et al. 2011). Other studies have, however, failed to find an association (in terms of statistically significant differences) between the two variables (Fischer et al. 1992; Splieth and Tachou 2013; Clayton et al. 2002; Flynn et al. 1985; Liu et al. 1998). The reported females' slightly higher prevalence may reflect their better oral hygiene awareness (Dababneh et al. 1999), their dietary habits in eating more healthy fruity food items which may also be erosive in nature (Splieth and Tachou 2013). Females also tend to visit the dentist more frequently which may result in an over representation and, therefore, introduce a classical selection bias if the study sample was recruited in dental practices. In addition, females often articulate health problems more willingly than men, which may lead to an added detection bias for females (Splieth and Tachou 2013). Other studies, however, have reported a greater occurrence of DH in males (Rane et al. 2013; Al-Khafaji 2013; Bamise et al. 2007), but again this may be due to differences in the demographics of the study populations.

2.2.6 Age

Dentine hypersensitivity is mostly prevalent among the young population in the third and fourth decades (Table 2.1). This could be linked to the increase in acidic food/drink intake and the influence of greater oral hygiene awareness and measures (Chabanski et al. 1997; Clayton et al. 2002; West et al. 2013). With ageing people in populations worldwide keeping their teeth longer, there may be an increased incidence of dentine hypersensitivity, gingival recession, and periodontal disease (Bahsi et al. 2012) (see Chap. 4).

2.3 Review of DH Prevalence Data

Dentine hypersensitivity is a prevalent clinical condition; however, studies evaluating its prevalence are not abundant and rather contradictory (Splieth and Tachou 2013, see also Favaro Zeola et al. 2019). A critical review of the published literature on DH clearly demonstrates a wide variation in the reported prevalence values of this condition (Table 2.1). This variation may be attributed to the differences in populations and sample selection, method of investigation, and dietary habits (Dababneh et al. 1999; Davari et al. 2013).

Uncertainty regarding the prevalence of DH may also have significant consequences for both patients and dental practitioners with a vague perception of prevalence comes uncertainty in diagnosis, the appropriate time to treat, and how aggressive the treatment should be (Cunha-Cruz et al. 2013). The extreme variation in the prevalence values reported in the published literature may be classified into three categories:

- DH prevalence using surveys (around 50%).
- DH prevalence diagnosed using combined surveys and clinical exams (1–20%).
- DH in patients who have periodontal disease or have been receiving periodontal treatment (60–90%).

A previous review on the burden of DH, however, by Cunha-Cruz and Wataha (2014) from the published studies in the literature would appear to suggest that the best estimate of the prevalence of DH was 10% with an average of 33% across the published studies accepted in their review.

2.4 Clinicians Awareness of DH

According to Gillam (2013), there has been limited data on the perception of clinicians in both identifying and treating DH, and previous studies and reviews have reinforced this observation indicating that clinicians have gaps in their understanding about the condition and its management (Schuurs et al. 1995; Gillam et al. 2002; Canadian Advisory Board on Dentin Hypersensitivity 2003; Cunha-Cruz et al. 2013; Kopycka-Kedzierawski et al. 2017; Exarchou et al. 2019) (Table 2.2). Although dental schools appear to include dentine hypersensitivity (DH) as part of a taught curriculum to educate undergraduates on the condition (Mosquim et al. 2024), it is evident that there are still concerns on whether dental professionals can identify and manage the condition effectively to benefit their patients (Doğan et al. 2023). Agheli et al. (2023), however, reported a more positive picture from a survey of 220 ADA (American Dental Association) members, in particularly among the more recently qualified clinicians.

2.5 Future Studies for the Prevalence of DH

DH is a condition with a relatively high prevalence among the different population groups. The presence of national surveys on the condition should help in forming a clear strategy for the prevention and treatment of this condition. Population-based representative samples are now needed (Splieth and Tachou 2013). Furthermore, given the changes in the definition of both DH and RS, investigators should undertake new studies with a view to capture more accurate prevalence values on the two conditions as currently these values are included under the term DH.

Data on the confounding and contributing factors may also need to be collected and analysed more carefully, as some of these factors have previously been disregarded in the reporting of prevalence values. In future, special attention should be taken in the design of study protocols to include the prevalence of NCCL and examining its association with DH given the increase in the prevalence of both erosive and abrasive intraoral lesions.

2.6 Conclusions

The prevalence reports of DH are not abundant and are somewhat contradictory. The wide variation in the prevalence values reported in the literature may be reduced by dividing the reporting of the condition into 3 categories: (1) DH prevalence using surveys (around 50%), (2) DH prevalence diagnosed using combined surveys and clinical exams (1–20%), and (3) DH in patients who have periodontal disease or have been receiving periodontal treatment (60–90%). Questionnaires have been commonly used for the evaluation of DH prevalence; however, when combined with clinical examination, these values were significantly reduced. Furthermore, investigators should undertake new studies with a view to capture more accurate prevalence values on

Table 2.2 Summary of selected awareness studies on DH by dental professionals

Authors	Country	Setting	Study type	n	Selected observations
Amarasena et al. (2010)	Australia	Practice	Questionnaire (postal)	284	800 questionnaires sent out, 295 responded. Perception of occurrence of DH was <20%. The main conclusion was that Australian dentists' perception of DH was generally consistent with the current scientific consensus on this subject
Cunha-Cruz et al. (2013)	USA	General practitioner setting (the Northwest Practice-based REsearch Collaborative in Evidence-based DENTistry) (PRECEDENT) t	On-line questionnaire (internet survey)	209	301 invitations, 209 responded. Clinicians rely on patients to assess the severity of DH. Modalities for the diagnosis and treatment of hypersensitivity were diverse in nature. The most successfully reported treatments were fluorides, glutaraldehyde/HEMA, bonding agents, potassium nitrates, and restorative treatments; clinical observation, advice regarding toothbrushing and diet, and laser therapy were the least successful treatments. The methods used to diagnose and treat DH in practice were challenging to justify
Afolabi et al. (2012)	Nigeria	176 Nigerian dentists attending a professional dental workshop	Questionnaire	176	73.3% of the responding dentists claimed to see patients with DH. 45.1% of the dentists mentioned cold as the commonest stimulus evoking pain in DH. 56.8% could correctly identify the hydrodynamic theory as the commonest theory of DH
Benoist et al. (2014)	Senegal	Private practice and public hospitals	Questionnaire (postal)	164	238 clinicians received the questionnaire and 68.9% returned the questionnaire. 83% had a good understanding of the pain characteristics related to DH with 92% recognizing chemical and thermal but not mechanical stimuli as triggering factors. Most responders (90.9%) failed to recognize the underlying mechanism for pain transmission across the dentine. 68% of the participants used mechanical stimuli to elicit DH pain as part of their diagnostic procedures. The use of a desensitizing toothpaste was recommended as was the professionally applied topical application. > 1/3rd of the participating dentists used root canal therapy to manage DH
Oderinu et al. (2017)	Nigeria	Dentists in six geographical zones	Cross-sectional study (questionnaire)	1057	92.8% of dentists described DH as a stimulated brief pain elicited from the tooth; 24.2% indicated that DH can be treated by altering the number of dentinal tubules (tubule occlusion?). Diagnostic measures included by tapping (20.6%) or scratching (73.4%). Extraction (24.7%) and root canal therapy (34.5%) were also indicated as part of the management of DH. Most dentists correctly identified the aetiological and predisposing factors (98.8%). Counselling was also recommended as part of the management of DH. The conclusions of the study indicated that practising dentists exhibited gaps in their knowledge of DH and its subsequent diagnosis and management.

(continued)

Table 2.2 (continued)

Authors	Country	Setting	Study type	n	Selected observations
Kopycka-Kedzierawski et al. (2017)	USA	National dental practice-based research network clinicians	On-line pre-clinical questionnaire	185	Majority of network practitioners used multiple methods to diagnose and manage DH. Desensitizing OTC potassium nitrate toothpaste and fluoride formulations are the most widely reported products used to manage DH in the practice setting. The majority reported that recessed gingiva (gingival recession), followed by the abrasion/erosion; abfraction/attrition lesions, and bruxism most likely contribute to DH
Pereira et al. (2018)	India	Mumbai region membership of IDA 500 dentists randomly selected	Questionnaire (e-mail)	206	Most of these respondents [90.2%]) indicated that half of their patients reported problems with DH; 78.2% respondents reported that the patients usually initiated the conversation on DH; and 83.4% indicated that up to 25% of patients considered DH to be a serious problem. 62.2% of the participants reported that the pain due to DH lasted ≤4 weeks. Most participants were aware of mechanisms underlying DH; majority of dentists (≥66%) reporting inadequate brushing of the teeth as an initiating cause with 50% suggesting that periodontal causes were implicated in DH. Desensitizing agents were recommended for home use. The conclusions from the study agree with previous studies and generally consistent with the current scientific consensus on the management of DH by dentists
Izhar et al. (2019)	Pakistan	Private and public clinics (Lahore)	Questionnaire	527/588	89.6% response. DH is a highly prevalent condition in dental practice. Recession of gums, aggressive brushing, and frequent use of tooth whitening procedures were identified as the predisposing factors. The application of air blast and spontaneous patient report confirmed by dental examination were the most frequently used diagnostic methods
Gillam et al. (2019)	Kuwait	A representative sample of Kuwaiti dentists who were randomly selected using the Kuwait dental association membership list	Questionnaire-based survey (Survey Monkey; hard copies)	190/318	59.7% response rate. Up to 25% of their patients reported DH. 10% of patients experiencing discomfort from DH which in some cases lasted up to 3 weeks. 66% (n = 100) of dentists indicated that the effect of DH on the QoL of their patients was moderate in nature. 51.9% (n = 84) indicating that toothbrushing had a major impact on the QoL. 'Gingival recession' and 'periodontal disease' were implicated as predisposing or aetiological factors of DH. Most dentists indicated that they were confident in recommending OTC products for home use

Exarchou et al. (2019)	Greece	Dentists in general dental practice or undertaking postgraduate studies in a dental school as well as a national conference	Questionnaire	191/230	83% response rate. 39.8% of dentists indicated that 1 in 10 of their patients experienced discomfort from DH. 76.4% of dentists indicating that their patients initiated the conversation on DH. 44% of the dentists indicated that they initiated the relevant conversation. 34.9% of dentists indicated that the duration of discomfort lasted up to 3 weeks. 76.4% indicated that DH had an impact on their patients' quality of life. Incorrect toothbrushing was considered a major etiological factor (68.6%). 'Air blast' (37.3%) and 'probing' (15%) were the main methods for identification. 83.6% of dentists indicated that they were confident in recommending over-the-counter products for home use
Favaro Zeola et al. (2019)	Brazil	Dental practice (private [70.5%] and public practice [29.5])	Questionnaire electronically sent using the Google forms tool	353	Response rate could not be determined. Prevalence was identified as a range (30–60%). Air blast and/or scratching with a dental probe was identified the main trigger for DH. First choice of management was the application of a dentine desensitizer (48.16%). The results of the study indicated that DH management was a challenge to clinicians in their daily practice
Hatton et al. (2020)	UK	Dental undergraduate (fourth and fifth year students (39%)) and dental staff (61%)	Questionnaire (by hand)		91 questionnaires (75.8% response rate) were returned; 37.5% of students indicated that 10% of patients suffered from DH, whereas 18.9% of dentists indicated that 25% of patients suffered from DH. Both dentists (22.6%) and 27.5% of students indicated that DH lasted >12 weeks. 18.9% of dentists considered that DH was a serious problem for patients although 32.5% of students were unsure. Dentists (66%) and students (62.5%) indicated that DH had a major impact on the quality of life (QOL) with 51.1% (dentists) and 56.3% (students) indicating that it was moderate in nature. Conclusion: The results of the present pilot study would suggest that in terms of knowledge and understanding of DH (e.g., hydrodynamic theory), both dentists (90.5%) and students (76.9%) were comparable, although in the assessment and subsequent management of DH, the results indicated that dentists were more confident than the students
Gillam et al. (2020)	UK	1100 dentists and 1100 dental hygienists/ therapists (DH/T)s in general and private dental practice	Questionnaire (postal)	346	346 questionnaires were returned (15.7%), of which 142 questionnaires were from dentists (12.9%) and 204 questionnaires were from DH/Ts (18.5%). The results were consistent with previous studies and would appear to suggest that, in terms of knowledge and understanding of DH (e.g., hydrodynamic theory), there is still some confusion concerning aspects of the diagnosis and management of the condition

(continued)

Table 2.2 (continued)

Authors	Country	Setting	Study type	*n*	Selected observations
Francisconi-Dos-Rios et al. (2021)	Brazil	Undergraduates and qualified dentists from a dental school	Questionnaire (by hand)	100	66.3% of participants indicated that up to 25% of their patients had DH; 41.7% indicated that the duration of discomfort was up to 8 weeks; 78.4% reported that they examined a patient with DH within the last 2–4 weeks; with 70.4% indicating that this was initiated following a conversation with the patient. Most of participants indicated DH affected the patients' quality of life. Attrition, exposed dentine, occlusal interference, gingival recession, and abrasion were factors identified in the aetiology of DH. The diagnostic procedures identifying or excluding DH included history of sensitivity, clinical examination, clinical testing, and probing. Differential diagnosis excluding conflicting clinical conditions such as fractured restoration, bleaching sensitivity, marginal leakage, chipped tooth, and periodontal disease. Most respondents indicated they were confident in diagnosing DH and providing advice to their patients. Only 38.8% of participants identified hydrodynamic theory as the underlying mechanism of DH. Methods to clinically evaluate DH included self-assessment, dental examination, dietary analysis, and thermal assessment. The use of desensitizing dentifrices, education on toothbrushing, in-office application of desensitizing products, and restorations were also recommended. From the results of this study, there appears to be confusion concerning the aetiology, diagnosis, and the subsequent management of DH
Mosquim et al. (2024)	Brazil	Undergraduate students and dentists (including postgraduates from all regions of Brazil, practicing dentists, academics)	On-line questionnaire	132 undergraduate students, 338 dentists	Most students and dentists reported that the prevalence of DH in their patients was between 21–30% and 31–40%, respectively Gingival recession and an acidic diet were the most frequent predisposing factors associated with the development of DH, followed by inappropriate hygiene habits (e.g., overzealous toothbrushing) and parafunctional habits. Majority of the questioned individuals were unable to differentiate DH from other causes of pain (e.g., sensitivity of caries or molar-incisor hypomineralization). Both undergraduate students and dentists showed a notable knowledge gap in the prevention, diagnosis, and management of DH

both DH/RS, gingival recession, and erosive tooth wear. The multiple confounding and contributing factors that are associated with DH including lifestyle habits and the impact of DH on the quality of life (QoL) should be evaluated more carefully in future research when investigators report on the prevalence of DH.

References

Afolabi AO, Ogundipe OK, Adegbulugbe IC, Shaba OP, Olojede ACO. Perception of dentine hypersensitivity and its management by a group of Nigerian dentists. Nig Q J Hosp Med. 2012;22:216–20.

Agheli N, De Faria NG, Maia RR, Siddanna GD, Inglehart MR. Dentists' education, knowledge, and professional behavior concerning the diagnosis and treatment of dentin hypersensitivity: an exploration. J Dent Educ. 2023;87:1705–17. https://doi.org/10.1002/jdd.13363.

Al-Khafaji H. Observations on dentine hypersensitivity in general dental practices in the United Arab Emirates. Eur J Dent. 2013;7(4):389–94. https://doi.org/10.4103/1305-7456.120634.

Al-Sabbagh M, Beneduce C, Andreana S, Ciancio SG. Incidence and time course of dentinal hypersensitivity after periodontal surgery. Gen Dent. 2010;58(1):e14–9.

Amarasena N, Spencer J, Ou Y, Brennan D. Dentine hypersensitivity—Australian dentists' perspective. Aust Dent J. 2010;55(2):181–7. doi. https://doi.org/10.1111/j.1834-7819.2010.01223.x.

Amarasena N, Spencer J, Ou Y, Brennan D. Dentine hypersensitivity in a private practice patient population in Australia. J Oral Rehabil. 2011;38(1):52–60. https://doi.org/10.1111/j.1365-2842.2010.02132.x.

Bahsi E, Dalli M, Uzgur R, Turkal M, Hamidi MM, Colak H. An analysis of the aetiology, prevalence and clinical features of dentine hypersensitivity in a general dental population. Eur Rev Med Pharmacol Sci. 2012;16(8):1107–16.

Bamise CT, Olusile AO, Oginni AO, Dosumu OO. The prevalence of dentine hypersensitivity among adult patients attending a Nigerian teaching hospital. Oral Health Prev Dent. 2007;5(1):49–53.

Benoist FL, Ndiaye FG, Faye B, Bane K, Ngom PI, et al. Knowledge of and management attitude regarding dentin hypersensitivity among dentists from a West African country. J Contemp Dent Pract. 2014;15:86–91.

Canadian Advisory Board on Dentin Hypersensitivity. Consensus-based recommendations for the diagnosis and management of dentin hypersensitivity. J Can Dent Assoc. 2003;69(4):221–6.

Chabanski MB, Gillam DG, Bulman JS, Newman HN. Prevalence of cervical dentine sensitivity in a population of patients referred to a specialist PeriodontologyDepartment. J Clin Periodontol. 1996;23(11):989–92. https://doi.org/10.1111/j.1600-051x.1996.tb00525.x. PMID: 8951625.

Chabanski MB, Gillam DG, Bulman JS, Newman HN. Clinical evaluation of cervical dentine sensitivity in a population of patients referred to a specialist periodontology department: a pilot study. J Oral Rehabil. 1997;24(9):666–72.

Chrysanthakopoulos NA. Prevalence of dentine hypersensitivity in a general dental practice in Greece. J Clin Exp Dent. 2011;3(5):e445–51.

Clayton DR, McCarthy D, Gillam DG. A study of the prevalence and distribution of dentine sensitivity in a population of 17–58-year-old serving personnel on an RAF base in the midlands. J Oral Rehabil. 2002;29(1):14–23.

Colak H, Aylikci BU, Hamidi MM, Uzgur R. Prevalence of dentine hypersensitivity among university students in Turkey. Niger J Clin Pract. 2012a;15(4):415–9. https://doi.org/10.4103/1119-3077.104514.

Colak H, Demirer S, Hamidi M, Uzgur R, Koseoglu S. Prevalence of dentine hypersensitivity among adult patients attending a dental hospital clinic in Turkey. West Indian Med J. 2012b;61(2):174–9.

Costa RS, Rios FS, Moura MS, Jardim JJ, Maltz M, Haas AN. Prevalence and risk indicators of dentin hypersensitivity in adult and elderly populations from Porto Alegre, Brazil. J Periodontol. 2014;85(9):1247–58. https://doi.org/10.1902/jop.2014.130728.

Cunha-Cruz J, Wataha JC. The burden of dentine hypersensitivity. In: Robinson PG, editor. Dentine hypersensitivity: developing a person-centred approach to oral health. Cambridge, MA: Academic Press; 2014. p. 34–44.

Cunha-Cruz J, Wataha JC, Heaton LJ, Rothen M, Sobieraj M, Scott J, Berg J. The prevalence of dentin hypersensitivity in general dental practices in the Northwest United States. J Am Dent Assoc. 2013;144(3):288–96. https://doi.org/10.14219/jada.archive.2013.0116.

Dababneh RH, Khouri AT, Addy M. Dentine hypersensitivity—an enigma? A review of terminology, mechanisms, aetiology and management. Br Dent J. 1999;187(11):606–611; discussion 603. https://doi.org/10.1038/sj.bdj.4800345.

Davari A, Ataei E, Assarzadeh H. Dentin hypersensitivity: etiology, diagnosis and treatment; a literature review. J Dent (Shiraz). 2013;14(3):136–45.

Demirci M, Karabay F, Berkman M, Özcan İ, Tuncer S, Tekçe N, Baydemir C. The prevalence, clinical features, and related factors of dentin hypersensitivity in the Turkish population. Clin Oral Investig. 2022;26(3):2719–32. https://doi.org/10.1007/s00784-021-04245-4. Epub 2022 Jan 27. PMID: 35083586.

Dhaliwal JS, Palwankar P, Khinda PK, Sodhi SK. Prevalence of dentine hypersensitivity: a cross-sectional study in rural Punjabi Indians. J Indian Soc Periodontol. 2012;16(3):426–9. https://doi.org/10.4103/0972-124X.100924.

Doğan Ç, Yıldırım S, Kuru L. Prevalence, etiology, diagnosis and treatment approaches of dentin hypersen-

sitivity from the perspective of dentists in Turkey: a survey study. Yeditepe Dent J. 2023;19:126–32. https://doi.org/10.5505/yeditepe.2023.66486.
Exarchou C, Betsani I, Sakellari D, Chatzopoulou D, Gillam D. A survey of dentists in the management of dentine hypersensitivity: a questionnaire-based study. Eur J Dent. 2019;13:383–90.
Favaro Zeola L, Soares PV, Cunha-Cruz J. Prevalence of dentin hypersensitivity: systematic review and meta-analysis. J Dent. 2019;81:1–6. https://doi.org/10.1016/j.jdent.2018.12.015. Epub 2019 Jan 11.
Fischer C, Fischer RG, Wennberg A. Prevalence and distribution of cervical dentine hypersensitivity in a population in Rio de Janeiro, Brazil. J Dent. 1992;20(5):272–6. https://doi.org/10.1016/0300-5712(92)90043-c.
Flynn J, Galloway R, Orchardson R. The incidence of 'hypersensitive' teeth in the West of Scotland. J Dent. 1985;13(3):230–6.
Francisconi-dos-Rios LF, Calabria MP, Pereira JC, Hatton J, Honório HM. Knowledge of Brazilian dentists and students in treating dentine hypersensitivity. Res Soc Dev. 2021;10(9):e28010917194.
Gillam DG. Current diagnosis of dentin hypersensitivity in the dental office: an overview. Clin Oral Investig. 2013;17(Suppl 1):S21–9.
Gillam DG, Seo HS, Bulman JS, Newman HN. Perceptions of dentine hypersensitivity in a general practice population. J Oral Rehabil. 1999;26(9):710–4. https://doi.org/10.1046/j.1365-2842.1999.00436.x.
Gillam DG, Seo HS, Newman HN, Bulman JS. Comparison of dentine hypersensitivity in selected occidental and oriental populations. J Oral Rehabil. 2001;28(1):20–5. https://doi.org/10.1046/j.1365-2842.2001.00631.x.
Gillam DG, Bulman JS, Eijkman MA, Newman HN. Dentists' perceptions of dentine hypersensitivity and knowledge of its treatment. J Oral Rehabil. 2002;29(3):219–25.
Gillam D, Dashti N, Chatzopoulou D. A survey of the professional opinions of Kuwaiti dentists for the treatment and management of dentine hypersensitivity: a questionnaire-based study. Jacobs J Dentistry Res. 2019;5:046.
Gillam DG, Chana B, Kumar K, Martin E. Knowledge of UK dental professionals in treating dentine hypersensitivity. JSM Dent. 2020;8:1130.
Hatton J, Kumar K, Gillam DG. Knowledge of UK dental undergraduates and dentists in treating dentine hypersensitivity. Dent Oral Biol Craniofac Res. 2020;3:1–6.
Haneet RK, Vandana LK. Prevalence of dentinal hypersensitivity and study of associated factors: a cross-sectional study based on the general dental population of Davangere, Karnataka, India. Int Dent J. 2016;66(1):49–57. https://doi.org/10.1111/idj.12206. Epub 2015 Nov 19. PMID: 26582076; PMCID: PMC9376521.
Izhar F, Nazir MA, Majeed A, Almas K. A study of dentists about their knowledge and practice of dentine hypersensitivity. Eur J Dent. 2019;13:540–6.
Kehua Q, Yingying F, Hong S, Menghong W, Deyu H, Xu F. A cross-sectional study of dentine hypersensitivity in China. Int Dent J. 2009;59(6):376–80.
Kopycka-Kedzierawski DT, Meyerowitz C, Litaker MS, Chonowski S, Heft MW, et al. Management of dentin hypersensitivity by national dental practice-based research network practitioners: results from a questionnaire administered prior to initiation of a clinical study on this topic. BMC Oral Health. 2017;17:41.
Lin YH, Gillam DG. The prevalence of root sensitivity following periodontal therapy: a systematic review. Int J Dent. 2012;2012:407023. https://doi.org/10.1155/2012/407023.
Liu HC, Lan WH, Hsieh CC. Prevalence and distribution of cervical dentin hypersensitivity in a population in Taipei, Taiwan. J Endod. 1998;24(1):45–7. https://doi.org/10.1016/S0099-2399(98)80213-6.
Mosquim M, Zabeu GS, Jacomine JC, Santin DC, Honório HM, Wang L. Brazilian undergraduates' and dentists' knowledge on preventing, diagnosing and managing dentin hypersensitivity: a cross-sectional questionnaire study. Int J Dent Hyg. 2024; https://doi.org/10.1111/idh.12833. Epub ahead of print.
Naidu GM, Ram K C, Sirisha NR, Sree Y S, Kopuri RK, Satti NR, Thatimatla C. Prevalence of dentin hypersensitivity and related factors among adult patients visiting a dental school in andhra pradesh, southern India. J Clin Diagn Res. 2014;8(9):ZC48–51. https://doi.org/10.7860/JCDR/2014/9033.4859. Epub 2014 Sep 20. PMID: 25386522; PMCID: PMC4225974.
Oderinu OH, Sede MA, Oginni AO, Adegbulugbe IC, Uti OG, et al. Knowledge, diagnosis, and management of dentine hypersensitivity: a national survey of dentists in Nigeria. Int Dent J. 2017;67:287–93.
Pereira R, Gillam DG, Bapatla S, Satyamurthy P. Awareness of dentine hypersensitivity among general dental practitioners in Mumbai, India. J Odontol. 2018;2:103.
Que K, Guo B, Jia Z, Chen Z, Yang J, Gao P. A cross-sectional study: non-carious cervical lesions, cervical dentine hypersensitivity and related risk factors. J Oral Rehabil. 2013;40(1):24–32. PMID: 22882712. https://doi.org/10.1111/j.1365-2842.2012.02342.x.
Ramlogan S, Raman V, Rees JS, Legall G. A cross-sectional study of dentine sensitivity in periodontitis patients in Trinidad and Tobago. Int J Dent Hyg. 2017;15(4):e69–77. https://doi.org/10.1111/idh.12202. Epub 2016 Feb 4.
Rane P, Pujari S, Patel P, Gandhewar M, Madria K, Dhume S. Epidemiological study to evaluate the prevalence of dentine hypersensitivity among patients. J Int Oral Health. 2013;5(5):15–9.
Rees JS, Addy M. A cross-sectional study of dentine hypersensitivity. J Clin Periodontol. 2002;29(11):997–1003. https://doi.org/10.1034/j.1600-051x.2002.291104.x. PMID: 12472992.
Rees JS, Addy M. A cross-sectional study of buccal cervical sensitivity in UK general dental practice and a summary review of prevalence stud-

ies. Int J Dent Hyg. 2004;2(2):64–9. https://doi.org/10.1111/j.1601-5029.2004.00068.x.

Savage KO, Oderinu OH, Oginni AO, Uti OG, Adegbulugbe IC, Dosumu OO. Dentine hypersensitivity and associated factors: a Nigerian cross-sectional study. Pan Afr Med J. 2019;33:272. https://doi.org/10.11604/pamj.2019.33.272.18056.

Scaramucci T, de Almeida Anfe TE, da Silva FS, Frias AC, Sobral MA. Investigation of the prevalence, clinical features, and risk factors of dentin hypersensitivity in a selected Brazilian population. Clin Oral Investig. 2014;18(2):651–7. https://doi.org/10.1007/s00784-013-1008-1.

Schuurs AH, Wesselink PR, Eijkman MA, Duivenvoorden HJ. Dentists' views on cervical hypersensitivity and their knowledge of its treatment. Endod Dent Traumatol. 1995;11:240–4.

Seong J, Bartlett D, Newcombe RG, Claydon NCA, Hellin N, West NX. Prevalence of gingival recession and study of associated related factors in young UK adults. J Dent. 2018;76:58–67. https://doi.org/10.1016/j.jdent.2018.06.005. Epub 2018 Jun 19

Splieth CH, Tachou A. Epidemiology of dentin hypersensitivity. Clin Oral Investig. 2013;17(Suppl 1):S3–8. https://doi.org/10.1007/s00784-012-0889-8.

Taani DQ, Awartani F. Prevalence and distribution of dentin hypersensitivity and plaque in a dental hospital population. Quintessence Int. 2001;32(5):372–6.

Teixeira DNR, Zeola LF, Machado AC, Gomes RR, Souza PG, Mendes DC, Soares PV. Relationship between noncarious cervical lesions, cervical dentin hypersensitivity, gingival recession, and associated risk factors: A cross-sectional study. J Dent. 2018;76:93–97. https://doi.org/10.1016/j.jdent.2018.06.017. Epub 2018 Jun 22. PMID: 29940290.

Tengrungsun T, Jamornnium Y, Tengrungsun S. Prevalence of dentine hypersensitivity among Thai dental patients at the Faculty of Dentistry, Mahidol University. Southeast Asian J Trop Med Public Health. 2012;43(4):1059–64.

Vijaya V, Sanjay V, Varghese RK, Ravuri R, Agarwal A. Association of dentine hypersensitivity with different risk factors - a cross sectional study. J Int Oral Health. 2013;5(6):88–92. Epub 2013 Dec 26. PMID: 24453451; PMCID: PMC3895724.

West NX, Sanz M, Lussi A, Bartlett D, Bouchard P, Bourgeois D. Prevalence of dentine hypersensitivity and study of associated factors: a European population-based cross-sectional study. J Dent. 2013;41(10):841–51.

Ye W, Feng XP, Li R. The prevalence of dentine hypersensitivity in Chinese adults. J Oral Rehabil. 2012;39(3):182–7. https://doi.org/10.1111/j.1365-2842.2011.02248.x.

3 The Impact of Dentine Hypersensitivity on Oral Health-Related Quality of Life

Katrin Bekes and Christian Hirsch

3.1 Quality of Life in Dentistry

3.1.1 Quality of Life and Health-Related Quality of Life

"Quality of life" (QoL) as a term was first introduced in 1920 by the British economist Arthur Cecil Pigou (1920), in a book about economics and welfare discussing governmental support for the lower class and its impact on their lives, as well as on national finances. Later, the expression "QoL" was defined in many ways and was used differently by various investigators, owing to its elusive nature. It became apparent that although one may intuitively know what it means, its abstract nature makes a clear definition difficult.

In medicine and dentistry, a paradigm shift has occurred in recent years, as patient-centered outcomes including QoL research have been receiving increasingly more attention (John et al. 2016a, b). Once regarded as a secondary outcome, occasionally useful to complement biologic and clinical markers of disease, it has been stated that "QoL issues are now at the forefront of public health policy" (Slade 2002). According to the World Health Organization, QoL can be defined as an individual's perception of his/her position in life, in the context of the culture and value systems in which he/she lives, and in relation to his/her expectations, goals, and concerns (World Health Organization 1993).

Health contributes to QoL, and the real impact of health and disease on QoL is known as health-related quality of life (HRQoL) (Naito et al. 2006). As with QoL, the concept of HRQoL is multifaceted and complex; therefore, defining it is a challenge (Cimprich and Paterson 2002). There is consensus that it captures people's perceptions about factors that are important in their everyday lives (Slade 2002). The definition of health by the World Health Organization as "a state of complete physical, mental, and social well-being, and not merely the absence of disease or infirmity" (World Health Organization 2006) implies that health is no longer seen as merely the absence of a disease but as a concept that focuses on the whole person (Absi et al. 1987). It is this idea of wholeness that led to the development of the concept of HRQoL.

K. Bekes (✉)
Department of Pediatric Dentistry, University Clinic of Dentistry, Medical University of Vienna, Vienna, Austria
e-mail: katrin.bekes@med.uniwien.ac.at

C. Hirsch
Clinic of Pediatric Dentistry, Department of Head Medicine and Oral Health, University of Leipzig, Leipzig, Germany
e-mail: christian.hirsch@medizin.uni-leipzig.de

D. G. Gillam (ed.), *Dentine Hypersensitivity*, https://doi.org/10.1007/978-3-031-74321-4_3

3.1.2 Oral Health-Related Quality of Life

3.1.2.1 What Is Oral Health-Related Quality of Life?

Oral health-related quality of life (OHRQoL) is a subset of HRQoL that focuses on oral health and orofacial concerns. OHRQoL is "a multidimensional construct that reflects (among other things) people's comfort when eating, sleeping, and engaging in social interaction; their self-esteem; and their satisfaction with respect to their oral health" (DHHS 2000). OHRQoL attempts to capture the subjective side of oral health. Thus, the concept of OHRQoL brings a new perspective to clinical dental care and research. It describes the way in which oral health affects a person's ability to function, psychological status, social factors, and pain or discomfort (Inglehart and Bagramian 2002). As Inglehart noted, "it shifts the focus of clinicians and researchers from the oral cavity alone to the patient as a whole" (Inglehart and Bagramian 2002).

OHRQoL has previously shown significant promise across various fields of dental research, spanning basic studies, clinical trials, and epidemiological surveys. Presently, there is a widespread recognition of the pivotal role of the patient's perspective in assessing the impact of diseases and treatment outcomes, arguably ranking as the foremost consideration. Although patient survival is not typically a concern in dentistry grasping, the patient's perception of disease effects is essential in elucidating diverse impacts.

3.1.2.2 Concepts of Oral Health

Following the traditional approach, oral health measures are based on clinical standards. Usually, oral health is described by using clinical oral-disease indicators (indices), as they provide a quantitative method for measuring, scoring, and analyzing dental conditions in individuals and groups. An index describes the status of individuals or groups with respect to the condition to be measured. For example, the severity of periodontal disease is documented by clinicians using parameters, for example, bleeding on probing, probing pocket depth, and clinical attachment level (Ng and Leung 2006). However, important as these objective measures are, these are surrogate measures and not the true end point of the process. They give no indication of the impact of the oral-disease processes or oral disorders on function or psychosocial well-being and provide little insight into the impact on daily living and quality of life (Allen 2003). To continue with this example, this means that other symptoms of periodontal disease, including those resulting from chronic inflammation and the destruction of tooth-supporting tissues (such as redness, bleeding on brushing, loosening of affected teeth, and persistent bad breath), are not normally documented by clinicians. However, such symptoms are highly relevant from the patient's point of view and often have a considerable adverse impact on their daily QoL (Locker 1988; Ng and Leung 2006).

On these grounds, Locker developed a conceptual framework for measuring oral health status (Locker 1988). It was based on the World Health Organization classification of impairment, disability, and handicap and attempted to capture all possible functional and psychosocial outcomes of oral disorders. Locker stated that disease can lead to impairment, which may then lead to a functional limitation or pain/discomfort, either physical or psychological. Any of these outcomes may lead to physical, psychological, or social disability, which was defined by Locker "as any limitation in or lack of ability to perform activities of daily living." As a final consequence, handicap can occur which is often characterized by social disadvantage (e.g., social isolation). Functional limitation may also lead directly to handicap.

In line with this, the FDI redefined the term oral health in 2016 (Glick et al. 2016): "Oral health is multifaceted and includes the ability to speak, smile, smell, taste, touch, chew, swallow, and convey a range of emotions through facial expressions with confidence and without pain, discomfort, and disease of the craniofacial complex." Other aspects of oral health were also mentioned, such as "it is a fundamental component of health and physical and mental well-being" and "it exists along a continuum influenced by the values and attitudes of people and communities." Furthermore, "it reflects the physiological, social, and psychological attributes that are essential to the quality of life" and "is influenced by the person's changing experiences, perceptions, expectations, and ability to adapt to circumstances."

3.1.2.3 How Can Oral Health-Related Quality of Life Be Measured?

As noted previously, OHRQoL is a multidimensional construct that cannot be observed directly. It needs to be visualized by means of suitable indicators. This could be done using a questionnaire approach. In dentistry, the patient perspective is evaluated using dental patient-reported outcome measures (dPROMs), which are increasingly acknowledged as crucial for understanding disease-related burdens and treatment effects (John 2018). The concept of oral health-related quality of life (OHRQoL) stands out as the foremost dPRO (Mittal et al. 2019). While dPROMs may consist of any number of items, often beginning with just one, OHRQoL instruments typically comprise multiple items that inquire about the impact of oral health on individuals' daily living. Several measurements to assess OHRQoL have been developed over time because of increased concern about the impact of oral conditions on a person's quality of life. Fundamentally, there are three categories of OHRQoL measure as indicated by Slade (2002): social indicators; global self-ratings of OHRQoL; and multiple-item questionnaires of OHRQoL. Multiple-item questionnaires are among the most widely used methods to assess OHRQoL (Al Shamrany 2006).

Given that the definitions of OHRQoL are vague, it is not surprising that there is a significant heterogeneity in focus, length, and format of the multiple-item questionnaires developed to evaluate OHRQoL. Nevertheless, all of them must fulfill a set of attributes and criteria for the assessment of health status and QoL measurement that were defined by the Scientific Advisory Committee of the Medical Outcomes Trust (Aaronson et al. 2002).

To enhance practicality and efficiency, streamlining the construct into the most pertinent and meaningful dimensions for patients is crucial. An international collaboration of experts in OHRQoL conducted a large secondary data analysis of four OHRQoL dimensions, namely: (1) oral function, (2) orofacial pain, (3) orofacial appearance, and (4) psychosocial impact (John et al. 2014a, b, 2016a, b). This is a concept that is valid worldwide and for all dental disciplines (John et al. 2020).

OHRQoL measures can be classified as either generic instruments that measure oral health overall or condition-specific instruments. In some instances, generic measures are too broad for accurate assessment of the links between specific oral conditions and OHRQoL, so that it is desirable to develop specialized instruments. For example, for dentine hypersensitivity (DH), a condition-specific patient-reported measure was developed (Boiko et al. 2010).

3.2 The Oral Health Impact Profile

A technically sophisticated and internationally widely used dPRO instrument is the Oral Health Impact Profile (OHIP), which was developed by Slade and Spencer (Fig. 3.1) (Slade and Spencer 1994). It differs from other OHRQoL measures in that it is based on both Locker's conceptual framework (Locker 1988) and input from dental patients with a variety of oral conditions (Slade and Spencer 1994). The questionnaire attempts to measure the effects of both the frequency and the severity of oral problems on functional and psychosocial well-being. It is a scaled index; it consists of 49 statements that have been rephrased as questions and grouped into seven domains (functional limitation, pain, psychological discomfort, physical disability, psychological disability, social disability, and handicap). For each OHIP item, the patient is asked how frequently he/she experienced the impact of that item during the last month. Responses concerning item impact are given using an ordinal rating scale (0 = never, 1 = hardly ever, 2 = occasionally, 3 = fairly often, 4 = very often). The summary score (sum of item responses resulting in a range of $0–4 \times 49 = 0–196$)

Question	Domain	Item
1	FL	Have you had difficulty chewing any foods because of problems with your teeth, mouth or dentures?
2	FL	Have you had trouble pronouncing any words because of problems with your teeth, mouth or dentures?
3	FL	Have you noticed a tooth which doesn't look right?
4	FL	Have you felt that your appearance has been affected because of problems with your teeth, mouth or dentures?
5	FL	Have you felt that your breath has been stale because of problems with your teeth, mouth or dentures
6	P1	Have you felt that your sense of taste has worsened because of problems with your teeth, mouth or dentures?
7	P1	Have you had food catching in your teeth or dentures?
8	P1	Have you felt that your digestion has worsened because of problems with your teeth, mouth or dentures?
9	P1	Have you had painful aching in your mouth?
10	P1	Have you had a sore jaw?
11	P1	Have you had headaches because of problems with your teeth, mouth or dentures?
12	P1	Have you had sensitive teeth, for example, due to hot or cold foods or drinks?
13	P1	Have you had toothache?
14	P1	Have you had painful gums?
15	P1	Have you found it uncomfortable to eat any foods because of problems with your teeth, mouth or dentures?
16	P1	Have you had sore spots in your mouth?
17	FL	Have you felt that your dentures have not been fitting properly?
18	P1	Have you had uncomfortable dentures?
19	P2	Have you been worried by dental problems?
20	P2	Have you been self conscious because of your teeth, mouth or dentures?
21	P2	Have dental problems made you miserable?
22	P2	Have you felt uncomfortable about the appearance of your teeth, mouth or dentures?
23	P2	Have you felt tense because of problems with your teeth, mouth or dentures?
24	D1	Has your speech been unclear because of problems with your teeth, mouth or dentures?
25	D1	Have people misunderstood some of your words because of problems with your teeth, mouth or dentures?
26	D1	Have you felt that there has been less flavor in your food because of problems with your teeth, mouth or dentures?
27	D1	Have you been unable to brush your teeth properly because of problems with your teeth, mouth or dentures?
28	D1	Have you had to avoid eating some foods because of problems with your teeth, mouth or dentures?
29	D1	Has your diet been unsatisfactory because of problems with your teeth, mouth or dentures?
30	D1	Have you been unable to eat with your dentures because of problems with them?
31	D1	Have you avoided smiling because of problems with your teeth, mouth or dentures?
32	D1	Have you had to interrupt meals because of problems with your teeth, mouth or dentures?
33	D2	Has your sleep been interrupted because of problems with your teeth, mouth or dentures?
34	D2	Have you been upset because of problems with your teeth, mouth or dentures?
35	D2	Have you found it difficult to relax because of problems with your teeth, mouth or dentures?
36	D2	Have you felt depressed because of problems with your teeth, mouth or dentures?
37	D2	Has your concentration been affected because of problems with your teeth, mouth or dentures?
38	D2	Have you been a bit embarrassed because of problems with your teeth, mouth or dentures?
39	D3	Have you avoided going out because of problems with your teeth, mouth or dentures?

Fig. 3.1 Oral Health Impact Profile (OHIP). (Acknowledgement to Slade and Spencer 1994). *FL* Functional limitation, *P1* Physical pain, *P2* Psychological discomfort, *D1* Physical disability, *D2* Psychological disability, *D3* Social disability, *H* Handicap

40	D3	Have you been less tolerant of your partner or family because of problems with your teeth, mouth or dentures?
41	D3	Have you had trouble getting along with other people because of problems with your teeth, mouth or dentures?
42	D3	Have you been a bit irritable with other people because of problems with your teeth, mouth or dentures?
43	D3	Have you had difficulty doing your usual jobs because of problems with your teeth, mouth or dentures?
44	H	Have you felt that your general health has worsened because of problems with your teeth, mouth or dentures?
45	H	Have you suffered any financial loss because of problems with your teeth, mouth or dentures?
46	H	Have you been unable to enjoy other people's company as much because of problems with your teeth, mouth or dentures?
47	H	Have you felt that life in general was less satisfying because of problems with your teeth, mouth or dentures?
48	H	Have you been totally unable to function because of problems with your teeth, mouth or dentures?
49	H	Have you been unable to work to your full capacity because of problems with your teeth, mouth or dentures?

Fig. 3.1 (continued)

represents a "problem index" that characterizes the OHRQoL. A "0" summary score indicates the absence of any problems, higher OHIP scores represent more impaired OHRQoL, and a summary score of "196" indicates that all problems were experienced very often in the last month. The patient's score can be evaluated by comparison to a table of standard values representative of different populations (John et al. 2003, 2004).

The 49-item version of the OHIP gives detailed information and is a sophisticated instrument when OHRQoL is the primary outcome in a clinical setting. However, it is rather time consuming and requires a substantial effort for the respondents. Consequently, short forms (21 items, 14 items, 5 items) have been developed (Slade 1997; Locker and Allen 2002) and proposed for use in settings where the time burden of a long OHRQoL questionnaire needs to be minimized. A version with 14 items is most frequently used (Baba et al. 2008).

3.3 A Condition-Specific Patient-Reported Measure: The Dentine Hypersensitivity Experience Questionnaire

In some instances, generic measures are insufficient in assessing the links between oral conditions and OHRQoL. For this reason, an OHRQoL measure specific for the impacts of DH was developed recently, based on interviews with people with DH (Boiko et al. 2010; Gibson et al. 2010): The Dentine Hypersensitivity Experience Questionnaire (DHEQ) (Fig. 3.2). This instrument aims to measure everyday impacts of DH on OHRQoL. The questionnaire was developed using a multi-staged impact approach and an explicit theoretical model. As a result, the DHEQ questionnaire has 48 items containing a description of the pain (6 items), a measurement of pain via visual analogue scale (3), a scale to capture subjective impacts of DH (34), a global oral

Question	Domain	Item
1	Restrictions	pleasure out of eating
2	Restrictions	cannot finish meal
3	Restrictions	longer to finish meal
4	Restrictions	problems eating ice-cream
5	Approach coping	modification in eating
6	Approach coping	careful when breathing
7	Approach coping	warming food/drinks
8	Approach coping	cooling food/drink
9	Approach coping	cutting fruit
10	Approach coping	putting a scarf over mouth
11	Approach coping	cold drinks/foods
12	Approach coping	hot drinks/foods
13	Approach coping	contact with certain teeth
14	Approach coping	change toothbrushing
15	Approach coping	biting in small pieces
16	Approach coping	other food
17	Social	longer than others to finish
18	Social	choose food with others
19	Social	hide the way of eating
20	Social	unable to take part in conversations
21	Social	painful at the dentist
22	Emotions	frustrated not finding a cure
23	Emotions	anxious of eating contributes
24	Emotions	irritating sensations
25	Emotions	annoyed I contributed
26	Emotions	guilty for contributing
27	Emotions	annoying sensations
28	Emotions	embarrassing sensations
29	Emotions	anxious because of sensation
30	Identity	difficult to accept
31	Identity	different from others
32	Identity	makes me feel old
33	Identity	makes me feel damaged
34	Identity	makes me feel unhealthy

Fig. 3.2 Impact scale of the Dentine Hypersensitivity Experience Questionnaire (DHEQ). (Acknowledgement to Boiko et al. 2010 and Baker et al. 2014)

health rating (1), and a scale to record effects on overall life (4).

The impact scale comprises 34 items and has five subscales based on the initial domains of the Wilson and Cleary model (Wilson and Cleary 1995): functional restrictions (4 items), coping (12), social impact (5), emotional impact (8), and identity (5). The items have coded responses on 7-point Likert scales (labeled strongly disagree, disagree, disagree a little, neither agree nor disagree, agree a little, agree, and strongly agree, coded 1–7, respectively). The summary measure ("total score") of the impact scale is calculated as the sum of the item scores per participant (possible range 34–238). The higher the total score of the DHEQ is, the more impaired the patient's OHRQoL is.

The DHEQ has been reported to demonstrate good psychometric properties (Boiko et al. 2010). It is longitudinally reliable, valid, and responsive and can discriminate between treatments of different efficacy (Baker et al. 2014). Moreover, a 10- and 15-item short form of the DHEQ has recently been derived (Machuca et al. 2014).

3.4 Dentine Hypersensitivity and Its Impact on Oral Health-Related Quality of Life

3.4.1 Dentine Hypersensitivity

As shown in the other chapters of this book, DH is a significant global clinical oral health problem in the adult population (Mantzourani and Sharma 2013) (Chap. 2) that is characterized by short or transient sharp pain arising from exposed dentine in response to an array of stimuli (such as thermal, mechanical, osmotic, or chemical elements) that cannot be ascribed to any other form of dental defect or pathology (Canadian Advisory Board on Dentin Hypersensitivity 2003) (Chaps. 4 and 5). The cold stimulus has been reported to cause the greatest problem to people affected by DH, as it increases the outward flow of fluid in the dentinal tubules, whereas a thermal hot stimulus produces contraction of the fluid in the tubules (Matthews and Vongsavan 1994).

Nevertheless, pain has extremely variable characteristics, ranging from discrete discomfort to extreme severity (McGrath 1986, 1994; Porto et al. 2009). In addition, not all people experiencing tooth sensitivity seek treatment to desensitize their teeth, because some do not perceive DH to be a severe oral health problem (Gillam et al. 1999). However, the influence of pain experienced can be considerable and can affect daily activities depending on the source of discomfort (for example, pain associated with consuming hot or cold foods and beverages [coffee, ice cream], during toothbrushing, or sometimes even while breathing) (Schuurs et al. 1995; Gillam et al. 2002). In these instances, these symptoms are highly relevant from the person's point of view and often have a considerable adverse impact on daily quality of life (Locker 1988).

3.4.2 Oral Health-Related Quality of Life in Patients with Dentine Hypersensitivity

To date, there has been some research conducted that has explored DH from a patient perspective (Douglas-de-Oliveira et al. 2018). Both general health-related quality of life measures, such as the EuroQol five-dimensional (EQ-5D) (Porritt et al. 2014), and specific OHRQoL measures, such as the Oral Health Impact Profile (OHIP) (Bekes et al. 2008, 2009; Idon et al. 2017; Lima et al. 2017; Masud et al. 2017; Sivaramakrishnan and Sridharan 2019; Bhowmik et al. 2021; Sgreccia et al. 2022), Oral Impacts on Daily Performance (OIDP) (Goh et al. 2016), and the Dentine Hypersensitivity Experience Questionnaire (DHEQ) (Boiko et al. 2010; He et al. 2012; Baker et al. 2014; Sufi et al. 2016a, b, Hall et al. 2017a, b, Basaran and Celik 2018; Krause et al. 2018; Guanipa Ortiz et al. 2019; Mason et al. 2019; Arheiam et al. 2022; Li et al. 2024), have been utilized in clinical trials and observational studies.

The first data that were published using an instrument that examined patients' self-perception of health and well-being to explore the impact of DH on OHRQoL came from a study that was conducted in Germany (Bekes et al. 2009). OHRQoL impairment was evaluated in 656 patients seeking care for their hypersensitive teeth in German dental offices. The study participants were asked to complete the adapted German version of the OHIP (OHIP-G) (John et al. 2002) prior to treatment. When their OHIP summary scores were analyzed and compared with those in a sample of the German general population ($n = 1541$) (John et al. 2003), the distribution of OHIP-G summary scores in patients with DH and in the general population was found to be different. The general-population participants had an OHIP-G median score of 5, compared to a median score of 30 in the patient group. The 10% of the subjects with the highest OHIP-G summary scores presented scores of 36 or higher (general population) and 66 or higher (patients). The mean OHIP-G summary score value of the study participants from the general population was 12.2 (±18.4), while the patients' mean OHIP-G summary score was 34.5 (±22.6). The difference in the mean values of 22.3 was clinically meaningful and statistically significant ($P < 0.001$). These results demonstrated that the patients with DH had impaired OHRQoL. The results also indicated that the influence of gender on OHRQoL depended on the population. In the general-population sample, female subjects had lower OHIP scores than male subjects ($P = 0.003$), whereas in the patient group, female patients had higher OHIP scores than male patients, but the difference was not statistically significant ($P = 0.27$). Lastly, age showed a curvilinear association with OHRQoL, with lower OHIP scores associated with younger and older adults, and higher OHIP scores (reporting more problems and indicating impaired OHRQoL) associated with middle-aged adults in both populations. The difference between younger (15–39 years) and older adults (40+ years) was statistically significant in the general population ($P < 0.001$). In the patient group, the difference was similar in magnitude to that and close to statistical significance ($P = 0.08$).

The results reflect findings for patients seeking care for their condition and certainly cannot be generalized to individuals experiencing DH but not seeking care. Moreover, the results relate to patients seen by general dentists and may not be generalized to those that could be obtained by health professionals who are more trained or calibrated in the assessment of DH. However, the setting is representative for typical patients who initially present in dental practice and where the general dentist is confronted with providing diagnosis and treatment for the challenging clinical problem of DH (Bekes et al. 2009).

The same investigators evaluated OHRQoL in 713 patients with DH before and after treatment intervention (Bekes et al. 2008). The treatment regimen was a 21-day home use of desensitizing dentifrice (elmex SENSITIVE toothpaste) in combination with a dental rinse (elmex SENSITIVE dental rinse) and a special toothbrush (elmex interX SENSITIVE toothbrush) twice a day for oral hygiene. The patients completed the OHIP-G before and after treatment intervention. Following the intervention, OHRQoL improved considerably, with a mean decrease in 13.5 OHIP-G units ($P < 0.001$). In particular, 50% of the patients showed a decrease in 11 or more OHIP-G units. No statistical significances, however, were observed for gender or age. The study had some limitations, as it was not randomized and did not include a control or placebo group. However, it was the first study undertaken to evaluate the effect of a DH treatment on OHRQoL and not solely from that of the clinician's perspective. Moreover, the study demonstrated that it is possible to measure the success of a treatment for DH with an OHRQoL instrument, the OHIP.

Further studies on the subject have since been carried out in recent years focusing on different treatment approaches and OHRQoL. They all show that dentin hypersensitivity has a negative impact on quality of life and that there is a significant improvement in the OHRQoL after treatment. For example, Douglas de Oliveira and colleagues noted significant statistical changes following treatment with surgical defect coverage on cervical dentin hypersensitivity across several dimensions of the OHIP-14, including physical pain, psychological comfort, physical disability, psychological disability, and the overall OHIP score (Douglas de Oliveira et al. 2013). Lima and co-authors similarly observed a significant improvement of OHRQoL in both the OHIP-14 total score and specific dimensions, such as physical pain, psychological disability, and social disability after interventions with laser and cyanoacrylate (Lima et al. 2017). Another study, focusing on laser treatment and potassium oxalate emphasizes the results by showing a reduction in the OHIP-14 score for all dimensions, indicating an improvement in patients' quality of life after the use of desensitizing therapies (Sgreccia et al. 2022). Likewise, Sivaramakrishnan and Sridharan (2019) were able to show that quality of life significantly improved in patients treated with either GLUMA or fluoride varnish (Sivaramakrishnan and Sridharan 2019).

The disease-specific DHEQ that was introduced in 2010 (Boiko et al. 2010) provides an alternative to the "generic" OHIP for assessing OHRQoL in patients with DH. It directly addressed the problems associated with sensitive teeth. Initial work with this newly developed measure examined whether it met the gold-standard guidelines for QoL instruments (Aaronson et al. 2002). For this initial analysis, the DHEQ was first applied in a general-population sample and in a sample of patients clinically diagnosed with DH (Boiko et al. 2010). The DHEQ instrument demonstrated good psychometric properties and was internally consistent (Cronbach's a = 0.86), reliable (ICC = 0.92), and demonstrated high validity scores. The DHEQ indicated that patients with DH had higher scores on the DHEQ (147.6 ± 5.98) than the general population (130.96 ± 35.06), indicating that these patients had impaired an OHRQoL. In particular, the DHEQ detected functional limitations (e.g., problems with eating ice cream), coping behaviors (e.g., careful when breathing, warming food/drinks, avoiding contact with certain teeth), emotional (e.g., annoying sensations), and social impacts (e.g., difficulties conversing) caused by DH.

These results were underlined and confirmed by a subsequent longitudinal study including three clinical trials with 311 participants (Baker et al. 2014). Each trial compared the efficacy of test and control dentifrices in providing relief from DH. Participants brushed at home twice daily for 8 or 12 weeks, respectively. The DHEQ was administered before and after treatment. The results demonstrated significant decreases in total DHEQ scores ($P < 0.001$), as well as all domain scores (except for identity and restriction once each), across all the trials. The coping domain showed the largest effect size, followed by the emotional domain; the identity domain showed the smallest decrease. In this analysis, the DHEQ was found to be highly useful for assessing changes in functional and personal experiences of DH, improvements in QoL status, and responsiveness to anti-sensitivity treatments.

Since then, further QoL studies have been undertaken using the DHEQ and these have confirmed the initial results. Two studies by Sufi et al. reported statistically significant changes in the DHEQ outcomes using two different dentifrices (Sufi et al. 2016a, b). In addition, Hall et al. were able to show significant improvements in almost all DHEQ endpoints, including intensity and bother some of sensations, total score, global oral health rating, adaptation, and emotional impact when using mouthwash containing 3% potassium nitrate (KNO_3) as an adjunct to brushing with fluoride toothpaste compared with use of the same toothpaste alone (Hall et al. 2017a, b). Statistically significant improvements in all DHEQ scores were also observed in a study by Lin et al. focusing on the treatment of DH with a stannous fluoride-containing dentifrice (Li et al. 2024).

In summary, it can be emphasized that regardless of the choice of instrument used to measure QoL, both condition-specific measure for measuring impacts of DH on OHRQoL may detect changes in functional and personal experiences of DH. DHEQ data may therefore be used to evaluate negative emotions specifically related to DH and aid in the development of effective interventions and health policies to address DH. It should be noted, however, a major drawback is the limited comparability of scores. This limitation restricts its application to evaluating the impact of dentin hypersensitivity and its treatment exclusively, without allowing for comparisons to other conditions like dental caries or tooth loss (Reissmann 2021). Consequently, oral disease-specific instruments offer limited utility. Conversely, the OHIP—which has relevance to determining the impact of DH as well—is not limited to this special patient group. For this reason, it has the advantage that it can be used in patients with other oral diseases and across conditions, therefore allowing DH to be compared with other oral conditions and enabling to the broader influence of hypersensitive teeth on patient's perceived health to be characterized.

3.5 Future Directions

Patient-reported outcomes and in particular the concept of OHRQoL have gained popularity in recent years. This new perspective on health suggests that the goal of dental care, which is good oral health, should no longer be seen as the absence of caries or periodontal disease, and that a patient's mental and social well-being also must be considered (Inglehart and Bagramian 2002). Evaluation of OHRQoL allows for this shift from traditional medical and dental criteria, as it captures the aim of this new perspective and focuses on subjective patient social and emotional experiences, as well as physical functioning, in defining appropriate treatment goals and outcomes (Sischo and Broder 2011).

In the future, it is desirable to evaluate OHRQoL in the clinical setting, as its measurement may identify issues on an individual level previously not recognized that could potentially be addressed through appropriate interventions; repeating the measurement after therapy would allow assessment of the efficacy of the intervention (Barnes and Jenney 2002). It could also guide choices and perhaps encourage new development. Regarding conditions such as DH, it may prove to be a valuable asset for clinicians when assessing their patients' quality of life before, during, and after treatment of various clinical conditions (Sixou 2013).

3.6 Conclusions

The concept of OHRQoL brings a new perspective to clinical dental care and research, as it allows insight into how a patient's oral health affects his/her well-being and quality of life at a given point in time. In patients with DH, limited data about OHRQoL are available, knowledge is still incomplete, and further research is desired. Nevertheless, preliminary data have shown that patients with DH report substantial OHRQoL impairment, and that the impact of this experienced oral pain on patients' perceived health is considerable. Thus, OHRQoL measurement provides additional information about the magnitude of the condition of DH and should be considered as a useful addition to clinical tests to assess the severity and impact of the reported problem.

References

Aaronson N, Alonso J, Burnam A, Lohr KN, Patrick DL, Perrin E, Stein RE. Assessing health status and quality-of-life instruments: attributes and review criteria. Qual Life Res. 2002;11:193–205.

Absi EG, Addy M, Adams D. Dentine hypersensitivity. A study of the patency of dentinal tubules in sensitive and non-sensitive cervical dentine. J Clin Periodontol. 1987;14:280–4.

Al Shamrany M. Oral health-related quality of life: a broader perspective. La Revue de Santé de la Méditerranée orientale. 2006;12:894–901.

Allen PF. Assessment of oral health related quality of life. Health Qual Life Outcomes. 2003;1:40. https://doi.org/10.1186/1477-7525-1-40.

Arheiam A, ELTantawi M, ELkadiki N, Elhashani A, Baker SR. Cross-cultural adaptation of the Arabic version of the DHEQ-15. Int J Dent Hyg. 2022;20:527–33. https://doi.org/10.1111/idh.12579.

Baba K, Inukai M, John MT. Feasibility of oral health-related quality of life assessment in prosthodontic patients using abbreviated Oral Health Impact Profile questionnaires. J Oral Rehabil. 2008;35:224–8. https://doi.org/10.1111/j.1365-2842.2007.01761.x.

Baker SR, Gibson BJ, Sufi F, Barlow A, Robinson PG. The dentine hypersensitivity experience questionnaire: a longitudinal validation study. J Clin Periodontol. 2014;41:52–9. https://doi.org/10.1111/jcpe.12181.

Barnes PM, Jenney MEM. Measuring quality of life. Curr Paediatr. 2002;2:476–80.

Basaran S, Celik C. Turkish adaptation of Dentine Hypersensitivity Experience Questionnaire (DHEQ). Community Dent Health. 2018;35:47–51. https://doi.org/10.1922/CDH_4151Basaran05.

Bekes K, Schaller HG, Hirsch C. [Verbesserung mundgesundheitsbezogener Lebensqualität durch die Anwendung von Mundhygieneprodukten für schmerzempfindliche und freiliegende Zahnhälse] Improvement of oral health-related quality of life in subjects with dentin hypersensitivity. ZWR. 2008;117:136–42.

Bekes K, John MT, Schaller HG, Hirsch C. Oral health-related quality of life in patients seeking care for dentin hypersensitivity. J Oral Rehabil. 2009;36:45–51. https://doi.org/10.1111/j.1365-2842.2008.01901.x.

Bhowmik E, Pawar Chandrashekhar D, Sharma Hareesha M. Comparative evaluation of fluorinol and calcium sodium phosphosilicate-containing toothpastes in the treatment of dentin hypersensitivity. Int J Dent Hyg. 2021;19:421–8. https://doi.org/10.1111/idh.12495.

Boiko OV, Baker SR, Gibson BJ, Locker D, Sufi F, Barlow AP, Robinson PG. Construction and validation of the quality of life measure for dentine hypersensitivity (DHEQ). J Clin Periodontol. 2010;37:973–80. https://doi.org/10.1111/j.1600-051X.2010.01618.x.

Canadian Advisory Board on Dentin Hypersensitivity. Consensus-based recommendations for the diagnosis and management of dentin hypersensitivity. J Can Dent Assoc. 2003;69:221–6.

Cimprich B, Paterson G. Health-related quality of life: conceptual issues and research applications. In: Inglehart MR, Bagramian RA, editors. Oral health-related quality of life. Chicago: Quintessence; 2002. p. 47–53.

DHHS. Oral health in America. A report of the Surgeon General. Rockville: US Department of Health and Human Services, National Institute of Dental and Craniofacial Research, National Institute of Health; 2000.

Douglas de Oliveira DW, Marques DP, Aguiar-Cantuaria IC, Flecha OD, Goncalves PF. Effect of surgical defect coverage on cervical dentin hypersensitivity and quality of life. J Periodontol. 2013;84:768–75. https://doi.org/10.1902/jop.2012.120479.

Douglas-de-Oliveira DW, Vitor GP, Silveira JO, Martins CC, Costa FO, Cota LOM. Effect of dentin hypersensitivity treatment on oral health related quality of life—a systematic review and meta-analysis. J Dent. 2018;71:1–8. https://doi.org/10.1016/j.jdent.2017.12.007.

Gibson B, Boiko O, Baker S, Robinson PG, Barlow A, Player T, Locker D. The everyday impact of dentine sensitivity: personal and functional aspects. Soc Sci Dent. 2010;1:11–20.

Gillam DG, Seo HS, Bulman JS, Newman HN. Perceptions of dentine hypersensitivity in a general practice population. J Oral Rehabil. 1999;26:710–4.

Gillam DG, Bulman JS, Eijkman MA, Newman HN. Dentists' perceptions of dentine hypersensitivity and knowledge of its treatment. J Oral Rehabil. 2002;29:219–25.

Glick M, Williams DM, Kleinman DV, Vujicic M, Watt RG, Weyant RJ. A new definition for oral health developed by the FDI World Dental Federation opens the door to a universal definition of oral health. Int Dent J. 2016;66:322–4. https://doi.org/10.1111/idj.12294.

Goh V, Corbet EF, Leung WK. Impact of dentine hypersensitivity on oral health-related quality of life in individuals receiving supportive periodontal care. J Clin Periodontol. 2016;43:595–602. https://doi.org/10.1111/jcpe.12552.

Guanipa Ortiz MI, Alencar CM, Freitas de Paula BL, Alves EB, Nogueira Araujo JL, Silva CM. Effect of the casein phosphopeptide-amorphous calcium phosphate fluoride (CPP-ACPF) and photobiomodulation (PBM) on dental hypersensitivity: a randomized controlled clinical trial. PLoS One. 2019;14:e0225501. https://doi.org/10.1371/journal.pone.0225501.

Hall C, Sufi F, Constantin P. Efficacy of an experimental 3% potassium nitrate mouthwash in providing long-term relief from dentin hypersensitivity: an 8-week randomized controlled study (Study 2). Am J Dent. 2017a;30:335–42.

Hall C, Sufi F, Wang N, Goyal CR. Efficacy of an experimental 3% potassium nitrate mouthwash in providing long-term relief from dentin hypersensitivity: an 8-week randomized controlled study (Study 1). Am J Dent. 2017b;30:27–34.

He SL, Wang JH, Wang MH. Development of the Chinese version of the dentine hypersensitivity experience questionnaire. Eur J Oral Sci. 2012;120:218–23. https://doi.org/10.1111/j.1600-0722.2012.00962.x.

Idon I, Esan TA, Bamise CT. Oral health-related quality of life in patients presenting with dentine hypersensitivity: a randomized controlled study of treatment effect. Eur J Gen Dent. 2017;6:99–105.

Inglehart MR, Bagramian RA. Oral health-related quality of life: an introduction. In: Inglehart MR, Bagramian RA, editors. Oral health-related quality of life. Chicago: Quintessence; 2002. p. 1–6.

John MT. Health outcomes reported by dental patients. J Evid Based Dent Pract. 2018;18:332–5. https://doi.org/10.1016/j.jebdp.2018.09.001.

John MT, Patrick DL, Slade GD. The German version of the oral health impact profile—translation and psychometric properties. Eur J Oral Sci. 2002;110:425–33.

John MT, LeResche L, Koepsell TD, Hujoel P, Miglioretti DL, Micheelis W. Oral health-related quality of life in Germany. Eur J Oral Sci. 2003;111:483–91.

John MT, Micheelis W, Biffar R. Reference values in oral health-related quality of life for the abbreviated version of the oral health impact profile. Schweiz Monatsschr Zahnmed. 2004;114:784–91.

John MT, Feuerstahler L, Waller N, Baba K, Larsson P, Celebic A, Kende D, Rener-Sitar K, Reissmann DR. Confirmatory factor analysis of the Oral Health Impact Profile. J Oral Rehabil. 2014a;41:644–52. https://doi.org/10.1111/joor.12191.

John MT, Reissmann DR, Feuerstahler L, Waller N, Baba K, Larsson P, Celebic A, Szabo G, Rener-Sitar K. Exploratory factor analysis of the oral health impact profile. J Oral Rehabil. 2014b;41:635–43. https://doi.org/10.1111/joor.12192.

John MT, Reissmann DR, Celebic A, Baba K, Kende D, Larsson P, Rener-Sitar K. Integration of oral health-related quality of life instruments. J Dent. 2016a;53:38–43. https://doi.org/10.1016/j.jdent.2016.06.006.

John MT, Rener-Sitar K, Baba K, Celebic A, Larsson P, Szabo G, Norton WE, Reissmann DR. Patterns of impaired oral health-related quality of life dimensions. J Oral Rehabil. 2016b;43:519–27. https://doi.org/10.1111/joor.12396.

John MT, Sekulic S, Bekes K, Al-Harthy MH, Michelotti A, Reissmann DR, Nikolovska J, Sanivarapu S, Lawal FB, List T, Persic Kirsic S, Strajnic L, Casassus R, Baba K, Schimmel M, Amuasi A, Jayasinghe RD, Strujic-Porovic S, Peck CC, Xie H, Haugaard Bendixen K, Simancas Pallares MA, Perez-Franco E, Naghibi Sistani MM, Valerio P, Letunova N, Nurelhuda NM, Bartlett DW, Oluwafemi IA, Dghoughi S, Ferreira J, Chantaracherd P, Rener-Sitar K. Why patients visit dentists—a study in all World Health Organization regions. J Evid Based Dent Pract. 2020;20:101459. https://doi.org/10.1016/j.jebdp.2020.101459.

Krause C, Lunau N, Sufi F. An exploratory clinical study to monitor clinical efficacy of an occluding technology dentifrice in providing short term relief from dentinal hypersensitivity. J Clin Dent. 2018;29:18–22.

Li R, Yang W, Grimaldi R, Zeng P, Smith G, Chen X. Efficacy of a stannous fluoride dentifrice for relieving dentinal hypersensitivity in Chinese population: an 8-week randomized clinical trial. Clin Oral Investig. 2024;28:230. https://doi.org/10.1007/s00784-024-05610-9.

Lima TC, Vieira-Barbosa NM, Grasielle de sa Azevedo C, de Matos FR, Douglas de Oliveira DW, de Oliveira ES, Ramos-Jorge ML, Goncalves PF, Flecha OD. Oral

health-related quality of life before and after treatment of dentin hypersensitivity with cyanoacrylate and laser. J Periodontol. 2017;88:166–72. https://doi.org/10.1902/jop.2016.160216.
Locker D. Measuring oral health: a conceptual framework. Community Dent Health. 1988;5:3–18.
Locker D, Allen PF. Developing short-form measures of oral health-related quality of life. J Public Health Dent. 2002;62:13–20.
Machuca C, Baker SR, Sufi F, Mason S, Barlow A, Robinson PG. Derivation of a short form of the dentine hypersensitivity experience questionnaire. J Clin Periodontol. 2014;41:46–51. https://doi.org/10.1111/jcpe.12175.
Mantzourani M, Sharma D. Dentine sensitivity: past, present and future. J Dent. 2013;41(Suppl 4):S3–17. https://doi.org/10.1016/S0300-5712(13)70002-2.
Mason S, Burnett GR, Patel N, Patil A, Maclure R. Impact of toothpaste on oral health-related quality of life in people with dentine hypersensitivity. BMC Oral Health. 2019;19:226. https://doi.org/10.1186/s12903-019-0919-x.
Masud M, Al-Bayat FH, Muhamed NAH, Alwi AS, Takiyudin Z, Hidayat MFH. Gingival recession and dentine hypersensitivity in periodontal patients: is it affecting their oral health related quality of life? J Int Dent Med Res. 2017;10:909–14.
Matthews B, Vongsavan N. Interactions between neural and hydrodynamic mechanisms in dentine and pulp. Arch Oral Biol. 1994;39(Suppl):87S–95S.
McGrath PA. The measurement of human pain. Endod Dent Traumatol. 1986;2:124–9.
McGrath PA. Psychological aspects of pain perception. Arch Oral Biol. 1994;39(Suppl):55S–62S.
Mittal H, John MT, Sekulic S, Theis-Mahon N, Rener-Sitar K. Patient-reported outcome measures for adult dental patients: a systematic review. J Evid Based Dent Pract. 2019;19:53–70. https://doi.org/10.1016/j.jebdp.2018.10.005.
Naito M, Yuasa H, Nomura Y, Nakayama T, Hamajima N, Hanada N. Oral health status and health-related quality of life: a systematic review. J Oral Sci. 2006;48:1–7.
Ng SK, Leung WK. Oral health-related quality of life and periodontal status. Community Dent Oral Epidemiol. 2006;34:114–22. https://doi.org/10.1111/j.1600-0528.2006.00267.x.
Pigou AC. The economics of welfare. London: MacMillan; 1920.
Porritt JM, Sufi F, Barlow A, Baker SR. The role of illness beliefs and coping in the adjustment to dentine hypersensitivity. J Clin Periodontol. 2014;41:60–9. https://doi.org/10.1111/jcpe.12177.
Porto IC, Andrade AK, Montes MA. Diagnosis and treatment of dentinal hypersensitivity. J Oral Sci. 2009;51:323–32.
Reissmann DR. Methodological considerations when measuring oral health-related quality of life. J Oral Rehabil. 2021;48:233–45. https://doi.org/10.1111/joor.12983.
Schuurs AH, Wesselink PR, Eijkman MA, Duivenvoorden HJ. Dentists' views on cervical hypersensitivity and their knowledge of its treatment. Endod Dent Traumatol. 1995;11:240–4.
Sgreccia PC, Dame-Teixeira N, Barbosa RES, Araujo PF, Zanatta RF, Garcia FCP. Assessment of the Oral Health Impact Profile (OHIP-14) improvement of different treatments for dentin hypersensitivity in noncarious cervical lesions-a randomized clinical study. Clin Oral Investig. 2022;26:6583–91. https://doi.org/10.1007/s00784-022-04610-x.
Sischo L, Broder HL. Oral health-related quality of life: what, why, how, and future implications. J Dent Res. 2011;90:1264–70. https://doi.org/10.1177/0022034511399918.
Sivaramakrishnan G, Sridharan K. Fluoride varnish versus glutaraldehyde for hypersensitive teeth: a randomized controlled trial, meta-analysis and trial sequential analysis. Clin Oral Investig. 2019;23:209–20. https://doi.org/10.1007/s00784-018-2428-8.
Sixou JL. How to make a link between oral health-related quality of life and dentin hypersensitivity in the dental office? Clin Oral Investig. 2013;17(Suppl 1):S41–4. https://doi.org/10.1007/s00784-012-0915-x.
Slade GD. Derivation and validation of a short-form oral health impact profile. Commun Dent Oral Epidemiol. 1997;25:284–90.
Slade GD. Assessment of oral health-related quality of life. In: Inglehart MR, Bagramian RA, editors. Oral health-related quality of life. Chicago: Quintessence; 2002. p. 29–45.
Slade GD, Spencer AJ. Development and evaluation of the Oral Health Impact Profile. Commun Dent Health. 1994;11:3–11.
Sufi F, Hall C, Mason S, Shaw D, Kennedy L, Gallob JT. Efficacy of an experimental toothpaste containing 5% calcium sodium phosphosilicate in the relief of dentin hypersensitivity: an 8-week randomized study (Study 1). Am J Dent. 2016a;29:93–100.
Sufi F, Hall C, Mason S, Shaw D, Milleman J, Milleman K. Efficacy of an experimental toothpaste containing 5% calcium sodium phosphosilicate in the relief of dentin hypersensitivity: an 8-week randomized study (Study 2). Am J Dent. 2016b;29:101–9.
Wilson IB, Cleary PD. Linking clinical variables with health-related quality of life. A conceptual model of patient outcomes. JAMA. 1995;273:59–65.
World Health Organization. Study protocol for the World Health Organization project to develop a Quality of Life assessment instrument (WHOQOL). Qual Life Res. 1993;2:153–9.
World Health Organization. Constitution of the World Health Organization. 2006; 45. Retrieved 2.5.2024, from https://cdn.who.int/media/docs/default-source/documents/publications/basic-documents-constitution-of-who179f0d3d-a613-4760-8801-811dfce250af.pdf?sfvrsn=e8fb384f_1&download=true.

4 Aetiology and Clinical Features of Dentine Hypersensitivity on all Tooth Surfaces and Including Non-Carious Cervical Lesions (NCCLs)

Ryan Olley and David Bartlett

4.1 Introduction

Dentine hypersensitivity (DH) is a common oral condition, which is typically short lasting, an intense pain located around teeth and often associated with cold stimuli. An innate problem with dentine hypersensitivity (DH) is that its clinical features are transient, and patients do not always present with DH at examination, even though they may suffer from it regularly. Indeed, the nature of DH appears to be cyclic, and most sufferers self-medicate and use desensitising toothpastes to control the condition. There are increasing suggestions from the published literature that DH supports the transient nature of the condition (Gillam 2013; West 2006; West et al. 2013b; Olley et al. 2015). The reasons for this trend, historically, have been unclear. Indeed, the cause/s of DH have been poorly understood and resulted in DH being termed an enigma decades ago, and this concept has been re-visited on a number of occasions (Johnson et al. 1982; Dababneh et al. 1999; Addy 2002; Markowitz and Pashley 2008). The apparent historical lack in the understanding of the aetiological processes in particular tooth wear often resulted in elusive treatment and preventive strategies which focused on the symptoms of DH rather than its cause/s (Markowitz and Pashley 2008). Nevertheless, our understanding of the condition is somewhat clearer today. This chapter therefore focuses attention on the clinical features of DH and in detail on the causes of DH and the associated clinical presentation.

R. Olley (✉)
Restorative Dentistry, School of Dentistry, College of Biomedical and Life Sciences, Cardiff University, Cardiff, UK
e-mail: OlleyR1@cardiff.ac.uk

D. Bartlett
Department of Prosthodontics, King's College London Dental Institute, London, UK

4.2 Clinical Features of DH

DH is a common clinical condition, and patients describe it as a short, sharp pain that affects the permanent dentition (Addy 2002). The clinical features are explained in the definition of DH. This was first suggested by Dowell and Addy in 1983 (Dowell and Addy 1983), later finalised by an international workshop on the design and conduct of clinical trials for DH (Holland et al. 1997), and most recently modified by the Canadian Advisory Board for Dentine Hypersensitivity (Canadian 2003). The definition stated that DH 'is characterised by short sharp pain arising from exposed dentine in response to stimuli typically thermal, evaporative, tactile, osmotic or chemical and which cannot be ascribed to any other form of defect or disease'. The clinical description of the condition is explained in the first part of this definition. The second part differentiates it from other clinical conditions that might have identical symptoms

D. G. Gillam (ed.), *Dentine Hypersensitivity*, https://doi.org/10.1007/978-3-031-74321-4_4

Table 4.1 Examples of clinical conditions that need to be excluded prior to a definitive diagnosis of DH

Dental caries
Cracked tooth
Fractured restoration
Post-restorative sensitivity
Medication sensitivity
Post-non-surgical/surgical periodontal sensitivity
Palatogingival groove
Non-odontogenic origin

but different management strategies (Dowell et al. 1985) and these are listed in Table 4.1.

In the definition of DH, the word 'disease' replaced the previously used word 'pathology' following the Canadian consensus. However, disease relates more to the clinical outcome of the condition, rather than its aetiology or pathology which will be discussed below.

4.3 Aetiology

DH can be associated with several aetiologies including most commonly post-surgical periodontal disease, erosion, and gingival recession. These are discussed in turn below together with some other rarer aetiologies.

4.3.1 Post-surgical Periodontal Disease (Recession-Induced by Management)

DH may occur iatrogenically and it has been reported to affect up to 57% of the general population in one subject reported study following scaling or root planning (Irwin and McCusker 1997). Another study of periodontal patients reported a prevalence of 85–95% (Chabanski et al. 1996). Several systematic reviews have also reported that postoperative sensitivity increases following the procedure and gradually reduces in intensity over 1–2 weeks (von Troil et al. 2002; Lin and Gillam 2012). In an early lab study, it was reported after root surface debridement, the dentine surface tubules were exposed after the removal of the surface covering or smear layer (in part). In health, a smear layer reforms and prevents 86% of fluid movement across the dentine (Pashley et al. 1978). The smear layer may be defined as a thin 'loose' layer consisting of organic collagen and glycosaminoglycans that form an adherent matrix over mineralised tissue arising from saliva and dentine particles that might occlude the dentine tubules (Brannstrom 1966; Pashley 1984). It has also been suggested that in periodontal disease and any treatment to exposing dentine, bacteria may colonise and break down the smear layer and penetrate into the root dentine (Adriaens 1989) to cause sensitivity and this might be another explanation for the mechanism of DH (Lundy and Stanley 1969; Brannstrom 1982; Dababneh et al. 1999). It is the bacterial products, however, rather than the bacteria, which are likely to diffuse towards the pulp. Initially, plasma proteins/immunoglobulins from the blood diffuse into the dentine tubules decreasing permeability (Pashley 1984). Following chronic periodontal disease and ongoing treatment, increases in pulpal pressures, nerve spouting, and more sensitive nerves, scar tissue, and reduced plasma proteins may worsen DH (Pashley 1984).

4.3.2 Tooth Whitening Procedures (Unknown or Not Understood Inter-Relationship)

Tooth whitening procedures often involve carbamide peroxide, which breaks down into hydrogen peroxide and urea and bleach the tooth. This causes dehydration within the tooth and symptoms of DH. However, the symptoms are often temporary and for the duration of treatment (Ferrari et al. 2007). Bleaching may involve a different mechanism to that of DH (Gillam et al. 2013) and therefore is not strictly an aetiology for DH and may require alternative management strategies (Markowitz 2010).

4.3.3 Developmental Lesions (Rare Conditions Where Surface Morphology of Teeth Change)

These can often affect the primary and later permanent dentition and can cause symptoms of DH. They include, for example, amelogenesis and dentinogenesis imperfecta as well other conditions of the enamel and/or dentine that cause hypomineralisation and hypoplasia such as molar incisor hypoplasia (MIH). As with bleaching, these symptoms may involve a mechanism different to that of DH (Gillam et al. 2013).

4.3.4 Dietary Factors (Erosive Diets) and Gingival Recession

DH is most associated with erosive dietary factors and gingival recession, and these will be discussed in more detail in the following sections of this chapter. Both authors contributed the largest clinical study to date, which investigated the presence or otherwise absence of DH in association with its various aetiologies, involving 3187 adults enrolled from general dental practices in France, Spain, Italy, the UK, Finland, Latvia, and Estonia (West et al. 2013b). The proportion of subjects who were examined clinically to have DH on at least one tooth surface was 42% following an evaporative stimulus in a clinical setting. The proportion of subjects who reported having DH in the previous 12 months was less (27%) and this might reflect the transient nature of the pain in addition to good coping mechanisms. Then, when the aetiology was investigated, there was a strong progressive relationship between clinically elicited DH and erosive tooth wear caused by dietary factors and gingival recession (West et al. 2013b). Amongst these subjects, 29% had signs of tooth wear recorded using the Basic Erosive Wear Examination (Bartlett et al. 2013). The prevalence figure of DH was relatively high compared to similar studies conducted in general dental practice, 2.8% (Rees and Addy 2004), 9.1% (Amarasena et al. 2011), and 5.3% (Bahsi et al. 2012), but DH has been reported in other studies and associated with erosive tooth wear (Lussi and Schaffner 2000; Fares et al. 2009) and gingival recession (Bamise et al. 2008) (see Chap. 2). In a population in the UK, the prevalence of DH examined clinically was observed to be over 40% and was associated with gingival recession (Olley et al. 2013). An investigation of the same group of patients also indicated that this population had 43% of tooth surfaces with tooth wear (Olley et al. 2014b. In a prospective study of randomly selected subjects in Switzerland, 34.8% of subjects reported DH; however, the prevalence of DH in those subjects with tooth wear was 84.6% (Lussi and Schaffner 2000). Subjects who recently consumed dietary acids were more likely to have DH when examined at their dental appointment and measures of tooth wear and DH severity were proportional (Olley et al. 2015). This supported previous suggestions that DH is a tooth wear phenomenon (Addy 2002). It often occurs with intact periodontal tissues when cervical enamel is removed, and coronal dentine exposed and in combination with non-carious cervical lesions (NCCLs) or following gingival recession (Veitz-Keenan et al. 2013). Therefore, it is important to recognise the clinical features of tooth wear, in particular erosion. These will be discussed in greater detail together with gingival recession and oral hygiene practices below.

4.3.5 Overzealous Brushing

This section has been added to highlight the importance of brushing force, especially in the initiation of DH. Previously, this process was poorly understood as it is difficult to quantify brushing force, but laboratory studies on dentine have since investigated the mode of action and shown that whilst overzealous brushing can easily remove the smear layer and expose dentine tubules, as would be expected, gentler brushing may re-create a smear layer gradually (over several weeks) and may therefore be therapeutic to preventing DH (Sehmi and Olley 2015). Brushing and NCCLs will further be explained in the section on abrasion, below.

4.4 Development of the DH Lesion

For the purposes of further understanding the aetiological processes involved in DH, the names 'lesion localisation' and 'lesion initiation' were proposed (Addy 2002). Lesion localisation involves dentine exposure, which may occur because of enamel or dentine wear or gingival recession. Lesion initiation may arise following lesion localisation and involves exposure of patent or un-occluded dentine tubules from the surface of dentine to the pulp. This often occurs following loss of the smear layer. It should be noted that in addition to the smear layer or other surface occlusion, the degree of sclerosis by peritubular dentine and the extent of occlusion by reparative dentine on the pulpal surface might also affect the capacity for fluid movement within the dentine tubules (Yoshiyama et al. 1996). Dentine exposure will not necessarily lead to DH if the dentine tubule system is not patent. Indeed, clinical observation studies show that DH can be uncommon even in cases where the pulp is visible through a thin bridge of dentine (Bartlett and Ide 1999), which is likely to consist of sclerotic or transparent dentine.

Tooth wear is the irreversible, non-traumatic loss of dental hard tissues due to aetiological processes classified as erosion, attrition, abrasion (Bartlett and Smith 2000; Ganss et al. 2006), and abfraction (Lee and Eakle 1984). Tooth wear may be considered a normal part of ageing, or a physiological process, from the anthropological perspective (Whittacker 2000). Historically, it has been suggested that the human dentition is designed to wear and that this process is important to optimise the functional capabilities of the dentition (Berry and Poole 1974). Within dentistry, Smith and Knight first distinguished physiological and active or pathological tooth wear (Smith and Knight 1984). Tooth wear may be defined as pathological as opposed as physiological if it appears in relatively younger patients and the rate of progression of tooth wear is fast. Crucially, physiological tooth wear allows time for the pulp to lay down reparative or secondary dentine, which could prevent fluid flow within dentine tubules and reduce DH (Krauser 1986). In contrast, pathological tooth wear may cause DH as well as other aesthetic and functional concerns (Smith and Knight 1984; Al-Omiri et al. 2006). During pathological tooth wear, the symptoms of DH are reported more frequently (Smith and Knight 1984; Absi et al. 1987; Addy and Pearce 1994; Dababneh et al. 1999; Addy 2000, 2002). As pathological tooth wear lesions progress into dentine, the radius of dentine tubules becomes larger and the distance to the pulp decreases. As a result, the hydraulic conductance of fluid within dentine (and DH symptoms) would be expected to increase (Pashley 1990). However, exposure of dentine (as a result of tooth wear or gingival recession) will not necessarily lead to the presence of DH per se (Absi et al. 1987; Yoshiyama et al. 1996; Addy 2002). Therefore, tools to measure tooth wear in terms of surface loss alone may not reflect the presence of DH.

4.5 Erosion and DH

Erosion continues to be considered the most common and important aetiological factor for tooth wear globally (Seligman et al. 1988; Deery et al. 2000; Addy and Hunter 2003; Grippo et al. 2004; Lussi 2006; Bartlett et al. 2013; Awad et al. 2019; Yu et al. 2021).

Erosion processes occur due to the superficial demineralisation of hard tissue and the chemical dissolution of the apatite crystals in enamel by an acid (Bartlett 2005) that is not produced by the oral flora, but from intrinsic or extrinsic sources (ten Carte et al. 2008), both of which are strongly associated with DH (West et al. 2013a; Olley et al. 2015). Typical sources of intrinsic acid are regurgitated stomach acid containing hydrochloric acid (HCL) due to vomiting or gastro-oesophageal reflux (Scheutzel 1996). Typical extrinsic sources are provided below (Zero 1996; Lussi 2006) (see Fig. 4.1):

- Diet (for example, acidic citrus and other fruits, carbonated beverages and sports drinks, beers and herbal teas, vinegars and pickles, candies)

- Medicaments (for example, non-encapsulated HCL replacement, chewing ascorbic acid tablets (vitamin C) and acetylsalicylic acid tablets (aspirin), iron tablets, salivary stimulants)
- Occupation (for example, jobs involving wine tasting or working near acidic industrial vapours)
- Sports (for example, improperly chlorinated swimming pools)

There is an increasing body of literature indicating that acid erosion caused by relatively small acidic challenges will lead to loss of enamel and dentine and expose the dentine tubules and initiate DH. This literature included laboratory research (Addy et al. 1987b; Absi et al. 1992; West et al. 1999; Vanuspong et al. 2002; Gregg et al. 2004; Ganss et al. 2009), review papers (Addy and Hunter 2003; Addy 2005; Zero and Lussi 2005; Lussi 2006), clinical research (Absi et al. 1992; Hughes et al. 1999; Hunter et al. 2000; Olley et al. 2012, 2014a, 2015; O'Toole and Bartlett 2017), and prevalence studies (Lussi and Schaffner 2000; Smith et al. 2008; West et al. 2013b).

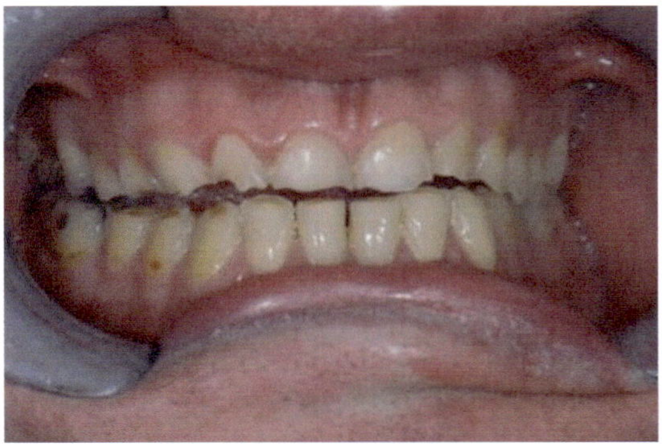

Fig. 4.1 An example of a patient with severe erosion, which has initiated a loss of crown height and an anterior open bite due to gastric erosion

Erosive acid challenges are important in removing the smear layer and pellicle (on the tooth surfaces exposed to saliva) and initiating DH. In two clinical studies, cavities were prepared in dentine, and hydrostatic pressures were applied to the exposed dentine. Patients reported sensations of short sharp pain in those lesions in which an acid challenge was used to remove the smear layer from the surface of the prepared cavity, but not in lesions in which the smear layer was present (Brannstrom 1965; Ahlquist et al. 1994). This can be easily demonstrated in the laboratory. Figure 4.2 shows a high-powered scanning electron microscopy image of the surface of root dentine taken from the buccal cervical region of a premolar tooth. Following treatment of the surface of the dentine with a 6% solution of citric acid under agitation, the smear layer was removed, and the dentine tubules become visible. This work is supported elsewhere (Pashley et al. 1981) (Addy et al. 1987a). Most of the dentine tubules are greater than 1 μm diameter post-acid challenge. This is greater than 0.83 μm, the minimum diameter reported as being required to elicit DH at the cervical area of

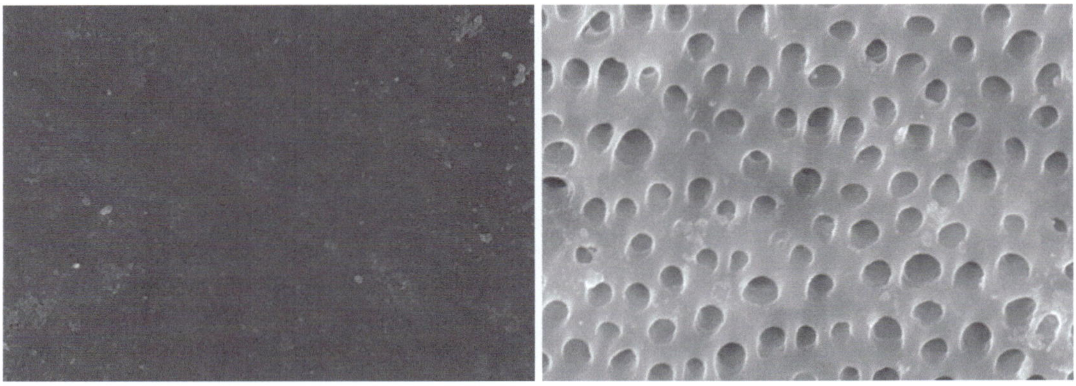

Fig. 4.2 Scanning electron micrograph (SEM) images (×2000) of untreated root surface (left) and root surface following a 1 minute 6% citric acid challenge with gentle agitation (right). Scale bar 2 μm

Table 4.2 Erosive products (with associated acids) available in the UK with pKa and pH values

Beverage	Acid	pKa (titratable acidity)	pH
Citric fruits including oranges, lemons, grapefruit	Citric acid	3.14	2.2
Apples, plums, and peaches	Malic acid	3.4	2.2
Grapes and wines	Tartaric acid	2.89	2.2
Fermented products and yogurt	Lactic acid	3.86	2.4
Preservative	Acetic acid	4.76	2.9
Rhubarb	Oxalic acid	4.14	1.3
Cola drink	Phosphoric acid	2.15	1.5

the tooth near the dentino-enamel junction (DEJ) (Absi et al. 1987). The effects of acids are to remove the smear layer and expose patent or unoccluded dentine tubules. It was concluded in these studies that the presence of these patent dentine tubules was related clinically to DH.

There are several food products that contain acids which are popular consumables in the UK. These are summarised, together with pH and pKa values (explained below) in Table 4.2.

Despite the acidity of these products, not all popular erosive beverages will initiate the exposure of the dentine tubules. This was demonstrated in an early study, which investigated the effect of various dietary beverages on dentine and reported that many of these popular erosive beverages of acidic or 'low' pH would not lead to exposure of the patent dentine tubules (Addy et al. 1987a). These beverages included a low pH carbonated drink, Coca-Cola, and Ribena (a fruit based soft drink). Instead, consumables, for example, red and white wine, citrus fruit juices, apple juice, and yogurt produced visible dentine tubules as observed by SEM (Addy et al. 1987a). Citric acid was also described at the time as most detrimental to human enamel (Meurman et al. 1987). Grenby et al. demonstrated that titratability was likely to be more important than pH in determining erosive potential (Grenby et al. 1989). For example, the Coca-Cola drink and Ribena were observed to have substantially lower titratable acidities in contrast to fruit juices (lemon, orange, and pineapple) and they were therefore less acidic. Titratable acidity or neutralisable acidity (pKa) is the volume of alkali required (typically 0.1 mol solution of sodium hydroxide) to raise the pH of a standardised volume of beverage (typically 25 ml) to pH 7 (Chadwick 2006). In dental erosion, titratability provides an indication of the actual concentration of hydrogen ions available to interact with a mineralised surface, which provides an indication of the erosive potential of a particular acid challenge (Zero 1996). In addition to a higher titratable acidity and lower pH, the severity of an erosive challenge is also likely to increase with the duration of the acid challenge, temperature, and ion concentration, frequency of acid challenge, and presence of chelating agents (Moss 1998; West et al. 2000; Wiegand et al. 2007). The latter is related to the calcium binding property of the acid. Acids, for example, citric, malic, and tartaric acid contain more than one carboxyl group in their chemical composition and this will result to the binding of more than one calcium ion at high pH (Meurman et al. 1987). Calcium binding from the saliva will result in loss of the ion effect of calcium in saliva, which will lead to more dissolution tendency. Also, if the calcium from saliva is bound, there may be a tendency for more dissolution of the dental tissue in order to replace the calcium lost in saliva (Meurman and tenCate 1996). This will result in further erosion of the surface layer, due to the gradual release of tooth mineral due to a buffering action (Grenby et al. 1989). As a result, fruit juices, for example, orange or pineapple juice, will result in more demineralisation than other popular erosive beverages such as the Coca-Cola and Lemonade drinks, which have lower levels of Ca and P (Grenby et al. 1989).

The importance of a mature salivary pellicle in providing a protective role during erosion must not therefore be underestimated; in particular, the phosphate, calcium, and fluoride content of an erosive challenge may prevent dental wear (Zero and Lussi 2005) and sleeping medications (which may reduce salivary flow) are associated with more reported DH (West et al. 2013a). Currently there is ongoing research in this area and clinical experiments have demonstrated that the salivary pellicle forms a protective layer against erosion (Moazzez et al. 2014).

Regarding the timing of erosion, clinical studies show that DH is more likely if acidic beverages are consumed more recently, within an hour (Olley et al. 2015). It has also been shown that contact time between the tooth and the acid leads to more DH, for example, patients who spent more than 10 min eating fruit per sitting or habits include sipping an erosive beverage or holding it in the mouth (O'Toole and Bartlett 2017).

4.6 Abrasion, NCCLs, and DH

Abrasion is a physical process, which occurs because of the mechanical wear of dental tissues by foreign bodies. Toothbrushing and dentifrices are common forms of dental abrasion (Addy and Hunter 2003; Addy and West 2013). Toothbrush abrasions are influenced by brushing habits, force applied, and the time spent brushing (Hooper et al. 2003). There are additional habits linked to abrasion, for example, onychophagia, clips, and other tools, which may contact the teeth. There is less data than erosion to support the role of abrasion in causing DH, but toothbrushing with a toothpaste has been implicated in the aetiology of DH (Addy and Hunter 2003; Abrahamsen 2005; Bartlett and Shah 2006; Ganss et al. 2009; Addy and West 2013), and more recent studies are identifying a greater role of toothbrushing force and filament type as being important in DH (Sehmi and Olley 2015; O'Toole and Bartlett 2017). A recent systematic review by Teixeira et al. (2020) demonstrates a high proportion of adults in the population with NCCLs and therefore exposed cervical dentine. This study reported that the average prevalence in the adult population for NCCLs is 46.7% and that older individuals were more likely to present with NCCLs (Teixeira et al. 2020). Enamel cervically on the tooth is thinner and hence in patients with extreme abrasion habits (perhaps in combination with erosion), the NCCL lesion will occur sooner, persist longer, and, with ongoing aetiology, continue to increase in size throughout life. Figure 4.3 shows a NCCL caused predominantly by excessive abrasion.

According to Addy (2005), the effects of normal toothbrushing on wear of enamel are negligible and unlikely to lead to exposure of the underlying dentine alone unless erosion is also occurring. Normal toothbrushing, even for extended periods of time (measured in years) will also cause limited wear of dentine and the wear may be limited to the smear layer, which would presumably have a subsequent effect on DH (Absi et al. 1992). Increasing the force of toothbrushing can, in addition, cause increased tooth surface loss in dentine. Manual, as opposed to electric toothbrushing has been demonstrated to cause more dentine wear because of the force applied with a manual toothbrush (Knezevic et al. 2010; Van der Weijden et al. 2011). However, studies have also demonstrated that electric toothbrushing causes more wear than manual brushing (Bartlett et al. 2013). Nonetheless, the type of toothbrush alone is not the only factor in dentine wear. Studies have shown that brushing

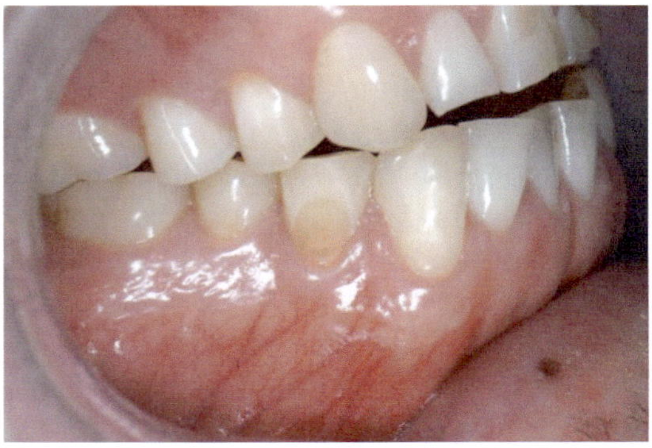

Fig. 4.3 An example of abrasion on the buccal cervical region commonly referred to as a non-carious cervical lesion (NCCL). Clinical features may include aesthetic concerns and perhaps DH

with medium and hard, rather than soft stiffness toothbrushes will cause more dentine wear (Smith et al. 2008). Furthermore, toothbrushing with a dentifrice adds an abrasive component. Nonetheless, normal toothbrushing with dentifrices (with the exception of non-hydrated alumina) in the absence of acid is likely to cause little or no wear of enamel and dentine (Hunter et al. 2002; Addy 2005). Abnormal or abusive use (for example, using excessive dentifrice) can however lead to pathological wear (Hunter et al. 2002; Hooper et al. 2003; Turssi et al. 2010). The filament stiffness of toothbrushes may also be important in dentine wear initiated by a dentifrice. Laboratory studies have demonstrated that smaller filament stiffness (decreasing diameter of filament) initiated more wear in dentine using various abrasives of dentifrice (post-acid erosion) and that the abrasivity of the dentifrice is more important than the filament stiffness (Wiegand et al. 2009). This would suggest that multifilament soft brushes may retain more toothpaste, which in turn might lead to more tooth wear. Following DH localisation through an NCCL, we next consider studies where the DH lesion may be initiated.

To initiate DH symptoms, the smear layer must be removed. Clinically, it has been reported that when greater forces are applied to healthy dentine using a manual toothbrush, patients are more likely to report pain that resembles DH (Addy 2005). Novel laboratory investigations into the mode of action of brushing force on the dentine surface studies have shown that when the brushing force is increased to 400 g (causing toothbrush filaments to easily bend), DH lesions are initiated, whereas with lighter brushing forces of 100 g (in which there is limited bend of filament), the smear layer is not removed and may even be recreated, over the equivalent period of brushing twice a day for 6–8 weeks (Sehmi and Olley 2015).

Clinically, softer toothbrushes have also been shown to cause more DH (O'Toole and Bartlett 2017). However, toothbrush filament type was differentiated only for manual and not electric toothbrushing (O'Toole and Bartlett 2017). It is therefore possible that because the brushing force with manual toothbrushes is much less standardised than with electric brushes, if built with an alert indicator when brushing too hard. Therefore, as mentioned above, the potentially greater contact with the tooth surfaces using a softer brush head and manual brushing (with unknown and possibly greater forces) may remove more smear layer and initiate greater DH.

Dentifrice abrasivity is normally measured using the RDA (relative dentine abrasivity), which has a numeric value. The International Organization for Standardization guidelines state that for dentine, the abrasivity of test formulation should not exceed 2.5 times the reference abrasive, e.g., RDA must not exceed 250 (International. Standards.Organisation.ISO.11609, 1995). Interestingly, the allowed pH range for dentifrice (pH 4–10) might be more cause for concern as this would suggest that some dentifrices of low pH could intrinsically lead to chemico-physical dental wear. Despite this, ISO standards ensure all products are above a pH that may cause demineralisation (pH 5.5 for enamel and pH 6.5 for dentine) or the contained fluoride balances the low pH effect (Hunter et al. 2002). Dentifrices saturated with dental mineral and in particular fluoride actively encourage remineralisation due to their buffering capacity and consequently abrasion is less (Betke et al. 2003; Zero and Lussi 2005). Interestingly, gently dabbing the surface of dentine (with a normal dentifrice containing NaF) can create occlusion of the dentine tubules (over the equivalent of rubbing the same surface for 10–12 weeks twice a day) (Olley et al. 2020b). However, the effect of NaF on tubule occlusion is therefore considerably longer compared with active ingredients specifically for DH that work quicker, within days, in occluding the dentine tubules and preventing DH symptoms (Olley et al. 2012). Nonetheless, this work reflects the importance of the action of dabbing and touch which may influence the smear layer and it is not unreasonable to suggest that some habits including overzealous scratching or rubbing tooth surfaces may also remove the smear layer and have been seen in practice to contribute DH symptoms.

Concerning dentifrices, although these are unlikely to cause DH lesion localisation, dentifrices of higher abrasiveness or overzealous use of brushing with dentifrice may initiate more dentine wear and DH lesion initiation by removal of the smear layer and establishment of patent dentine tubules (Addy and Hunter 2003; Sehmi and Olley 2015). Some dentifrices, especially those containing silica, may have a therapeutic effect in preventing DH by partially occluding the dentine tubules over time (Addy and Mostafa 1989; West et al. 2002) and may also contain active ingredients capable of increasing this effect over shorter periods (Olley et al. 2012, 2014a). Due to a reduction in DH symptoms, it has been shown that dentifrices with active ingredients to occlude the dentine tubules may reduce DH irrespective of brushing force applied (Mullan et al. 2017). In these situations, overzealous brushing aetiology may continue, unidentified, to increase the size of the NCCL lesion over time.

4.7 Attrition and DH

Attrition is the physical wear of dental hard tissues due to tooth-to-tooth contact on occlusal or incisal tooth surfaces. In normal function, the teeth only contact for a short period of time for eating or swallowing. However, when this contact occurs at other times, it is termed parafunction or bruxism. This often occurs nocturnally as a form of stress relief (Bartlett and Smith 2000). Although DH is more common on buccal tooth surfaces in association with gingival recession, prevalence studies which have also investigated occlusal surfaces show that the occlusal surfaces also demonstrate DH (Bamise et al. 2008; Olley et al. 2013) (Fig. 4.4). The severity of DH on occlusal surfaces is associated with the severity of tooth wear clinically (Olley et al. 2015).

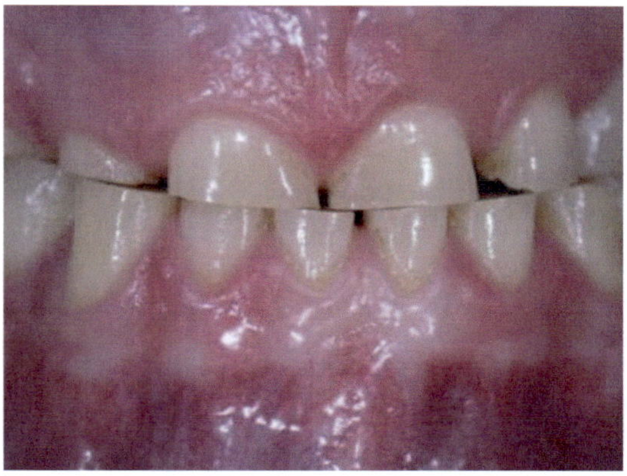

Fig. 4.4 An example of severe attrition associated with bruxism. Note the incisal surfaces are flattened

4.8 Abfraction and DH

Abfraction (later named in 1991) was first suggested by Lee and Eakle (1984) and Grippo (1991). Abfraction was attributed to those tooth wear lesions that could not be explained due to erosion and/or abrasion and which occurred due to occlusal stress, often occurring near to the cervical margin of teeth (Nascimento et al. 2016). As a cause of NCCLs, they have been associated with DH (Addy 2002). Limited inconclusive data, however, supports the correlation between occlusal stress, abfraction, and NCCLs (Nascimento et al. 2016), which will be further explained in relation to the multifactorial aetiology of NCCLs, below. Sarode and Sarode (2013) also challenged the theory behind abfraction lesions in a review indicating that the theory is not proven and that there is evidence against the theory. Some papers globally continue to utilise the term abfraction, perhaps as a multifunctional tooth wear umbrella term for NCCLs. It is therefore important to be aware of the term. Anecdotally, occlusal stress may become more important for lesions that are extremely deep (Nascimento et al. 2016). Here, there is so little tooth remaining cervically due to tooth wear/ NCCL (perhaps initially caused by erosion and abrasion) that any excessive occlusal stress, may

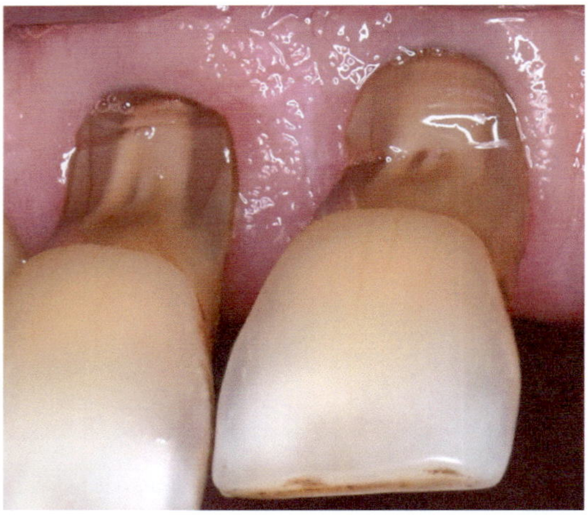

Fig. 4.5 Example of the 'abfraction' lesion misnomer, likely caused initially by Erosion - Abrasion (and referred to commonly as an NCCL). Due to little tooth structure now, occlusal forces may pose a risk for future de-coronation

now not simply be a difficult to prove aetiology of cervical wear, but more likely a risk factor for future de-coronation (see Fig. 4.5).

4.9 Multifactorial Aetiologies of Tooth Wear and DH

In tooth wear, it is unusual that attrition, abrasion, or erosion occur individually and it may be more accurate to describe them, as in a previous review, through dental tribology terminology as two body, three body, and chemico-physical wear, respectively (Addy 2000, 2005). For patients, these wear processes may include oral hygiene practices, dietary habits, stress, and their effects on the occlusion (Bartlett and Shah 2006; Bartold 2006; Shah et al. 2009).

A common multifactorial lesion that may present with aesthetic concerns and/or DH is the NCCL. These often occur on labial or buccal tooth surfaces perhaps due to anatomy and/or effects and degree of brushing force. It has been broadly suggested that NCCLs may be due to chemical degradation of enamel and/or dentine as well as flexural biomechanical loading forces originating from some location distant from the actual point of loading (Glossary of Prosthodontic Terms. 2018). The impact of occlusal forces as a predominant concern in NCCL aetiology might be true, for example, in a deep buccal cervical NCCL with limited cervical tooth tissue remaining and excessive occlusal loading (see also Fig. 4.5). Such a lesion may warrant restoration due to the force from occlusal loading. However, in the case of most NCCLs, such as the one shown in Fig. 4.3, the principal early aetiologies are toothbrushing and toothpaste abrasion often combined with erosion. Indeed, the evidence for predominant aetiologies involved in NCCLs and DH in the published literature have evolved over the last few decades. In 1984, a case study and review reported that the predominant aetiologies were more likely to be due to abfraction, erosion, and abrasion (Lee and Eakle 1984). Subsequently, in 1996, a prevalence study on 1007 dental hospital patients attributed the main aetiologies as erosion and abrasion (Smith and Robb 1996) and erosion has been described as the predominant aetiology (Addy and Hunter 2003). A further recent review of the literature continues to support the notion that NCCLs are multifactorial in nature with erosion and abrasion, as well as perhaps some occlusal forces in particular eccentric loading having an effect in some situations (Bhundia et al. 2019). However, the role of occlusal loading is not fundamental, and the important aetiologies are therefore now more likely to be erosion and abrasion (Bartlett and Shah 2006; Smith et al. 2008). The term abfraction is, as explained previously, misleading, considering the multidisciplinary nature of NCCLs.

Overall, the research would suggest that erosion is most important for DH in both the exposure of dentine and initiation of a DH lesion. If these aetiologies are to be avoided, then the protection afforded to the dentine by the acquired pellicle and the smear layer must play an important role in the transient nature of DH in both NCCL and post-surgical recession. For example, dental erosion often works in synergy with abrasion, in the aetiology of NCCLs and DH (Lussi 2006) and toothbrushing will at the very least remove the acquired pellicle, which has been shown to offer protection against erosion in vitro (Wetton et al. 2006). Combinations of toothbrushing with an erosive acid challenge will also enhance the removal of the smear layer and it was suggested in an early in vitro study that brushing should therefore be avoided immediately after meals (Absi et al. 1987). Another in vitro study reported that toothbrushing alone may take several years to remove the smear layer and expose the dentine tubule system, but this exposure occurred more readily if followed by an erosive acid challenge (Absi et al. 1992). Clinically, it has also been shown that toothbrushing immediately post-acid challenge can lead to more DH like symptoms (Ahlquist et al. 1994; Addy 2005). Evidence therefore supports the role of multiple factors, in particular erosion and abrasion, in the aetiology of DH, even though one factor may be dominant in the process.

The synergy between the various aetiologies is partially reflected in the current clinical suggestion from the dental profession to avoid toothbrushing immediately after acidic food or drink consumption (Dababneh et al. 1999). Whilst it has been shown that the time between erosive attack and brushing may not be a particular concern in tooth wear (Hong et al. 2020), it is recommended to avoid brushing after vomiting and anecdotally may be sensible to continue to avoid brushing immediately after an erosive beverage due to the time taken for the pH in the mouth to recover. Moreover, the time since erosion has since been shown as perhaps more important when considering DH, with greater DH being reported clinically closer to an acidic consumable (Olley et al. 2015). Therefore, allowing time before brushing would be reasonable to enable the smear layer to reform and reduce the chances of DH symptoms whilst brushing (Olley et al. 2015).

4.10 Oral Hygiene, Gingival Recession, and DH

Teeth with good oral hygiene, less bleeding on probing and where dentine is exposed through gingival recession are more likely to have DH (Olley et al. 2013) (Addy et al. 1987b, c, d) (Olley et al. 2013). Furthermore, periodontal disease has been linked previously to DH indirectly through gingival recession (Chabanski et al. 1996; Madhu et al. 2006). Tobacco is a significant risk factor for periodontal disease throughout Europe (Olley and Gallagher 2010), and European prevalence studies have also demonstrated an association between tobacco usage and DH (West et al. 2013b). Therefore, oral hygiene, periodontal status, and tobacco use are all relevant factors in the aetiology of DH. Good oral hygiene and tobacco control must therefore be encouraged by clinicians, but unfortunately the caveat is that patients who have DH may be less likely to brush their teeth due to pain. This increases the level of plaque on their dentine, which may paradoxically reduce DH but may increase their likelihood of periodontal disease. The evidence for this is entirely anecdotal, but it is now known that good oral hygiene is linked to a higher prevalence of DH (Olley et al. 2013) and thus patients with DH are likely to brush their teeth normally.

Gingival recession and in turn DH may also be initiated iatrogenically due to abnormal oral hygiene procedures (Addy and Hunter 2003) or as a result of dental practice following placement of indirect restorations, even those situated away from the biological width, slowly over time (Olley et al. 2018). Inappropriate brushing techniques (too hard or frequent) may cause dentine exposure and lesion localisation as a result of gingival recession (Chabanski et al. 1996; Addy and Hunter 2003; Hooper et al. 2003; McCracken et al. 2003; Smith et al. 2008) and DH initiation (Sehmi and Olley 2015), and there is an association between toothbrushing habits, gingival recession, and DH (Addy et al. 1987b, c, d; Olley et al. 2013).

4.11 Future Trends

This chapter has first recognised the importance of tooth wear, in particular erosion, but also overzealous brushing in the aetiology of NCCLs, occlusal/incisal wear, and DH, and it is important that future treatment strategies consider the importance of the aetiology of DH. Tooth wear (attrition, abrasion, and erosion), unlike DH, are diseases recognised by WHO. The severity of DH has been reported to affect the quality of life (Boiko et al. 2010) (see Chap. 3). Both tooth wear and/or DH should be identified together with the associated aetiologies as these will also be important in the subsequent management of the condition (Olley and Sehmi 2017) (see Chap. 10). Although the aetiology of DH is a surface phenomenon, the action of specific desensitising dentifrices that work sub-surface may potentiate their effects for DH management (Mullan et al. 2017). Sometimes, it is helpful to know DH is present. DH may be a useful clinical indicator of an active tooth wear process, as demonstrated by the first novel study to investigate this specifically (Olley et al. 2015).

Erosion remains the primary concern in DH aetiology. In 1997, a report demonstrated that UK soft drinks consumption had risen by 56% in the previous 10 years and was predicted to continue rising 2–3% each year thereafter (Zenith-International-Ltd 1997). This predicted increase was subsequently confirmed by a subsequent report from the British Soft Drinks Association in 2011 (BSDA 2011). Although there have been some reassuring overall decreases in consumption of other acidic beverages between 2010 and 2021 (BSDA 2021), it is concerning that the amounts have remained higher overall than in 2004 and have not decreased considerably over the last decade. The consumption of sports and energy drinks and bottled (including sparkling) water consumption has continued to increase in the UK. This may be common amongst those individuals wishing to follow a healthy active lifestyle, but as with the other acidic beverages, they are strongly associated with patient reported DH (West et al. 2013a; Olley et al. 2015). Table 4.3 shows the UK soft drink consumption in 2004, 2010, and 2021.

This data clearly indicates the importance of prevention, counselling, and management of DH (see Chap. 10). For example, the progression of tooth wear and associated DH may be measured (at various time points) using clinical photographs or study models for monitoring purposes by the clinician (Bartlett 2003). Furthermore, clinical indices, for example, the Basic Erosive Wear Examination for tooth wear (Bartlett et al. 2008; Olley et al. 2014b) and the CHI score, may be used to measure the severity of DH (Olley et al. 2013). The BEWE, as a screening tool to monitor tooth wear, is recommended in practice following recent UK Government publications (Delivering better oral health: an evidence-based toolkit for prevention 2021). Furthermore, surface roughness in dentine has recently been related to the degree of tubule patency and therefore provides a further useful scientific tool to help measure the DH indirectly in the laboratory (Olley et al. 2020a).

In the future, the UK population is projected to continue growing and ageing. From 2020 to 2030, it is predicated that the size of the population will increase from 67.1 million to 69.2 million. The numbers of older people will increase the fastest, with those aged 85 years and over expected to double from 1.7 million in 2020 to 3.1 million by 2045 (Robards 2022).

The proportion of adults with total tooth loss in the Adult Dental Health Surveys (conducted within the UK) fell from 37% in 1968 to 6%, in England, Wales, and Northern Ireland, by 2009 (Adult Dental Health Survey 2009). By 2009,

Table 4.3 UK soft drink consumption between 2004, 2010, and 2021

	Million litres consumed in the UK		
UK soft drinks	2004	2010	2021
Carbonates	6195	6400	5345
Powdered soft drinks and dilutables	3125	3500	3303
Bottled water (including sparkling)	2060	2055	2514
Still and juice drinks	1090	1450	914
Fruit juice	1040	1180	956
Sports and energy drinks	320	600	906

over half of individuals aged 85 or more retained some natural teeth in England (Adult Dental Health Survey 2009). It was estimated in 2009 that ongoing individuals under 45 would retain most of their teeth throughout their life (Adult Dental Health Survey 2009), supporting earlier estimates from 1998 that by 2028 total tooth loss will be eliminated in those under 65 years and significantly reduced in those under 75 years of age (Kelly et al. 1998).

The population in the UK is ageing, retaining their teeth for longer, and tooth wear, in particular erosion, has been described as increasing with age (Van't Spijker et al. 2009; Cunha-Cruz et al. 2010; Steele and O'Sullivan 2011; Olley and Sehmi 2017), together with ongoing aetiologies such as abrasion and the high proportions of NCCLs, especially as older age groups (Teixeira et al. 2020). It is therefore suggested that the prevalence of tooth wear and DH in the future will remain high and continue as we age (Olley and Sehmi 2017). The largest cross-sectional study to investigate the prevalence of DH was conducted in young individuals (aged 18–35) and showed that the prevalence of DH in the young European population was high with over 41% patients reporting a history of DH (West et al. 2013b). A further study, of the same population, revealed 29% tooth wear on buccal and lingual surfaces with exposed dentine and it also demonstrated that the consumption of erosive acidic food and drinks and other risk factors, including but not limited to acid regurgitation and vomiting, were risk factors for tooth wear (Bartlett et al. 2013). Tooth surfaces with DH may also be occlusal (Olley et al. 2015). Furthermore, cross-sectional studies in China show that the greatest DH or NCCLs were seen in individuals in their sixties (Que et al. 2013). The increasing tooth wear and DH will create greater treatment complexities in an ageing population in dental practice (Olley and Frost Bem 2019).

Unfortunately, awareness of the aetiology of tooth wear globally continues to vary and can be low, even in some dental centres, and more erosion is identified in individuals who are less aware (Al-Ashtal et al. 2015; Skalsky Jarkander et al. 2018; Schmidt and Huang 2022). The importance of the awareness amongst the population of tooth wear and its links to DH cannot, therefore, be underestimated.

In summary, it remains important for epidemiological researchers and dental care professionals to be aware that DH is increasingly prevalent in all ages, on all tooth surfaces and that DH is a clinical sign of an active tooth wear process.

References

Abrahamsen TC. The worn dentition—pathognomonic patterns of abrasion and erosion. Int Dent J. 2005;55(4 Suppl 1):268–76.

Absi EG, Addy M, Adams D. Dentine hypersensitivity. A study of the patency of dentinal tubules in sensitive and non-sensitive cervical dentine. J Clin Periodontol. 1987;14(5):280–4.

Absi EG, Addy M, Adams D. Dentine hypersensitivity—the effect of toothbrushing and dietary compounds on dentine in vitro: an SEM study. J Oral Rehabil. 1992;19(2):101–10.

Addy M. Dentine hypersensitivity: definition, prevalence, distribution and aetiology. In: Addy M, Embery G, Edgar WM, Orchardson R, editors. Tooth Wear and sensitivity. Martin Dunitz: London; 2000. p. 239–48.

Addy M. Dentine hypersensitivity: new perspectives on an old problem. Int Dent J. 2002;52(5):367–75.

Addy M. Tooth brushing, tooth wear and dentine hypersensitivity—are they associated? Int Dent J. 2005;55(4 Suppl 1):261–7.

Addy M, Hunter ML. Can tooth brushing damage your health? Effects on oral and dental tissues. Int Dent J. 2003;53(Suppl 3):177–86.

Addy M, Mostafa P. Dentine hypersensitivity. II. Effects produced by the uptake in vitro of toothpastes onto dentine. J Oral Rehabil. 1989;16(1):35–48.

Addy M, Pearce N. Aetiological, predisposing and environmental factors in dentine hypersensitivity. Arch Oral Biol. 1994;39(Suppl):33S–8S.

Addy M, West NX. The role of toothpaste in the aetiology and treatment of dentine hypersensitivity. Monogr Oral Sci. 2013;23:75–87.

Addy M, Absi EG, Adams D. Dentine hypersensitivity. The effects in vitro of acids and dietary substances on root-planed and burred dentine. J Clin Periodontol. 1987a;14(5):274–9.

Addy M, Griffiths G, Dummer P, Kingdom A, Shaw WC. The distribution of plaque and gingivitis and the influence of toothbrushing hand in a group of South-Wales 11–12 year-old children. J Clin Periodontol. 1987b;14(10):564–72.

Addy M, Mostafa P, Newcombe R. Dentine hypersensitivity: a comparison of five toothpastes used

during a 6-week treatment period. Br Dent J. 1987c;163(2):45–51.
Addy M, Mostafa P, Newcombe RG. Dentine hypersensitivity: the distribution of recession, sensitivity and plaque. J Dent. 1987d;15(6):242–8.
Adriaens PA. Bacterial invasion in periodontitis, is it important in periodontal treatment? Rev Belge Med Dent (1984). 1989;44(2):9–30.
Adult Dental Health Survey (2009) Summary report and thematic series. https://digital.nhs.uk/data-and-information/publications/statistical/adult-dental-health-survey/adult-dental-health-survey-2009-summary-report-and-thematic-series.
Ahlquist M, Franzen O, Coffey J, Pashley D. Dental pain evoked by hydrostatic pressures applied to exposed dentin in man: a test of the hydrodynamic theory of dentin sensitivity. J Endod. 1994;20(3):130–4.
Al-Ashtal A, Johansson A, Omar R, Johansson AK. Awareness and knowledge of dental erosion among Yemeni dental professionals and students. BMC Oral Health. 2015;15(1):119. https://doi.org/10.1186/s12903-015-0103-x.
Al-Omiri MK, Lamey PJ, Clifford T. Impact of tooth wear on daily living. Int J Prosthodont. 2006;19(6):601–5.
Amarasena N, Spencer J, Ou Y, Brennan D. Dentine hypersensitivity in a private practice patient population in Australia. J Oral Rehabil. 2011;38(1):52–60.
Awad MA, et al. Prevalence, severity, and explanatory factors of tooth wear in Arab populations. J Dent. 2019;80:69–74. https://doi.org/10.1016/j.jdent.2018.09.011.
Bahsi E, Dalli M, Uzgur R, Turkal M, Hamidi MM, Colak H. An analysis of the aetiology, prevalence and clinical features of dentine hypersensitivity in a general dental population. Eur Rev Med Pharmacol Sci. 2012;16(8):1107–16.
Bamise CT, Olusile AO, Oginni AO. An analysis of the etiological and predisposing factors related to dentin hypersensitivity. J Contemp Dent Pract. 2008;9(5):52–9.
Bartlett DW. Retrospective long term monitoring of tooth wear using study models. Br Dent J. 2003;194(4):211–3. discussion 204
Bartlett D. The implication of laboratory research on tooth wear and erosion. Oral Dis. 2005;11(1):3–6.
Bartlett DW, Ide M. Dealing with sensitive teeth. Prim Dent Care. 1999;6(1):25–7.
Bartlett DW, Shah P. A critical review of non-carious cervical (wear) lesions and the role of abfraction, erosion, and abrasion. J Dent Res. 2006;85(4):306–12.
Bartlett DW, Smith BGN. Definition, classification and clinical assessment of attrition, erosion and abrasion of enamel and dentine. In: Addy M, Embery G, Edgar WM, Orchardson R, editors. Tooth wear and sensitivity—clinical advances in restorative dentistry. London: Martin Dunitz; 2000. p. 87–93.
Bartlett D, Ganss C, Lussi A. Basic Erosive Wear Examination (BEWE): a new scoring system for scientific and clinical needs. Clin Oral Investig. 2008;12(Suppl 1):S65–8.
Bartlett DW, Lussi A, West NX, Bouchard P, Sanz M, Bourgeois D. Prevalence of tooth wear on buccal and lingual surfaces and possible risk factors in young European adults. J Dent. 2013;41(11):1007–13.
Bartold PM. Dentinal hypersensitivity: a review. Aust Dent J. 2006;51(3):212–8; quiz 276.
Berry DC, Poole DF. Masticatory function and oral rehabilitation. J Oral Rehabil. 1974;1(2):191–205.
Betke H, Schick U, Buchalla W, Hellwig E, Attin T. [Influence of the buffer capacity of amine fluoride-containing toothpastes and gels in enamel erosion]. Schweiz Monatsschr Zahnmed. 2003;113(11):1158–64.
Bhundia S, Bartlett D, O'Toole S. Non-carious cervical lesions—can terminology influence our clinical assessment? Br Dent J. 2019;227(11):985–8. https://doi.org/10.1038/s41415-019-1004-1.
Boiko OV, Baker SR, Gibson BJ, Locker D, Sufi F, Barlow AP, Robinson PG. Construction and validation of the quality of life measure for dentine hypersensitivity (DHEQ). J Clin Periodontol. 2010;37(11):973–80.
Brannstrom M. The surface of sensitive dentine. An experimental study using replication. Odontol Revy. 1965;16(4):293–9.
Brannstrom M. Sensitivity of dentine. Oral Surg Oral Med Oral Pathol. 1966;21(4):517–26.
Brannstrom M. Dentin and pulp in restorative dentistry. London: Wolfe Medical Publications Ltd; 1982.
BSDA. The 2011 soft drinks report. London: B. S. D. Association; 2011. Publications (britishsoftdrinks.com).
British Soft Drinks Association 2021 https://www.britishsoftdrinks.com
Canadian, Advisory, board, on, dentine and hypersensitivity. Consensus-based recommendations for the diagnosis and management of dentin hypersensitivity. J Can Dent Assoc. 2003;69(4):221–6.
Chabanski MB, Gillam DG, Bulman JS, Newman HN. Prevalence of cervical dentine sensitivity in a population of patients referred to a specialist Periodontology Department. J Clin Periodontol. 1996;23(11):989–92.
Chadwick RG. Dental Erosion. London: Quintessence Publishing Co. Ltd; 2006.
Cunha-Cruz, J., H. Pashova, J. D. Packard, L. Zhou, T. J. Hilton and P. for Northwest (2010). Tooth wear: prevalence and associated factors in general practice patients. Community Dent Oral Epidemiol 38(3): 228–234.
Dababneh RH, Khouri AT, Addy M. Dentine hypersensitivity—an enigma? A review of terminology, mechanisms, aetiology and management. Br Dent J. 1999;187(11):606-611; discussion 603.
Deery C, Wagner ML, Longbottom C, Simon R, Nugent ZJ. The prevalence of dental erosion in a United States and a United Kingdom sample of adolescents. Pediatr Dent. 2000;22(6):505–10.
Delivering Better Oral Health: an evidence-based toolkit for prevention (fourth edition). 2021. https://www.bascd.org/latest-delivering-better-oral-health-an-

evidence-based-toolkit-for-prevention-fourth-edition-published/.
Dowell P, Addy M. Dentine hypersensitivity—a review. Aetiology, symptoms and theories of pain production. J Clin Periodontol. 1983;10(4):341–50.
Dowell P, Addy M, Dummer P. Dentine hypersensitivity: aetiology, differential diagnosis and management. Br Dent J. 1985;158(3):92–6.
Fares J, Shirodaria S, Chiu K, Ahmad N, Sherriff M, Bartlett D. A new index of tooth wear. Reproducibility and application to a sample of 18- to 30-year-old university students. Caries Res. 2009;43(2):119–25.
Ferrari M, Cagidiaco MC, Monticelli F, Kugel G, Barker ML, Gerlach RW. Daytime use of a custom bleaching tray or whitening strips: initial and sustained color improvement. Am J Dent. 2007;20 Spec No A:19A–22A.
Ganss C, Klimek J, Lussi A. Accuracy and consistency of the visual diagnosis of exposed dentine on worn occlusal/incisal surfaces. Caries Res. 2006;40(3):208–12.
Ganss C, Hardt M, Blazek D, Klimek J, Schlueter N. Effects of toothbrushing force on the mineral content and demineralized organic matrix of eroded dentine. Eur J Oral Sci. 2009;117(3):255–60.
Gillam DG. Current diagnosis of dentin hypersensitivity in the dental office: an overview. Clin Oral Investig. 2013;17(Suppl 1):S21–9.
Gillam D, Chesters R, Attrill D, Brunton P, Slater M, Strand P, Whelton H, Bartlett D. Dentine hypersensitivity—guidelines for the management of a common oral health problem. Dent Update. 2013;40(7):514–6, 518–20, 523–4.
Gregg T, Mace S, West NX, Addy M. A study in vitro of the abrasive effect of the tongue on enamel and dentine softened by acid erosion. Caries Res. 2004;38(6):557–60.
Grenby TH, Phillips A, Desai T, Mistry M. Laboratory studies of the dental properties of soft drinks. Br J Nutr. 1989;62(2):451–64.
Grippo JO. Tooth flexure. J Am Dent Assoc. 1991;122(7):13.
Grippo JO, Simring M, Schreiner S. Attrition, abrasion, corrosion and abfraction revisited: a new perspective on tooth surface lesions. J Am Dent Assoc. 2004;135(8):1109–18. quiz 1163–5
Holland GR, Narhi MN, Addy M, Gangarosa L, Orchardson R. Guidelines for the design and conduct of clinical trials on dentine hypersensitivity. J Clin Periodontol. 1997;24(11):808–13.
Hong D, Lin X, Wiegand A, Yu H. Does delayed toothbrushing after the consumption of erosive foodstuffs or beverages decrease erosive tooth wear? A systematic review and meta-analysis. Clin Oral Investig. 2020;24(12):4169–83. https://doi.org/10.1007/s00784-020-03614-9.
Hooper S, West NX, Pickles MJ, Joiner A, Newcombe RG, Addy M. Investigation of erosion and abrasion on enamel and dentine: a model in situ using toothpastes of different abrasivity. J Clin Periodontol. 2003;30(9):802–8.
Hughes JA, West NX, Parker DM, Newcombe RG, Addy M. Development and evaluation of a low erosive blackcurrant juice drink. 3. Final drink and concentrate, formulae comparisons in situ and overview of the concept. J Dent. 1999;27(5):345–50.
Hunter ML, West NX, Hughes JA, Newcombe RG, Addy M. Erosion of deciduous and permanent dental hard tissue in the oral environment. J Dent. 2000;28(4):257–63.
Hunter ML, Addy M, Pickles MJ. The role of toothpastes and toothbrushes in the aetiology of toothwear. Int Dent J. 2002;52:399–405.
Irwin CR, McCusker P. Prevalence of dentine hypersensitivity in a general dental population. J Ir Dent Assoc. 1997;43(1):7–9.
The glossary of prosthodontic terms: ninth edition. J Prosthet Dent. 2018;117(5S):e1–e105. https://doi.org/10.1016/j.prosdent.2016.12.001.
Johnson RH, Zulqar-Nain BJ, Koval JJ. The effectiveness of an electro-ionizing toothbrush in the control of dentinal hypersensitivity. J Periodontol. 1982;53(6):353–9.
Kelly M, Steele J, Nuttall N, Bradnock G, Morris J, Nunn J. Adult dental health survey. Oral Health in the United Kingdom; 1998. p. 257–88.
Knezevic A, Nyamaa I, Tarle Z, Kunzelmann KH. In vitro assessment of human dentin wear resulting from toothbrushing. J Calif Dent Assoc. 2010;38(2):109–13.
Krauser JT. Hypersensitive teeth. Part I: etiology. J Prosthet Dent. 1986;56(2):153–6.
Lee WC, Eakle WS. Possible role of tensile stress in the etiology of cervical erosive lesions of teeth. J Prosthet Dent. 1984;52(3):374–80.
Lin YH, Gillam DG. The prevalence of root sensitivity following periodontal therapy: a systematic review. Int J Dent. 2012;2012:407023. https://doi.org/10.1155/2012/407023. Epub 2012 Oct 31.
Lundy T, Stanley HR. Correlation of pulpal histopathology and clinical symptoms in human teeth subjected to experimental irritation. Oral Surg Oral Med Oral Pathol. 1969;27(2):187–201.
Lussi A. Dental erosion from diagnosis to therapy. Karger; 2006.
Lussi A, Schaffner M. Progression of and risk factors for dental erosion and wedge-shaped defects over a 6-year period. Caries Res. 2000;34(2):182–7.
Madhu PS, Setty S, Ravindra S. Dentinal hypersensitivity?-Can this agent be the solution? J Dent Res. 2006;17:178–84.
Markowitz K. Pretty painful: why does tooth bleaching hurt? Med Hypotheses. 2010;74(5):835–40.
Markowitz K, Pashley DH. Discovering new treatments for sensitive teeth: the long path from biology to therapy. J Oral Rehabil. 2008;35(4):300–15.
McCracken GI, Janssen J, Swan M, Steen N, de Jager M, Heasman PA. Effect of brushing force and time on plaque removal using a powered toothbrush. J Clin Periodontol. 2003;30(5):409–13.

Meurman JH, tenCate JM. Pathogenesis and modifying factors of dental erosion. Eur J Oral Sci. 1996;104(2):199–206.

Meurman JH, Rytomaa I, Kari K, Laakso T, Murtomaa H. Salivary pH and glucose after consuming various beverages, including sugar-containing drinks. Caries Res. 1987;21(4):353–9.

Moazzez RV, Austin RS, Rojas-Serrano M, Carpenter G, Cotroneo E, Proctor G, Zaidel L, Bartlett DW. Comparison of the possible protective effect of the salivary pellicle of individuals with and without erosion. Caries Res. 2014;48(1):57–62.

Moss SJ. Dental erosion. Int Dent J. 1998;48(6):529–39.

Mullan F, Paraskar S, Bartlett DW, Olley RC. Effects of tooth-brushing force with a desensitising dentifrice on dentine tubule patency and surface roughness. J Dent. 2017;60:50–5. https://doi.org/10.1016/j.jdent.2017.02.015.

Nascimento M, Dilbone D, Pereira P, Geraldeli S, Delgado A, Duarte W. Abfraction lesions: etiology, diagnosis, and treatment options. Clin Cosmet Investig Dent. 2016:79. https://doi.org/10.2147/CCIDE.S63465.

O'Toole S, Bartlett D. The relationship between dentine hypersensitivity, dietary acid intake and erosive tooth wear. J Dent. 2017;67:84–7. https://doi.org/10.1016/j.jdent.2017.10.002.

Olley RC, Frost Bem PM. Clinical and academic recommendations for primary dental care prosthodontics. Br Dent J. 2019;227(6):451–5. https://doi.org/10.1038/s41415-019-0785-6.

Olley RC, Gallagher JE. Tobacco usage and control: information and advice for primary dental care practitioners. Dent Update. 2010;37(1):40–2, 45–6, 49–50 passim.

Olley RC, Sehmi H. The rise of dentine hypersensitivity and tooth wear in an ageing population. Br Dent J. 2017;223(4):293–7. https://doi.org/10.1038/sj.bdj.2017.715.

Olley RC, Pilecki P, Hughes N, Jeffery P, Austin RS, Moazzez R, Bartlett D. An in situ study investigating dentine tubule occlusion of dentifrices following acid challenge. J Dent. 2012;40(7):585–93.

Olley RC, Wilson R, Moazzez R, Bartlett D. Validation of a Cumulative Hypersensitivity Index (CHI) for dentine hypersensitivity severity. J Clin Periodontol. 2013;40(10):942–7.

Olley RC, Parkinson CR, Wilson R, Moazzez R, Bartlett D. A novel method to quantify dentine tubule occlusion applied to in situ model samples. Caries Res. 2014a;48(1):69–72.

Olley RC, Wilson R, Bartlett D, Moazzez R. Validation of the basic erosive wear examination. Caries Res. 2014b;48(1):51–6.

Olley RC, Moazzez R, Bartlett D. The relationship between incisal/occlusal wear, dentine hypersensitivity and time after the last acid exposure in vivo. J Dent. 2015;43(2):248–52. https://doi.org/10.1016/j.jdent.2014.11.002.

Olley RC, Andiappan M, Frost PM. An up to 50-year follow-up of crown and veneer survival in a dental practice. J Prosthet Dent. 2018;119(6):935–41. https://doi.org/10.1016/j.prosdent.2017.06.009.

Olley RC, Alhaij S, Mohsen BM, Appleton PL, Chadwick RG, Ball G. Novel Confocal-Laser-Scanning-Microscopy and conventional measures investigating eroded dentine following dentifrice dab-on and brushing abrasion. Heliyon. 2020a;6(3):e03282. https://doi.org/10.1016/j.heliyon.2020.e03282.

Olley RC, Mohsen BM, Alhaij S, Appleton PL. Measurement of eroded dentine tubule patency and roughness following novel dab-on or brushing abrasion. J Dent. 2020b;98:103358. https://doi.org/10.1016/j.jdent.2020.103358.

Pashley DH. Smear layer: physiological considerations. Oper Dent Suppl. 1984;3:13–29.

Pashley DH. Mechanisms of dentin sensitivity. Dent Clin N Am. 1990;34(3):449–73.

Pashley DH, Livingston MJ, Reeder OW, Horner J. Effects of the degree of tubule occlusion on the permeability of human dentine in vitro. Arch Oral Biol. 1978;23(12):1127–33.

Pashley DH, Michelich V, Kehl T. Dentin permeability: effects of smear layer removal. J Prosthet Dent. 1981;46(5):531–7.

Que K, Guo B, Jia Z, Chen Z, Yang J, Gao P. A cross-sectional study: non-carious cervical lesions, cervical dentine hypersensitivity and related risk factors. J Oral Rehabil. 2013;40(1):24–32. https://doi.org/10.1111/j.1365-2842.2012.02342.x.

Rees JS, Addy M. A cross-sectional study of buccal cervical sensitivity in UK general dental practice and a summary review of prevalence studies. Int J Dent Hyg. 2004;2(2):64–9.

Robards, J. 2022. Statistical bulletin: 2020-based national population projections. https://www.ons.gov.uk/.../nationalpopulationprojections/2020basedinterim.

Sarode GS, Sarode SC. Abfraction: a review. J Oral Maxillofac Pathol. 2013 May;17(2):222–7. https://doi.org/10.4103/0973-029X.119788.

Scheutzel P. Etiology of dental erosion—intrinsic factors. Eur J Oral Sci. 1996;104(2):178–90.

Schmidt J, Huang B. Awareness and knowledge of dental erosion and its association with beverage consumption: a multidisciplinary survey. BMC Oral Health. 2022;22(1) https://doi.org/10.1186/s12903-022-02065-w.

Sehmi H, Olley RC. The effect of toothbrush abrasion force on dentine hypersensitivity in-vitro. J Dent. 2015;43(12):1442–7. https://doi.org/10.1016/j.jdent.2015.10.014.

Seligman DA, Pullinger AG, Solberg WK. The prevalence of dental attrition and its association with factors of age, gender, occlusion, and TMJ symptomatology. J Dent Res. 1988;67(10):1323–33.

Shah P, Razavi S, Bartlett DW. The prevalence of cervical tooth wear in patients with bruxism and other causes of wear. J Prosthodont. 2009;18(5):450–4.

Skalsky Jarkander M, Grindefjord M, Carlstedt K. Dental erosion, prevalence and risk factors among a group of adolescents in Stockholm County. Eur Arch Paediatr Dent. 2018;19(1):23–31. https://doi.org/10.1007/s40368-017-0317-5.

Smith BG, Knight JK. A comparison of patterns of tooth wear with aetiological factors. Br Dent J. 1984;157(1):16–9.
Smith BG, Robb ND. The prevalence of toothwear in 1007 dental patients. J Oral Rehabil. 1996;23(4):232–9.
Smith WA, Marchan S, Rafeek RN. The prevalence and severity of non-carious cervical lesions in a group of patients attending a university hospital in Trinidad. J Oral Rehabil. 2008;35(2):128–34.
Steele J, O'Sullivan I. Executive summary adult dental health survey 2009. London: The Stationary Office; 2011.
Teixeira DNR, Thomas RZ, Soares PV, Cune MS, Gresnigt MMM, Slot DE. Prevalence of noncarious cervical lesions among adults: a systematic review. J Dent. 2020;95:103285. https://doi.org/10.1016/j.jdent.2020.103285. Epub 2020 Jan 30. PMID: 32006668.
ten Carte JM, Larsen MJ, Pearce E, Fejerskov O. Chemical interactions between the tooth and oral fluids. In: Fejerskov O, Kidd EAM, editors. Dental caries: the disease and its clinical management. Oxford/Amres/Iowa: Blackwell Munksgaard; 2008.
Turssi CP, Messias DC, Hara AT, Hughes N, Garcia-Godoy F. Brushing abrasion of dentin: effect of diluent and dilution rate of toothpaste. Am J Dent. 2010;23(5):247–50.
Van der Weijden FA, Campbell SL, Dorfer CE, Gonzalez-Cabezas C, Slot DE. Safety of oscillating-rotating powered brushes compared to manual toothbrushes: a systematic review. J Periodontol. 2011;82(1):5–24.
Van't Spijker A, Rodriguez JM, Kreulen CM, Bronkhorst EM, Bartlett DW, Creugers NHJ. Prevalence of tooth wear in adults. Int J Prosthodont. 2009;22(1):35–42.
Vanuspong W, Eisenburger M, Addy M. Cervical tooth wear and sensitivity: erosion, softening and rehardening of dentine; effects of pH, time and ultrasonication. J Clin Periodontol. 2002;29(4):351–7.
Veitz-Keenan A, Barna JA, Strober B, Matthews AG, Collie D, Vena D, Curro FA, Thompson VP. Treatments for hypersensitive noncarious cervical lesions: a Practitioners Engaged in Applied Research and Learning (PEARL) network randomized clinical effectiveness study. J Am Dent Assoc. 2013;144(5):495–506. https://doi.org/10.14219/jada.archive.2013.0152.
von Troil B, Needleman I, Sanz M. A systematic review of the prevalence of root sensitivity following periodontal therapy. J Clin Periodontol. 2002;29 Suppl 3:173–7; discussion 195-6. https://doi.org/10.1034/j.1600-051x.29.s3.10.x. PMID: 12787217.
West NX. Dentine hypersensitivity. Monogr Oral Sci. 2006;20:173–89.
West NX, Hughes JA, Parker DM, Newcombe RG, Addy M. Development and evaluation of a low erosive blackcurrant juice drink. 2. Comparison with a conventional blackcurrant juice drink and orange juice. J Dent. 1999;27(5):341–4.
West NX, Hughes JA, Addy M. Erosion of dentine and enamel in vitro by dietary acids: the effect of temperature, acid character, concentration and exposure time. J Oral Rehabil. 2000;27(10):875–80.
West NX, Hughes JA, Addy M. Dentine hypersensitivity: the effects of brushing toothpaste on etched and unetched dentine in vitro. J Oral Rehabil. 2002;29(2):167–74.
West NX, Lussi A, Seong J, Hellwig E. Dentin hypersensitivity: pain mechanisms and aetiology of exposed cervical dentin. Clin Oral Investig. 2013a;17 Suppl 1:S9–19.
West NX, Sanz M, Lussi A, Bartlett D, Bouchard P, Bourgeois D. Prevalence of dentine hypersensitivity and study of associated factors: a European population-based cross-sectional study. J Dent. 2013b;41(10):841–51.
Wetton S, Hughes J, West N, Addy M. Exposure time of enamel and dentine to saliva for protection against erosion: a study in vitro. Caries Res. 2006;40(3):213–7.
Whittacker DK. Historical and forensic aspects of tooth wear. In: Addy M, Emberry G, Edgar R, Orchardson R, editors. Tooth wear and sensitivity—clinical advances in restorative dentistry. London: Martin Dunitz; 2000.
Wiegand A, Stock A, Attin R, Werner C, Attin T. Impact of the acid flow rate on dentin erosion. J Dent. 2007;35(1):21–7.
Wiegand A, Kuhn M, Sener B, Roos M, Attin T. Abrasion of eroded dentin caused by toothpaste slurries of different abrasivity and toothbrushes of different filament diameter. J Dent. 2009;37(6):480–4.
Yoshiyama M, Suge T, Kawasaki A, Ebisu S. Morphological characterization of tube-like structures in hypersensitive human radicular dentine. J Dent. 1996;24(1–2):57–63.
Yu T, Tao DY, Lu HX, Zhu JL, Xie CY, Bartlett D, Feng XP. Prevalence and associated factors of tooth Wear in Shanghai. Chin J Dent Res. 2021;24(2):95–103. https://doi.org/10.3290/j.cjdr.b1530421.
Zenith-International-Ltd. The 1997 sucralose soft drinks report. Reading: T. a. L. I. Ltd.; 1997.
Zero DT. Etiology of dental erosion—extrinsic factors. Eur J Oral Sci. 1996;104(2 (Pt 2)):162–77.
Zero DT, Lussi A. Erosion—chemical and biological factors of importance to the dental practitioner. Int Dent J. 2005;55(4 Suppl 1):285–90.

Further Reading

The Royal College of Surgeons England (2021) have provided clinical guidelines for dental erosion, its diagnosis, prevention, and management.

5 The Physiological Basis of Dentin Hypersensitivity

Kenneth Markowitz and David Pashley

5.1 Introduction

For over 100 years, dentists have known that enamel is not sensitive to drilling. However, as soon as a bur in a dental handpiece passes through the dentino-enamel junction (DEJ), patients immediately experience a sharp, well-localized pain. It was clear to dentists and histologists that the dentino-enamel junction represented a boundary between a secreted tissue (the enamel) and dentin, a living tissue possessing the intrinsic biological property of irritability (Verworn 1913). This property of dentin could be readily explained if pulpal nerve fibres extended from pulpal soft tissues and passed through the dentinal tubules to the DEJ. Histological studies, however, failed to conclusively reveal the presence of nerves in the sensitive, outer portion of the dentin. When present, nerves in the dentin are restricted to the inner half of the tissue, close to the densely innervated dental pulp (Fig. 5.1a) (Byers 1984).

Odontoblasts, the principal cellular element at the dentin–pulp boarder, have a process extending approximately one-third the distance to the dentino-enamel junction (Byers and Sugaya 1995). Recent physiological and gene expression studies have demonstrated that these dentin-forming cells respond to pain-provoking stimuli in a way that was similar to sensory receptors (Fig. 5.1b) (Magloire et al. 2010; El Karim et al. 2011; Chung et al. 2013). Until recently, it was not clear whether odontoblasts could activate the intradental nerves since conventional synaptic structures have not been identified linking these cells.

Some earlier evidence even shed doubt on the notion that odontoblasts are necessary for dentin sensitivity. Trauma to the dentin that destroys the odontoblast layer fails to abolish dentin hypersensitivity (DH). Odontoblasts then may play a role but not necessarily critical to tooth sensitivity (Brännström 1963, 1968; Lundy and Stanley 1969; Lilja et al. 1982). In this chapter, we will explore new insights into the role odontoblasts play in dentin sensitivity and the mechanism used by odontoblasts to communicate with nerves in more detail. The view that there are three competing theories to explain dentin sensitivity, namely (i) the nerve receptor, (ii) odontoblast receptor, and (iii) hydrodynamic theories (Aminoshariae and Kulild 2021), featured in classic textbooks, has been made obsolete since all three mechanisms appear to contribute and act together.

Gysi (1900) was the first to speculate that the sensitivity of dentin was due to stimulus-evoked fluid shifts in the dentin tubules. Brännström and his colleagues systematically studied fluid move-

K. Markowitz (✉)
Rutgers School of Dental Medicine, Rutgers the State University of New Jersey, Newark, NJ, USA
e-mail: markowkj@sdm.rutgers.edu

D. Pashley
Dental College of Georgia, Augusta University, Augusta, GA, USA

D. G. Gillam (ed.), *Dentine Hypersensitivity*, https://doi.org/10.1007/978-3-031-74321-4_5

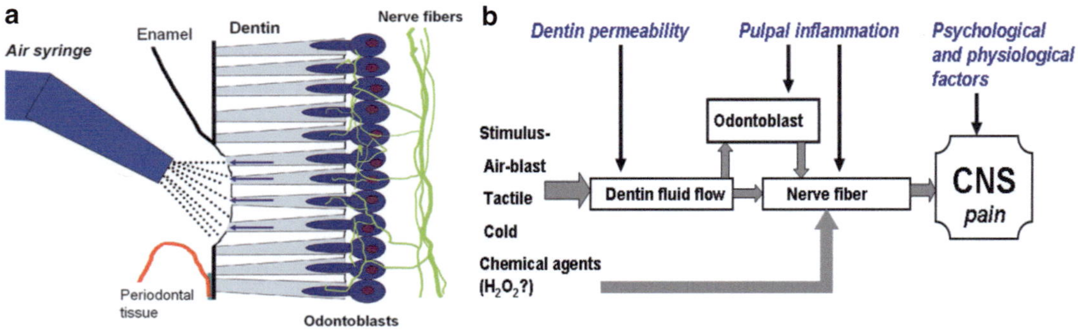

Fig. 5.1 (**a**) Diagram of sensitive dentin showing exposed tubules in an area of dentin erosion or gingival recession. Stimuli, for example, air blasts directed towards the dentin surface, induce outward fluid shifts in the tubules which activate nerve ending located in deep dentin and pulp. The odontoblasts respond to various forms of pain-producing stimuli and activate intradental nerve fibres by ATP release. Treatments for sensitive teeth can act by reducing the dentine permeability or by reducing the excitability of the intradental nerves. (Reprinted with permission from: Markowitz (2010, 2013)). (**b**) Schematic diagram showing the physiological processes leading to pain-associated DH. Fluid flow in the dentin tubules triggers nerve responses which lead to pain perception in the central nervous system (CNS). The odontoblasts also respond to fluid flow and other pain-provoking stimuli. Some stimuli, for example, cold, may also cause pain by directly activating the nerve endings. The relationship between the magnitude of a stimulus applied to the dentin and pain perception is by no means fixed. Dentin permeability, the biological environment of the dental pulp, and central psychological and physiological factors are variables that can alter pain processing. (Reprinted with permission from: Markowitz (2009))

ment in dentin in vitro, which occurred in response to thermal, evaporative, tactile, and osmotic stimuli (Brännström 1962, 1965, 1966, 1986, 1992; Brännström et al. 1967). In general, stimuli that elicit pain when applied to exposed dentin also induce fluid shifts that can be studied in laboratory experiments. Brännström's theory is referred to as the hydrodynamic hypothesis. Later animal experiments that directly linked transdentin fluid movements with excitation of the intradental nerves (Matthews and Vongsavan 1994) gave credence to the view that intradental nerves act as mechanoreceptors that are activated by dentin fluid shifts. Recent work confirmed that the odontoblasts also act as mechanosensitive cells capable of exciting the intradental nerves (Shibukawa et al. 2015). The hydrodynamic mechanism in teeth represents a novel adaptation of fluid flow-sensing mechanoreceptors to the unique anatomical environment of the dentin–pulp complex.

Fluid shifts, however, are not the only way that pain can be evoked. As with the other parts of the body, intradental nerves can respond directly to pain-producing stimuli regardless of the dentin fluid shifts evoked by those stimuli (Chung et al. 2013). Cold foods and beverages and hyperosmotic solutions stimulate nerves directly by activating thermal receptors located on intradental nerve endings (Park et al. 2006, Lee, Lee et al. 2020). Even where the intensity of the pain response does not correlate with the magnitude of the dentin fluid shifts, the dentin tubules act as conduits whereby the external stimuli reach the pain transduction mechanism (Chidchuangchai et al. 2007).

Although considered "pathological", DH may serve important physiologic functions in humans and other animals. The intradental nerves participate in the sensation of biting force and in this way may protect the teeth from fracture (Olgart et al. 1988). Dentin sensation arising in the elongated tusk of the Narwhal whale appears to contribute to the animal's ability to sense the tonicity in its immediate environment. This tusk has cementum channels connecting dentin tubules to the tooth's surface. This sensory input is important in the artic marine environment over time (noting changes in the environment) since it helps the animal avoid being trapped by ice as well as sensing variations in the water's salinity (Nweeia et al. 2014).

Understanding pain plasticity is critical to appreciating the impact of disease states, therapy, and host factors in modulating this experience (Pashley 2013). Dentin permeability and intradental nerve excitability are peripheral loci where disease processes can upregulate pain and where therapeutic strategies seek to interrupt the events leading to pain transmission. Analysis of these peripheral factors highlights the relationship of DH to patient behaviour and other dental health issues, for example, tooth wear, erosion, caries, and periodontal disease (see Chaps. 4 and 8). Less well understood, but equally important, however, is the role of central nervous system plasticity in explaining the large degree of variability observed in the intensity of DH symptoms and the impact of this type of pain on quality of life (QoL) (Sessle 2000; Bekes and Hirsch 2013; Sixou 2013) (see Chap. 3).

5.2 The Anatomical Substrates of Dentin Hypersensitivity

Intense cold can elicit pain in healthy intact teeth. This form of stimulation is generally used to determine pulp vitality in clinical examinations. Hot foods and beverages can also elicit pain in healthy teeth. Cold, however, has been observed to be a more reliable modality for pulp vitality testing (Fuss et al. 1986). In intact teeth, dentin is covered coronally by enamel and by cementum on the root surfaces. These external coverings seal the tubules so well that there are little intratubular fluid shifts in response to the application of hydrodynamic stimuli (evaporative, tactile, or osmotic). Once the peripheral coverings of dentin are removed by abrasion, erosion, caries processes, or scaling procedures, dentin becomes hyper-conductive, compared to its previous unexposed condition. In this state, hydrodynamic stimuli elicit large fluid shifts that evoke pain (Pashley 2013).

5.3 Dentin

Compared to non-sensitive dentin, sensitive areas have exposed, patent tubules (Absi et al. 1987, 1989; Yoshiyama et al. 1989). In human subjects, the severity of sensitivity symptoms correlated with the number of open tubules/dentin surface area and the diameters of those tubules (Kontturi-Nahri and Närhi 1993). Root scaling and restorative procedures leave the dentin surface covered by a layer of burnished cutting debris called the smear layer (Pashley 1984) (Fig. 5.2). This cutting debris is forced into the tubule orifices approximately 1 μm (the smear plug) and then covered by further 1 μm of smear layer. The smear layer reduces the hydraulic conductance (the capacity of dentin

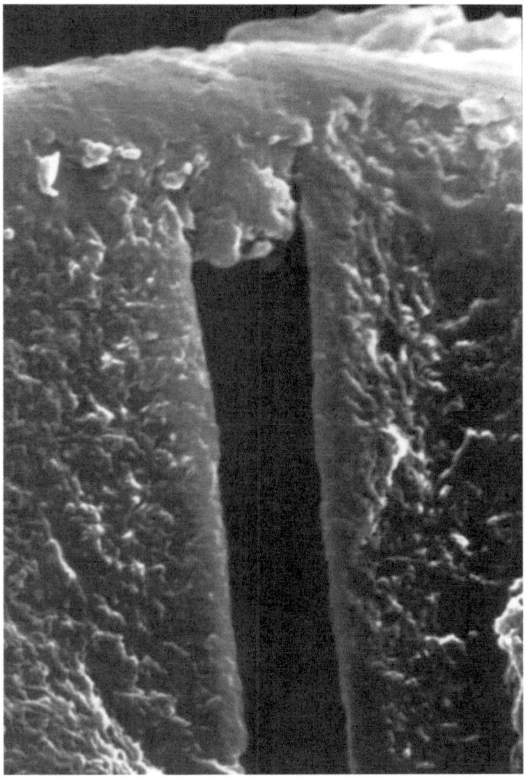

Fig. 5.2 Smear layer covering dentin cut with a high-speed carbide bur. Note that cutting debris extends into the dentin tubule about 1–2 μm. The combination of smear layer/smear plugs reduces fluid flow across dentin by 90%. Loss of smear layers and smear plugs increases dentin fluid flow and hence DH. (Used with permission from Pashley (1992b))

for pressure-driven, convective flow), about 10–30 times compared to what it would be in the absence of this surface covering (Pashley et al. 1981; Carrilho et al. 2007). When the smear layer and smear plugs are dissolved by the organic acids present in the diet or produced by plaque microorganisms, the exposed dentin can become sensitive (Pashley 1986).

Dentine is essentially a bioactive extracellular matrix where the dental pulp is surrounded by mineralized dentin (Smith et al. 2012). Measurements of the tissue pressure of pulpal soft tissues show that its hydrostatic pressure is positive, rather than being negative as is common in skin (Guyton and Hall 2000). Intraocular, intramedullary, intracranial, and intrapulpal tissue pressures are all positive, ranging from 14 to 16 mmHg (Matthews and Vongsavan 1994; Ciucchi et al. 1995; Heyeraas and Berggreen 1999; Guyton and Hall 2000). Positive pulpal tissue pressure is probably the result of the average capillary hydrostatic pressure exceeding the oncotic pressure of the plasma proteins and the relatively meagre lymph drainage of the pulp (Pashley 1992a; Heyeraas and Berggreen 1999). This positive tissue pressure in the pulpal soft tissues is responsible for the slow outward seepage of dentinal fluid whenever the outer coverings (enamel or cementum) are lost (Ciucchi et al. 1995). The rate of this outward fluid flow that is present in the absence of hydrodynamic stimulation is not sufficient to activate pulpal sensory nerves in the pulp. This was shown definitively in cat teeth by Vongsavan and Matthews (1992) and by Matthews and Vongsavan (1994).

Stimuli-induced fluid shifts occur when the baseline outward convective flow accelerates or reverses in response to probing, air blasts or thermal changes (Anderson et al. 1967; Matthews et al. 1993; Pashley et al. 1996; Andrew and Matthews 2000; Vongsavan et al. 2000). Experiments using hydrostatic pressure stimuli on human and animal teeth (Fig. 5.3a) demonstrate that the intradental nerves are more sensitive to outward flow than to inward fluid displacements (Fig. 5.3b, c) (Matthews and Vongsavan 1994; Andrew and Matthews 2000; Charoenlarp et al. 2007; Vongsavan and Matthews 2007).

Both tactile stimulation and air blasts are commonly used stimuli in DH clinical studies (Gillam et al. 2000) (see Chap. 7). Intradental nerve responses to these stimuli may also be evoked when the smear layer is removed from dentin and not in its presence (Hirvonen et al. 1984). Abrading the dentin to form a smear layer or applying agents to the dentin that occlude the dentin tubules abolished these responses.

Pressing the dentin with a sharp explorer induces sufficient inward fluid shift to exceed the pain threshold (Fig. 5.4a). When the pressure is removed, an outward fluid shift occurs due to the elastic recoil of the dentin surface that also activates the intradental nerves (Fig. 5.4b) (Camps et al. 2003).

Air blasting is a very effective provocation of tooth sensitivity pain that acts by inducing rapid outward fluid shifts (Fig. 5.4c) (Matthews et al. 1993; Pashley et al. 1996; Andrew and Matthews 2000). Air blasts evaporate fluid from the dentin tubules. This, in turn, produces cooling of the dentin and an outward fluid shift caused by capillary action. Evaporative fluid movement may occur through small or incompletely occluded tubules. It is commonly experienced in clinical practice that superficial dentin, for example, in a cavity preparation extending to the dentin-oenamel junction (DEJ), is quite sensitive. Superficial dentin has

Fig. 5.3 (**a**) Experimental arrangement used to examine the effect of hydrostatic pressure application to an etched dentin surface on transdental fluid flow and intradental nerve activity in animal experiments. Intradental nerve activity was recorded from single fibres isolated from the inferior alveolar nerve and from multiple units in the dentin. (**b**) Following the application of positive pressure to the dentin surface, there is inward dentin fluid flow. This results in little activation of the intradental nerves. In contrast, negative pressure induces outward flow; this is associated with a vigorous nerve response recorded from both dentin and the single unit recordings. (**c**) Relationship between transdentin flow rates produced in response to pressure applications and number of nerve impulse recorded from the dentin. Inward flow evoked little in the way of nerve responses. Outward transdentin flow above approximately 0.75 $nL/s/mm^2$ evoked nerve responses. The magnitude of the nerve response appeared to be positively associated with the outward flow rate. (Vongsavan and Matthews (2007) reproduced with permission)

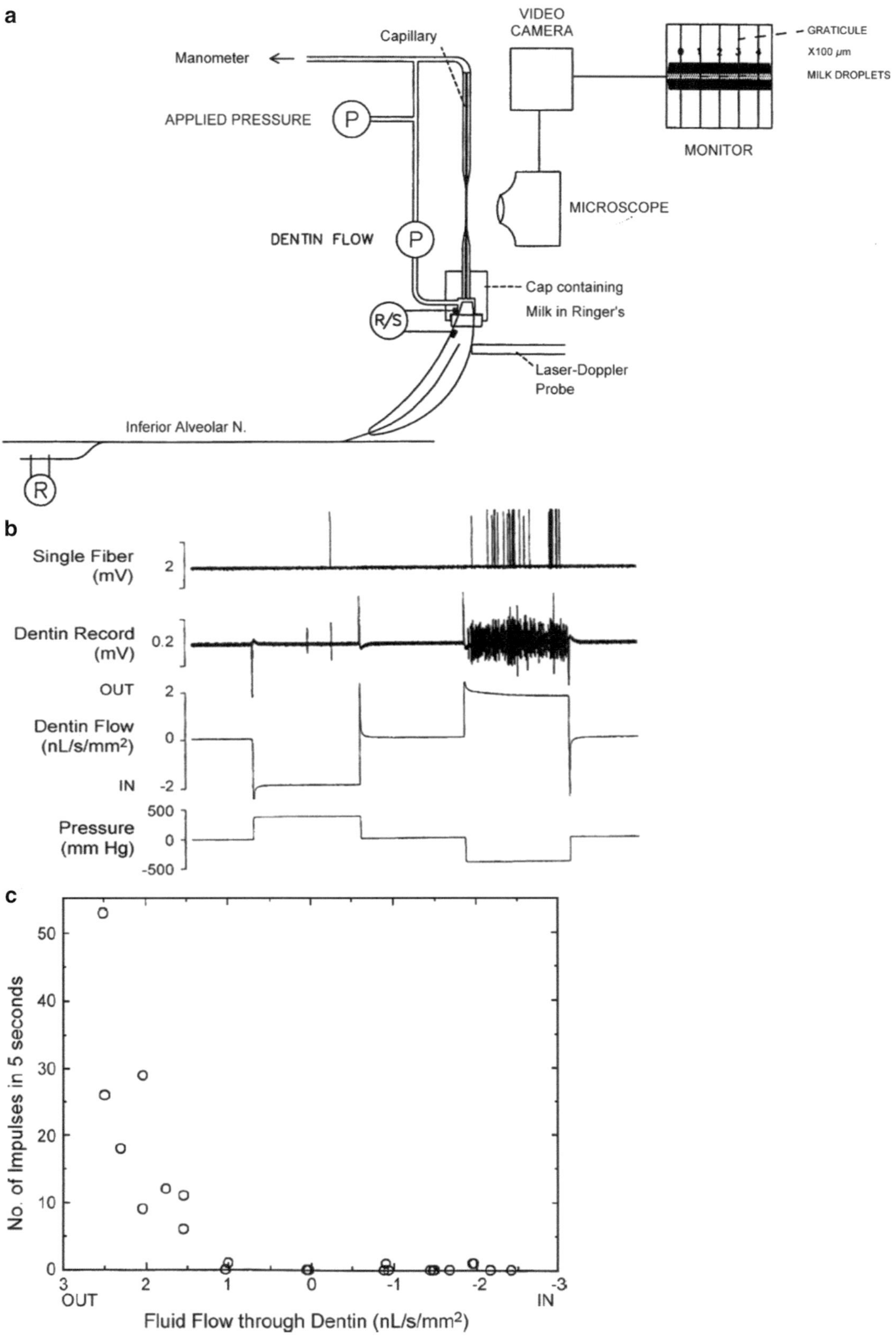
a
VIDEO CAMERA
Capillary
Manometer
GRATICULE
X100 μm
MILK DROPLETS
APPLIED PRESSURE
P
MONITOR
MICROSCOPE
DENTIN FLOW
P
Cap containing
Milk in Ringer's
R/S
Laser-Doppler
Probe
Inferior Alveolar N.
R
b
Single Fiber
(mV)
2
Dentin Record
(mV)
0.2
OUT
2
Dentin Flow
(nL/s/mm²)
0
IN
-2
500
Pressure
(mm Hg)
0
-500
c
No. of Impulses in 5 seconds
50
40
30
20
10
0
3
OUT
2
1
0
-1
-2
-3
IN
Fluid Flow through Dentin (nL/s/mm²)

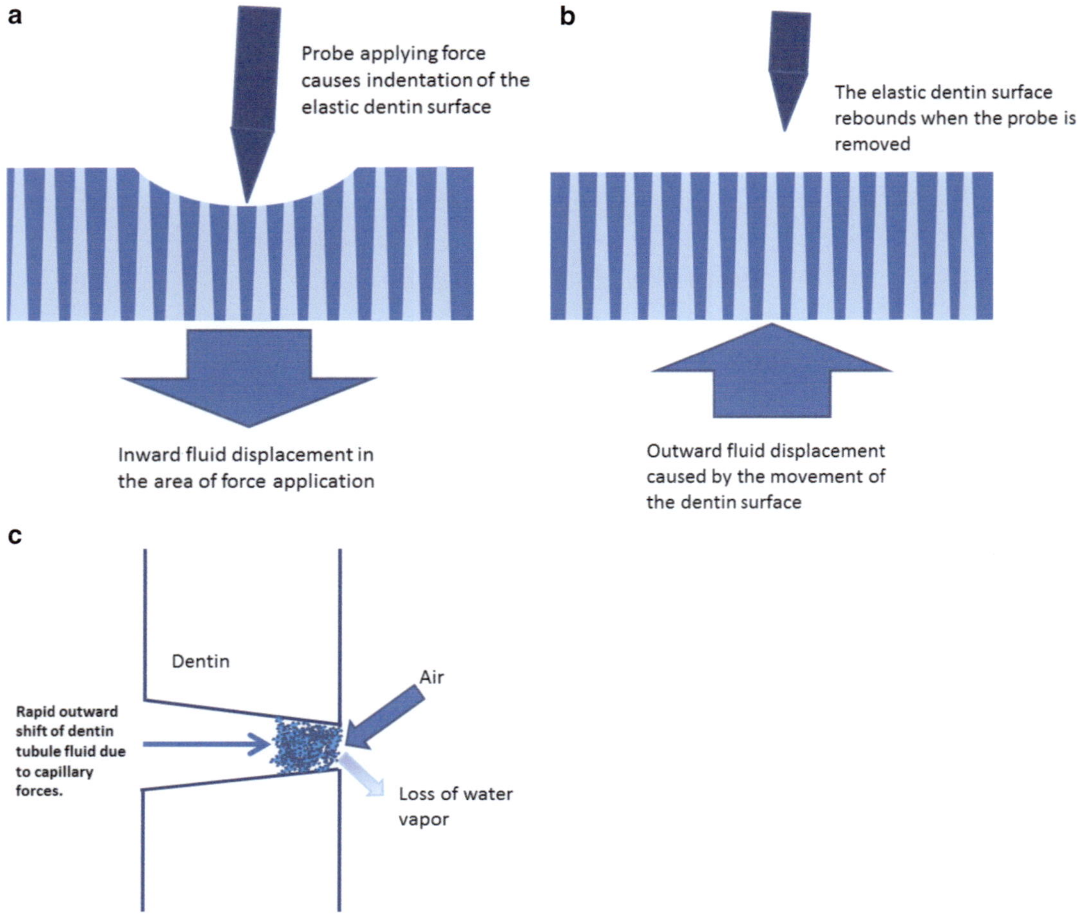

Fig. 5.4 Mechanism by which tactile and air blasts stimulation cause pain in sensitive teeth. (**a**) Tactile stimulation with a sharp probe may cause both plastic (scratching) and elastic (reversible) deformation of the exposed, possibly demineralized, dentin surface. When tactile forces are applied with a sharp probe, the dentin surface indents. Since the dentinal tubules widen towards the pulp, this causes an inward fluid shift that may be of sufficient magnitude to stimulate the intradental nerves in the deep dentin and pulp (not shown). (**b**) Removal of the probe from the dentin surface causes the surface to recoil. This recoil triggers outward dentin fluid flow that is highly excitatory to the intradental nerves (Camps and Pashley 2003; Camps et al. 2003). (**c**) Air blasts convert fluid in the exposed open ends of the dentinal tubules into water vapour that escapes under the influence of the air current. This causes an immediate outward movement of dentin fluid due to capillary forces. The evaporative action of air blasts can also cause cooling of the dentin surface that can induce pain as well. Occlusion of the dentinal tubules by a porous substance, such as the smear layer, may result in a near complete blockage of convective fluid movements but has considerably less impact on fluid shifts induced by air blasts since evaporation of fluid from the tubule orifice will still occur. (Matthews et al. 1993)

been reported to possess narrow tubules that have a lower hydraulic conductance than deep dentin (Fogel et al. 1988). The dentin tubules do, however, have extensive branching near the DEJ that makes this tissue porous and can sustain evaporative fluid movements (Mjör and Nordahl 1996).

5.4 Physiological Factors Altering Dentin Permeability and Sensitivity

Fluid flow is generally expressed as the ease with which fluid can flow across dentin or its hydraulic conductance (Eq. 5.1). That is, hydraulic conductance is simply the measured fluid flow rate (Q) divided by the difference in hydrostatic pressure across dentin forcing the fluid through 1 cm^2 of dentin surface area per min (Eq. 5.2).

$$Q = \pi \Delta P N r^4 / 8 \eta L \quad \text{(Hagen - Poiseuille law for capillary flow)} \qquad (5.1)$$

where

Q = volumetric fluid flow (μL min^{-1}) in a unit area
N = number of pores (i.e., tubules per unit area)
ΔP = hydrostatic pressure difference across dentin (cm H_2O)
r = radius of dentinal tubules
η = viscosity of fluid
L = length of dentinal tubules (cm)

$$\mathrm{Lp} = Q / \Delta P A t \qquad (5.2)$$

where

Lp = hydraulic conductance (μL cm^{-2} min^{-1} cm H_2O^{-1})
Q = volumetric fluid flow (μL min^{-1})
ΔP = hydrostatic pressure difference across dentin (cm H_2O)
A = area of dentin (cm^2)
t = time in min.

Being a system of tubules arranged approximately parallel (in the mid-coronal dentin), flow and diffusion through dentin follow certain physical laws. Both convective fluid flow and diffusion are proportional to the number of exposed tubules and inversely proportional to their length. Diffusion across dentin varies with the square of the tubule radius, while convective fluid flow through dentinal tubules varies with the fourth power of the radius (Eq. 5.1). The steep relationship between radius and convective flow is because intratubular fluid flow is laminar (Merchant et al. 1977). That is, concentrically smaller cylinders of fluid slip beneath larger more stationary cylinders adjacent to the walls of the tubules. This causes frictional resistance to fluid flow. If a tubule occluding agent can reduce tubule radii anywhere throughout the length of the tubule by one-half, the resistance to fluid flow increases not by ½ squared, as in diffusion, but by ½ to the fourth power. Thus, reductions in tubule radius by one-half reduce diffusion to one-fourth of its original value but restrict convective fluid flow to one-sixteenth of its original value. This relationship predicts that dentin tubules need not necessarily be completely sealed in order to reduce DH (Reeder Jr et al. 1978). The dependence of fluid flow on tubule radius, density, and length also explains the anatomic variations that are observed in the permeability of dentin from different sites within a tooth. In general, the deep dentin above pulp horns of posterior teeth or above the pulp tip in an anterior tooth has the highest permeability of any area of exposed dentin (Pashley et al. 1978, 1987). These areas of dentin also have the highest innervation density (Byers 1984). These anatomical factors explain why these regions of the tooth are very sensitive.

If one compared the convective flow measured through a dentin specimen of known tubule diameter, thickness, and density with the expected flow calculated for that specimen, the calculated flow is usually an order of magnitude greater than the actual flow (Michelich et al. 1978). Dentin tubules have irregular walls and contain collagen fibres and other structures that partially obstruct flow.

The hydraulic conductance of a porous solid is a measure of the ease with which a pressure gradient generates flow through the material (Eq. 5.2). In experiments where dentin flow is measured, hydraulic conductance reflects the dentin's permeability to convective flow (Reeder et al. 1978). As described above, removal of the smear layer and smear plug increases dentin's hydraulic conductance. Hydraulic conductance measurements are used to screen the ability of agent to treat DH by reducing dentin permeability.

When solutes are applied to permeable dentin surfaces, they diffuse through the tubules, in proportion to their concentration gradient. The physiological outward flow of dentin fluid reduces the inward flux of solutes by its rinsing action (Pashley and Matthews 1993). Due to the different dependencies of diffusion and flow on tubule radius, partial tubule occlusion can reduce this outward rinsing action of flow and enhance inward diffusion (Pashley et al. 2002). The opposing action of outward flow on inward diffusion is an important factor in limiting transdentin drug delivery, the interaction of restorative materials with dentin, and the effect of bacterial toxins on the dental pulp. The outward flow may also transport host-derived proteins, for example, clotting factors (Pashley et al. 1984) and immunoglobulins into the dentin tubules (Hahn and Overton 1997). These macromolecules may interact with one another or the tubules themselves forming obstructions that subsequently reduce fluid flow.

Solutes applied to the dentin surface also initiate outward osmotic water movements. For example, pellets soaked in saturated calcium chloride can draw sufficient fluid through dentin to elicit pain. This may be used as a clinical test to detect defective restoration margins (Pashley et al. 1996). In general, osmotic water movements through dentin are limited since the tubules are permeable to most low molecular weight solutes (Pashley and Whitford 1980). Large molecular weight solutes, such as proteins, have a limited ability to diffuse into dentin, particularly in the presence of the smear layer. Under conditions where the penetration of the solutes into dentin are restricted, outward osmosis is favoured (Pashley et al. 1979).

The dentin tubules provide the pathway that links dentin stimulation with nerve responses. The dentin tubules are also the routes by which pain can be facilitated by bacterial factors or relieved by therapeutic agents that either reduce dentin permeability or inhibit the activation of the intradental nerves (Markowitz and Pashley 2008; Pashley 2013). Although dentin does not remodel in the same way as bone, the formation of smear layers, tertiary dentin, peritubular dentin, and intratubular mineral can reduce dentin permeability and DH (Mjör 2001). The susceptibility of this hard tissue to acid dissolution and abrasion are important factors in understanding DH aetiological factors and designing preventive strategies that are critical to patient management (Addy 1992) (see Chaps. 4 and 8). In Chap. 6, we will consider how partial tubule occlusion can enhance the delivery of potassium salts to the innervated deep dentin.

5.5 Nerve Activation

The densely innervated teeth give rise to a spectrum of pain experiences ranging from the agony of acute pulpitis to the sensations encountered by DH sufferers. Clinical research, together with evidence from in vivo studies where the nerve responses to dentin stimulation are recorded, has been useful in determining which of the various sensory nerve fibre types present in the pulp, respond to dentin stimulation, and in determining the role of dentin permeability in altering the capacity of stimuli to evoke nerve responses (Markowitz and Pashley 2008). Information concerning the sensory function of odontoblasts have been investigated in vitro and using animal models.

Stimulation of exposed dentin in healthy teeth results in a sharp, well-localized pain that does not last beyond the duration of the stimulus (Anderson et al. 1967; Anderson and Matthews 1976; Ahlquist and Franzén 1994). This corresponds to pain associated with A-fibre type nociceptor activation evident in other parts of the body. The identity of the nerve fibre type responding to dentin stimulation was confirmed in physiological experiments. In these experiments, the nerve units responding to air blasts, probing, and other stimuli applied to etched dentin were observed to have low electrical thresholds and rapid conduction velocities consistent with A-fibres (Närhi et al. 1982a, 1992b; Närhi 1985). These A-fibres are myelinated throughout most of their course but lose myelination as they reach the superficial pulp and dentin. This loss of myelination has, however, made characterization of the distal portions of the afferents difficult when viewing histological sections. Recently, it has been demonstrated using immunohistochemical markers that most of the unmyelinated nerve fibres present in the superficial pulp tissue are the extensions of myelinated axons (Henry et al. 2012). In contrast to the intradental A-fibres, narrow diameter, slowly conducting pulpal C-fibres are unmyelinated throughout their entire course. These units do not respond to the types of innocuous dentin stimuli that evoke DH pain, but they do respond to direct injurious stimuli, for example, noxious heat, directed to the pulp tissue. Capsaicin, the active ingredient in hot peppers, stimulates C-fibres via the same receptor as is activated by heat but has little effect on the rapidly conducting intradental A-fibres (Närhi et al. 1992a; Ikeda et al. 1997).

The relationship between the activation of intradental nerve fibre types and people's pain experience was studied in experiments conducted on human volunteers (Ahlquist and Franzén 1994). In these experiments, the electrophysiological responses of the intradental nerves to tooth stimulation were recorded from dentin cavities at the same time as the experimenters recorded the subject's pain rating and description. The authors observed that cold stimulation evoked pain described as sharp and evoked A-fibre impulses recorded from the dentin (Ahlquist et al. 1984). For a series of cold stimulus applications, the intensity of the pain was proportional to the frequency of the nerve response (Fors et al. 1984). In contrast to cold, the application of several algesic (pain-producing) chemicals to deep dentin or exposed pulp evoked dull aching pain and did not produce nerve responses that could be recorded through dentin cavities (Ahlquist et al. 1994). This type of pain was probably due to small diameter C-fibre activation. These human and animal studies have established a functional classification of the intradental nerves and relate people's pain experiences to activation of afferent type and relate tooth sensitivity to other forms of sharp well-localized pain.

Several characteristics of DH are unique. Pain is the only sensory modality experienced when teeth are stimulated. In conducting experiments using electrical tooth stimulation, human subjects report a tingling (rather than painful) sensation when the threshold is reached. This observation suggested that not all tooth stimulation resulted in pain (McGrath et al. 1983). Several lines of evidence indicate the relationship of this "pre-pain" sensation to pain. For example, temporal (increasing the frequency) and spatial (simultaneous administration of the stimulus to adjacent teeth) summation result in this liminal stimulus being perceived as painful, indicating that the tingling sensation is in fact a brief, low amplitude pain sensation (Närhi et al. 1984; Virtanen et al. 1987).

5.6 Cellular Analysis of Pulpal Afferents

Nociceptive afferents may be classified by histochemical markers, as well as according to the types of receptors, ion channels, and transmitters present in the neuron (Chung et al. 2013). Mammalian trigeminal afferents are a heterogeneous population of sensory neurons, most of which convey non-painful mechanosensory information arising in the exquisitely sensitive skin and hairs of the face (Catania 2011), as well as sensation from the mucosa (Sessle and Greenwood 1976). In order to examine the properties of pulpal afferents, histological examination of pulp tissue is performed, or the cell bodies of pulpal afferents are examined in the trigeminal ganglion (Byers et al. 1982, 1987; Pan et al. 2000). Pulpal afferents can be traced to their cell bodies by placing certain rapidly diffusing tracers into dentin cavities and following a period to allow for the transport of these tracers. The cell bodies in the pulpal neurons can be visualized (Eckert et al. 1997; Pan et al. 2003). Using the appropriate histochemical technique, these labelled cell bodies can be examined for the presence of various receptors and other markers of neuronal phenotype (Henry and Hargreaves 2007). The labelled pulpal afferent cell bodies can also be isolated, maintained in tissue culture, and harvested for physiological or biochemical analysis (Kim et al. 2011; Chung et al. 2013). Using this approach to isolate pulpal afferent cell bodies, the gene expression of various receptor types and ion channels can be characterized (Chung et al. 2013).

Although the electrophysiological responses of isolated cell bodies to various chemicals and thermal stimulation can be recorded, this approach does not allow for the responses of afferents to natural dentin stimuli to be examined, and since disaggregated neuronal stomata lack long axons, the cells' conduction velocity cannot be determined (Kim et al. 2011). Because of these limitations, we cannot with certainty assign the various ion channels, transmitters, and receptors observed in pulpal afferents to belonging to A or C-fibres. Recent methods for examining histochemical markers and analysis of cell size have allowed pulpal afferent cell bodies to be classified in a manner that approximates axon classification based on response to dentin stimulation and axon conduction velocity.

Most pulpal afferent cell bodies that were isolated in culture were observed to respond to heat and the heat sensation-inducing chemical agent capsaicin. This population of cells also binds the plant isolectin IB4. Electrophysiological recordings revealed that these IB4+ and capsaicin-responsive cells had action potentials having inflections (humps) on their repolarizing phase (Kim et al. 2011). Most pulpal afferents also expressed mRNA for TRPV1—the heat/capsaicin receptor. This population of neurons probably corresponds to C-fibre nociceptors. In contrast, approximately 20% of the pulpal afferent cell bodies examined lacked responses to capsaicin, lacked IB4 binding, and had action potentials that did not have a hump on the repolarizing phase. A similar proportion of afferents were TRPV1 mRNA negative (Kim et al. 2011). Some pulpal afferent cell bodies also respond to cold and cold sensation-inducing chemicals, for example, menthol (Park et al. 2006). Histochemical, electrophysiological, and pharmacological methods have determined that the pulpal primary afferents possess many types of receptors and respond directly (in in vitro experiments without dentin) to a variety of stimuli (Lee et al. 2020). RNA transcription can also be analysed in single cells to determine receptor gene transcription. Using these approaches, a hyperosmotic stimuli receptor has been identified (Lee et al. 2020).

These and other results clearly demonstrate that pulpal afferents possess the ability to respond directly to thermal stimulation. Noxious heat stimulates responses in intradental C-fibres (Närhi et al. 1982a, b; Jyväsjärvi and Kniffki 1992). The sharp abrupt pain responses observed when cold stimuli are applied to teeth are possibly a combined effect of cold-induced dentin fluid flow and direct action of cold on receptors on intradental nerve endings (Jyväsjärvi and Kniffki 1987; Park et al. 2006; Chidchuangchai et al. 2007).

When viewed within the intact trigeminal ganglion, a slightly different neuronal pattern emerges. Many pulpal afferents were IB4- and contained the vasoactive neuropeptide, calcitonin gene-related peptide (CGRP) (Fried et al. 2011). Capsaicin stimulation of isolated pulp tissue induces release of this neuropeptide, indicating that this neuronal population possesses the thermally activated TRPV1 receptor and plays a role in controlling the pulpal vasculature (Fehrenbacher et al. 2009). One population of non-neuropeptide containing afferents was observed to account for few trigeminal ganglion cell bodies but formed a dense network of nerve fibres in the superficial pulp, indicating a role in dentin sensation (Chung et al. 2012). This population may include the cell bodies that give rise to the intradental A-fibres since this population is known to be relatively unresponsive to capsaicin (Närhi et al. 1992a).

In many respects, the intradental nociceptors resemble low-threshold mechanoreceptors (LTM) known to mediate non-painful mechanosensation in other parts of the body (Fried et al. 2011). The conduction velocities of some of the pulpal afferents classify these units as Aß-fibres (Närhi et al. 1983). This type of afferent is not normally associated with pain but with non-painful mechanosensation. Examination of pulpal afferent cell bodies in the trigeminal ganglion indicated that many express markers and have cytological feature, for example, cell size that resembles LTM rather than typical nociceptors. The stimuli that trigger pain in sensitive teeth are innocuous in that they do not damage tissue without forceful or repeated application. These features of DH have led investigators to consider the intradental nerves responding to hydrodynamic forces—"low-threshold algoneuron" as opposed to true nociceptors. The reason that activation of these algoneurons results in pain has to do more with their connections in the central nervous system than to the intrinsic response properties of these cells (Fried et al. 2011).

The transduction of hydrodynamic forces into nerve responses implies that these intradental algoneurons possess receptors that are activated by mechanical forces. The preferential sensitivity of intradental nerves to outward fluid displacements indicates that these mechanoreceptors respond best to a tugging type of force application (Vongsavan and Matthews 2007) (Fig. 5.3). Mechanosensitive ion channels are found widely in nature and underlie nerve responses to several modalities in addition to touch, including osmotic stimulation and sound. In mechanoreceptors, a transmembrane transduction channel is anchored by intracellular and extracellular elements to the cytoskeleton of the receptor or nerve and to an extracellular structure (Fig. 5.5). The transduction channel responds to tension or shear opening or closing, and it is this action that gates ion conductance (Gillespie and Walker 2001; Tsunozaki and Bautista 2009).

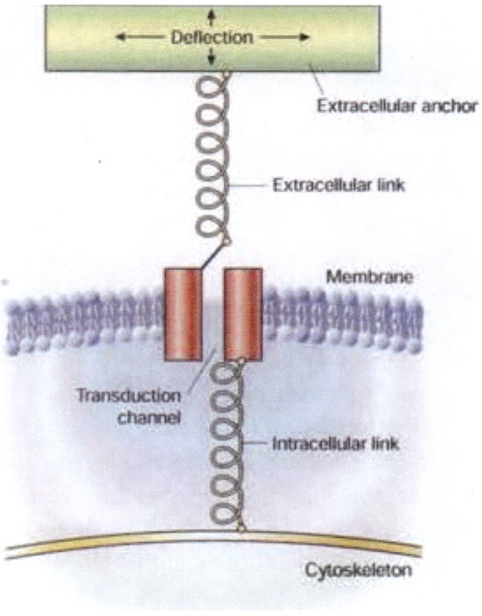

Fig. 5.5 Schematic of a hypothetical mechanosensitive receptor anchored at one end in a nerve membrane and, at the other end, in an extracellular surface. Deformation would open an ion-sensitive channel (Gillespie and Walker (2001) used with permission)

The experiments of Vonsavan, Matthews, and co-workers reviewed above suggest that dentin stimulation activates pulpal A-fibres through mechanical forces. Many ion channels have been proposed as putative mechanoreceptors (Delmas and Coste 2013) in sensory neurons. Some of these channels also mediate responses to other stimuli such as cold and low pH. It has been difficult to prove a mechanosensory function for several candidates' ion channels; since genetic knock-out animals lacking these channels occasionally appear to retain some mechanically mediated sensations (Kang et al. 2012).

Gene expression of a number of proposed mechanosensory ion channels has been examined in rat trigeminal ganglion cells, including labelled pulpal afferents (Hermanstyne et al. 2008). Trigeminal neurons expressed mRNA for many putative mechanosensory channels, most of which were not expressed in pulpal afferents. Using polymerase chain reaction probes to know channels, only one, the acid-sensing ion channel 3 (ASIC3) was found in pulpal afferents. ASIC3 was expressed in 67% of the pulpal afferents sampled. In this study, most pulpal afferents also expressed TRPA1, a chemoreceptive channel that may also be activated by cold (McKemy 2005). Based on the observation that TRPA1 is also activated by oxidizing compounds, it has been hypothesized that this receptor is responsible for the pain that accompanies tooth bleaching (Markowitz 2010).

The percent of neurons expressing ASIC3 was not altered by the induction of pulp inflammation, indicating that ASIC3 is constitutively expressed in the nerve fibres of intact healthy teeth (Hermanstyne et al. 2008). This observation that intradental mechanoreceptors are present in healthy intact teeth was expected since freshly exposed dentin, as would occur in fractured or chipped teeth, is sensitive to both cold air and other stimuli. Physiological experiments examining the nerve responses induced by hydrodynamic stimulation in animals lacking ASIC3 (knockouts) are therefore needed to definitively establish the role of this, and other, ion channels in mediating nerve responses to hydrodynamic stimulation.

Electrophysiological and anatomical studies have identified a promising mechanosensitive channel candidate. The piezo family of channels mediates both nociceptive and non-pain mechanical nerve activation. Like other mechanosensitive ion channels, piezo channels connect the cell's cytoskeleton with extracellular structures causing movement or stretch of the cell membrane to open a nonselective cation channel (Fig. 5.5) (Lin et al. 2022). Pulpal afferents that were histochemically labelled for piezo responded to mechanical stimulation are IB4- and do not respond to capsaicin. These neurons also have cell bodies in the larger range for pulpal afferents indicating that they would give rise to A-fibre type myelinated axons (Won et al. 2017). In the pulp, piezo has been identified to be principally in myelinated axons in the radicular and central coronal pulp and in the nonmyelinated terminal branches of the axons as they ascend to the peripheral pulp and dentin (Cho et al. 2022). Transcriptomic analysis of dentin labelled trigeminal ganglion neurons identified piezo2, a piezo variant observed in non-nociceptive mechanosensitive afferents (Emrick et al. 2020). This highlights the role of intradental nerves in bite force perception and the nature of these neurons as low-threshold algo-receptors (Fried et al. 2011).

To activate pain or other forms of conscious sensation, nerves responding to stimuli transmit all-or-none impulses to the central nervous system. In pain fibres, activation of one of the sensory receptors described above depolarizes the nerve cell membrane; if a threshold is reached, voltage-gated ion channels open (Armstrong and Hille 1998), resulting in an action potential that is transmitted to the central nervous system. The pattern and frequency of action potentials encodes information concerning the perceived intensity of the stimulation. Several types of cation selective ion channels mediate the initiation and termination of the action potential, with voltage-gated sodium channels (VGNa) being responsible for the action potential's rising phase (Amir et al. 2006). In myelinated pulpal afferents, the distribution of VGNa channels is restricted to nodes of Ranvier in the myelinated segment of the fibre and spread out in the peripheral unmyelinated portion of the axon (Henry et al. 2012).

5.7 The Odontoblast Hydrodynamic Hypothesis

In the past, several lines of evidence yielded conflicting information on the role of odontoblasts in dentin sensitivity. Dentin overlying a disrupted odontoblast layer may be sensitive. This observation challenges the notion that the odontoblasts are a critical cellular participant in DH (Lilja et al. 1982) (Fig. 5.1). However, odontoblast do possess an assortment of nerve-like receptors that enable these cells to respond to various chemical, thermal, and mechanical stimuli (Magloire et al. 2010; El Karim et al. 2011; Chung et al. 2013; Tsumura et al. 2013). They also express various voltage-gated Na and K channels depending on the location within the tooth and the tooth's developmental stage (Davidson 1994; Allard et al. 2006; Byers and Westenbroek 2011; Ichikawa et al. 2012).

Pulpal afferents possess purinergic receptors (Cook and McCleskey 2002). When pulpal cells are damaged, cytoplasmic ATP is released into the extracellular fluid. ATP is a potent excitant of nociceptors. Odontoblast ATP release may contribute to nerve activation by hydrodynamic forces since the odontoblast cell bodies are often aspirated into the tubules and destroyed during air blasting or traumatic restorative procedures (Brännström 1963). Recent evidence shows that cell-to-cell ATP signalling provides a means whereby odontoblast can sense hydrodynamic and other stimuli and transmit excitatory signals to the intradental nerves.

Conventional chemical synapses linking odontoblasts with intradental nerves have not been identified (Byers 1984), odontoblasts have an impact on intradental nerve function. These cells control the environment of the intradental nerve endings by determining the dentin fluid's ionic composition, and they also provide the structural support needed for the mechanosensitive nerve endings to detect dentin fluid flow

(Magloire et al. 2010). In response to dentin stimulation, damage to the odontoblasts may also result in prostaglandin formation and as noted above, release of cytoplasmic ATP and potassium ions into the extracellular fluid (Cook and McCleskey 2002).

Recent experiments have clarified the important role of odontoblasts in dentin sensitivity and largely settled the century-long debate on the role of these cells. In experiments where odontoblasts and trigeminal neurons were maintained in culture together, mechanical stimulation of the odontoblasts evoked an excitatory calcium conductance not only in the mechanically stimulated cell but in other nearby odontoblasts and neurons. The mechanically stimulated odontoblast released ATP into the extracellular medium through specialized membrane pores. The responses of the neighbouring odontoblasts and neurons to this mechanically induced ATP release are mediated by various purinergic receptors (Shibukawa et al. 2015). It has been proposed that odontoblasts participate in mediating the response to hydrodynamic dentin stimulation not by conventional synapses but rather by autocrine/paracrine types of signalling involving ATP and other transmitters such as glutamate (Shibukawa et al. 2015; Nishiyama et al. 2016). Inflammatory processes can sensitize this process (Utreras et al. 2013).

Immunohistochemical and pharmacological tools have been used to demonstrate that odontoblasts have piezo mechanoreceptors that trigger ATP release when odontoblasts are mechanically stimulated (Sato et al. 2018; Sun et al. 2022). These studies confirm earlier observations that ATP activated sensory afferents but did not investigate odontoblast-nerve transmission directly in vivo. The role of odontoblast piezo channels and members of the transient receptor potential receptor family was investigated in a rat model where sensitive teeth were generated by cavity preparation and the animal's pain score was measured using a behavioural scale. In this experiment, animals with odontoblast deletions could be generated by a genetic manipulation where odontoblast death was triggered by diphtheria toxin administration. Although this and other manipulations such as genetic knockouts occasionally result in "collateral damage" making interpretation difficult, this study revisited a question raised by earlier clinical research, e.g., are the odontoblasts necessary for dentin sensitivity (Lilja et al. 1982)? Analysis of pain responses following the administration of various pharmacological antagonists indicates that piezo receptors are important in generating pain when exposed dentin is exposed to cold. In animals where the odontoblasts were deleted, cold stimulation of exposed dentin failed to evoke pain behaviour, indicating that odontoblasts are necessary for the transduction of pain following dentin stimulation. Using pharmacological tools and electrophysiology, the investigators provided evidence supporting the role of ATP in odontoblast-nerve signalling. As indicated by previous studies, this is accomplished by an ATP efflux pore, pannexin-1, and ATP receptors (P2X3) on the nerve endings (Ohyama et al. 2022). It is interesting that these investigators used tubule sealing with restorative resin as the "positive control" when testing the actions of agonists and antagonists on dentin stimulus evoked pain. This highlights the overarching importance of dentin permeability in dentin sensitivity.

As is the case for the intradental nerves, direct activation of odontoblasts by cold and other stimuli occurs without dentin fluid shifts. In odontoblasts, cold activates TRPC5 receptors, which directly activate odontoblast in isolated cells, where there is no contact with dentin (Bernal et al. 2021). As shown in Fig. 5.1b, dentin fluid flow and thermal stimuli can activate the intradental nerves directly or through the odontoblast. The odontoblasts provide a site for dentin stimulus transduction that is closer to the dentin surface than the interdental nerve endings (Lee et al. 2019).

It is also possible that the physiological responses of odontoblasts, like those of osteocytes in bone, have non-nociceptive functions such as in dentin formation. Osteocytes respond to the mechanical stimulation of bone by boosting their metabolic activity and maintaining the mineralization of the bone matrix (Cowin 2007). In the case of odontoblasts, electrophysiological responses to dentin damage and stimulation may be involved in tertiary dentin formation (Byers and Westenbroek 2011). Reactionary dentin formation frequently occurs in response to dentin wear and as such it is possible that sensory transduction by odontoblasts triggers reactionary dentin formation (Xu et al. 2024). The fact that odontoblasts and nerves engage in two-way communication makes it possible for responses to dentin exposure and stimulation to occur in regional patches of pulp tissue activating tertiary dentin formation involving a region of the tooth as is observed (Nishiyama et al. 2016). Sensory activation may regulate rather than simply activate tertiary dentin formation. Piezo channels may inhibit mineralized tissue formation, preventing excessive tertiary dentin formation following dentin exposure (Matsunaga et al. 2021). Further research is needed to determine the sensory function of these versatile cells.

5.8 Pain and the Pulp Environment

Symptoms, including a decrease in the pain threshold, and an increase in the intensity of pain, accompany inflammation (Park et al. 2001). Pulpal inflammation may be responsible for exposed dentin becoming hypersensitive (Pashley 2013). Inflammation-related plasticity has a major impact on the excitability and pharmacological sensitivity of nociceptors during pathological states (Gold and Flake 2005; Henry and Hargreaves 2007; Chung et al. 2013). Pulp inflammation may also be triggered by trauma to the tooth or bacterial invasion of the pulp or dentin.

Oral microorganisms invade and colonize the dentin tubules when caries spreads into dentin (Love et al. 2000). Bacterial products, enzymes, and antigens diffuse through relatively intact dentin layers into the pulp where they can produce an inflammatory response (Brännström 1962; Lundy and Stanley 1969; Goldberg et al. 2008). In acute pulpitis, inflammatory mediators accumulate in the pulp, resulting in sensitization and eventual activation of the nociceptors leading to spontaneous pain (Bowles et al. 2003). This process may also be triggered by bacteria products invading the dentin (Warfvinge et al. 1985; Jontell et al. 1998; Fouad 2012), by chronic dentin exposure or the trauma of restorative procedures (Olgart et al. 1991; Mjör 2001). As the pulp's most superficial cell, odontoblasts participate with antigen-presenting dendritic cells in initiating the immune response to caries and other antigenic challenges to the dental pulp (Yumoto et al. 2018).

In caries, the type and intensity of the pulp's inflammatory response are dependent on the depth of bacterial invasion into dentin (Izumi et al. 1995; Cooper et al. 2011). Considerable variability exists in the symptoms experienced by people with carious teeth. Teeth with deep carious lesions, heavily infected with *Lactobacillus* species, were observed to be relatively asymptomatic. In contrast, teeth with lesions infected with predominantly anaerobic organisms were more likely to present with thermal sensitivity and other symptoms (Hahn et al. 1993).

Various by-products of bacterial metabolism, for example, amines, are highly excitatory to intradental nerves (Panopoulos 1992). Organic acids, the principal metabolic by-product of sugar fermentation by *Lactobacillus* and other caries-associated bacteria have complex effects on pain. Organic acids have an inhibitory effect on intradental nerve activity induced by chemical stimulation (Panopoulos 1992). Acids also enhance dental pain by activating certain receptors and sensitizing other receptors, e.g., TRPV1, to heat stimulation (Goodis et al. 2006). Variations in the bacterial population of a carious lesion may also influence the type of lesion metabolism and the inflammatory response that develops in the pulp, which in turn may determine the degree to which pain sensitization occurs (Hahn and Liewehr 2007).

Even without directly invading the pulp, bacteria can influence the function of the intradental nerves. Lipopolysaccharide (LPS) is an important toxin released by gram negative anaerobic bacteria, which initiate both local pulpal and systemic inflammatory responses (Okiji et al. 1992; Chattipakorn et al. 2002; Bletsa et al. 2006). This toxin can trigger shock and systemic organ damage (Quan et al. 2001). Direct exposure of the pulp to LPS induces severe inflammation and pain facilitation-associated changes in the central nervous system areas that receive input from pulpal nociceptors (Chattipakorn et al. 2005). LPS may diffuse through dentin and facilitate the actions of thermally activated ion channels (Nissan et al. 1995; Chung et al. 2011; Diogenes et al. 2011). These changes would be expected to make the tooth very sensitive to hot and cold.

There are numerous links that exist between the activation of the immune system, inflammation, and pain facilitation (Bletsa et al. 2009; Kress 2010). For example, trigeminal neurons possess toll-like receptors and other components of the innate immune system (Byers et al. 1992; Byers and Närhi 1999; Veerayutthwilai et al. 2007; Horst et al. 2009). These receptors are part of the body's early warning system that responds to LPS and other bacterial products. This mechanism may help explain the algesic effect of anaerobic bacteria (Wadachi and Hargreaves 2006). Nociceptors are also sensitized by lipid-based oxidation by-products in tissue. These substances form in tissue having severe inflammatory responses due to the action of neutrophils (Hargreaves and Ruparel 2016). Direct activation of oxidation receptors in odontoblasts and intradental nerves may be responsible for the pain experienced by people whose teeth are exposed to high peroxide concentrations during tooth bleaching procedures (Markowitz 2010; Chen et al. 2021). Peroxide exposure caused pulpal cells to produce inflammatory mediators.

Inflammatory mediators appear to induce phosphorylation of TRPV channels, causing them to become more sensitive than normal to thermal stimulation (Jeske et al. 2006). Nitric oxide (NO), an oxidative-free radical generated by the enzyme nitric oxide synthetase (NOS), has been implicated in inflammatory processes in the dental pulp. Because NO is rapidly destroyed, investigators follow increases in NOS enzyme activity in normal versus inflamed rat pulps (Law et al. 1999; Fujita et al. 2004). The exact role of NO in DH remains to be discovered.

Inflammation and pain are intimately linked, with nociceptor activation being an initiating factor in triggering inflammation and inflammation sensitizing and activating nociceptors (Kim 1990). Painful stimuli, for example, tooth preparation, result in an increase in pulpal blood flow, as well as increases in intrapulpal pressure and outward dentin fluid flow. These effects can also be evoked by activation of the intradental sensory nerves by electrical, chemical, or hydrodynamic stimuli (Pertl et al. 1993; Heyeraas et al. 1994; Olgart 1996; Andrew and Matthews 2002). Stimulus-evoked release of vasoactive peptides, for example, substance P and CGRP, from the pulpal terminals of intradental nerve endings initiates vasodilatation and increases vascular permeability, which are the early vascular manifestations of inflammation (Kerezoudis et al. 1993; Fehrenbacher et al. 2009). This phenomenon is referred to as "neurogenic inflammation".

Compared to acute pulpitis, the role of bacteria and pulp inflammation in DH is less clear. Although healthy, freshly exposed dentin can be sensitive and sensitive cervical abrasions are frequently plaque-free (Addy et al. 1987), sensitization of intradental nerve responses can occur due to interactions between the pulp and plaque covering the tooth's root surface (Tammaro et al. 2000). However, bacteria do not pass through the intact dentin boundary separating the pulp from the tooth surface in sensitive teeth (Michelich et al. 1980). Although dentin tubules observed in SEMs appear to have a diameter of about 1 μm, their functional diameter is only about one-twentieth of that value due to the presence of intratubular material, such as collagen fibres, mineral concretions, etc. (Michelich et al. 1978). The functional consequences of this restricted tubule diameter are that dentin does not permit bacteria to reach the pulp. That is, the dentinal fluid that reaches the pulp chamber is sterile (Michelich et al. 1980). Dentin acts in a similar manner to a 0.2 μm Millipore filter in keeping oral microorganisms from infecting pulpal soft tissue.

Inflammation can exacerbate DH symptoms by making the intradental nerve endings more responsive to dentin fluid flow. Serotonin (5-HT) is an inflammatory mediator that is released by platelets and mast cells into damaged tissue. It is involved in a number of pain conditions, including migraine headache (Sommer 2004). 5-HT application to exposed dentin also lowers the threshold of A-fibre units to hydrodynamic dentin stimulation (Ngassapa et al. 1992). Prior to 5-HT application, these units failed to respond to a weak osmotic stimulant, glucose solution application, to exposed etched dentin. Following application of 5-HT to the dentin, glucose application evoked an excitatory response indicting a lowering of the hydrodynamic threshold. This observation may explain the sensitivity to sweets often experienced during pulpitis. Serotonin sensitizes trigeminal nociceptors to both thermal and chemical stimulation, enhancing stimulation-evoked CGRP release (Loyd et al. 2013).

Inflammatory mediators frequently act synergistically in potentiating the response to excitation (Hirafuji and Ogura 1987; Bletsa et al. 2009). For example, bradykinin enhances the capsaicin-evoked CGRP release from intradental nerve endings (Goodis et al. 2000). In these experiments, prostaglandin-E application enhanced this action of bradykinin.

There are also structural changes in the intradental nerves that are a consequence of injury and inflammation (Byers and Närhi 1999). Following traumatic cavity preparation, sprouting of CGRP-containing nerve fibre terminals was observed in the superficial pulp tissue (Taylor et al. 1988). Because of this response, there may be a large increase in the innervation density of the superficial pulp tissue following injury, especially in the normally sparsely innervated cervical and radicular pulp. The timing of sprouting follows the general time course of increases in post-operative DH symptoms encountered following restorative or periodontal procedures. Nerve sprouting is at its maximum 1 week following injury and then the anatomic pattern returns to normal by 3 weeks after injury (Byers 1994; Byers and Närhi 1999; Rodd and Boissonade 2001). Post-operative symptoms tend to be at their worst 1 week after any restorative procedure and generally abate during the following weeks. Nerve sprouting has also been observed in human teeth with deep caries (Rodd and Boissonade 2001).

Injury and inflammation also may initiate the partial demyelination of afferents and changes in the type and spatial pattern of the VGNa channels (Henry et al. 2009). Demyelination can result in abnormal electrical interactions between the axons that allow impulses in one afferent to excite adjacent neurons. These alterations make the afferents more excitable. The specific type of VGNa channels expressed in nerve fibres may be altered by inflammation and nerve injury (Renton et al. 2005; Henry et al. 2009; Luo et al. 2010). The VGNa channels expressed in neurons exposed to inflammation have altered pharmacological sensitivities compared to neurons innervating healthy tissue (Lai et al. 2004). It is hypothesized that this altered pharmacological susceptibility is responsible for the difficulties encountered in obtaining local anaesthesia in inflamed teeth (Hargreaves and Keiser 2002). Investigating the ability of anti-inflammatory drugs to reverse the actions of inflammation on local anaesthetic efficacy is ongoing but has not yielded conclusive results (Parirokh and Abbott 2022).

A mild inflammatory response can be induced in human teeth by preparing dentin cavities and restoring the teeth with defective temporary restorations that allow bacterial leakage. Following 1 week, the inflamed teeth exhibited enhanced pain responses to cold stimulation compared to intact teeth. These changes in thermal sensitivity are not initiated by an increase in dentin permeability (Ajcharanukul et al. 2011). These experiments demonstrate that the pain response in sensitive teeth may be enhanced by inflammation, making the teeth hypersensitive. When sensitive teeth are evaluated clinically, teeth exhibiting dental caries, defective restorations, and tooth fractures should also be considered in the differential diagnosis process and corrected, since in the presence of these conditions, DH is unlikely to resolve with standard topical desensitizing treatments (Orchardson and Gillam 2006) (Fig. 5.6) (see Chap. 8).

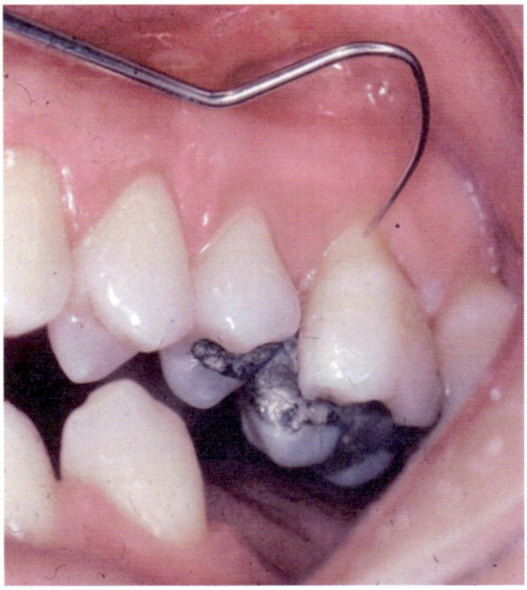

Fig. 5.6 Clinical photograph of a super-erupted, sensitive first molar showing the relationship between DH and defective restorations. The tooth was sensitive to cold liquids, air blasts, and probing of the exposed mesial buccal root with a dental explorer as shown. The patient's sensitivity symptoms were longstanding and failed to improve following the application of an oxalate-based topical desensitizer to the exposed root surface. Following the replacement of the existing amalgam restoration, the sensitivity symptoms resolved, and the tooth remained asymptomatic and vital. Pulpal inflammation caused by bacterial leakage around the restoration is presumed to have sensitized the intradental nerves to stimuli. In this sensitized state, usually effective topical desensitizing agents fail to provide pain relief. Replacement of the defective restoration allows the inflammatory process and the pain sensitization to resolve. (From Markowitz K, unpublished photograph)

5.9 Central Representation of Tooth Sensitivity

Using advanced imaging and electrophysiological methods, it is possible to localize the areas of the brain activated by tooth stimulation (Kubo et al. 2008; Meier et al. 2012). Repeated or intense activation of nociceptors may facilitate the pain transmission in the central nervous system. Activation of pulpal afferents by noxious heat stimulation has been reported to induce an enhancement of the responses to those same thermal stimuli by second-order neurons in the brainstem's trigeminal nuclear complex (Ahn et al. 2012). Intense activation of the intradental nerves or the induction of pulpal inflammation by the administration of noxious chemicals may also induce alterations in gene expression in the trigeminal nuclear complex and enhanced nociception in other facial areas, e.g., the lip (Park et al. 2001; Chattipakorn et al. 2005). The role of central plasticity in DH is, however, unclear at present. The role of physiological and psychological factors as well as gender in dental pain perception is being investigated (Parirokh and Abbott 2022). The concept that a "pain phenotype" may exist in the population with persons requiring special care in the management of DH, local anesthesia, and other considerations is under investigation. It is possible that nociceptor activation accompanying periodontal procedures that precede episodes of DH sensitize the central pathways, resulting in more pain being triggered by dentin stimulation.

5.10 Dentin Plasticity

Oral microorganisms also have profound effects on the permeability of exposed dentin. Despite the capacity for excessive tooth brushing to cause dentin surface loss, plaque-control has an important role in preventing DH following periodontal therapy (Wallace and Bissada 1990; Tammaro et al. 2000). Plaque-covered exposed dentin surfaces were observed to have widened tubules compared to surfaces that were kept plaque-free (Suge et al. 2006). The acid-liability of smear layers is responsible for the frequently observed lack of DH in patients immediately after root scaling and the onset of DH that appeared up to 7–14 days following scaling procedures (pocketdentistry.com, Chap. 3). This time delay presumably enables the plaque to form on the root surface and for the microorganisms to dissolve the smear layer/smear plug combination (Kerns et al. 1991).

Dentin is a biological composite consisting of mineral and an organic phase that is mostly collagen. In addition to collagen, the organic matrix of dentin also contains several non-collagenous proteins that play an important role in dentin mineralization (Tay and Pashley 2009; Kim et al. 2010). These proteins are highly acidic and contain calcium-binding phosphate groups that pattern mineral formation (Boskey et al. 1990). The odontoblasts trigger mineralization by secreting these proteins into the predentin at the mineralization front (Veis 1993). The link between the sensory function of odontoblasts and dentin formation is being investigated (Matsunaga et al. 2021).

The composition of dentin influences its susceptibility to damage and its capacity for repair. As with dentin from which it is derived, dentin smear layers also contain mineral and organic components (Pashley 1992b).

In order to degrade dentin, both the organic and inorganic phases of the tissue must be attacked by the caries process (Love 2002). Plaque-derived acids dissolve the mineral component of the smear layer and underlying dentin; bacterial and host-derived enzymes can attack the organic phase of the dentin (Chaussain-Miller et al. 2006). Host-derived collagen degrading enzymes, for example, the matrix metalloproteinases (MMPs), originate in the crevicular fluid, saliva, and dentin itself. In dentin, these enzymes can be activated by acid exposure, and these enzymes are believed to contribute to erosive tooth structure loss (Buzalaf et al. 2012). In restored teeth, the long-term action of MMPs and other enzymes may also weaken the dentin-restoration bond by degrading resin-infiltrated collagen fibrils (Tjäderhane et al. 2013a). Dentin treatment with chlorhexidine or other cationic compounds preserves bond strength by inhibiting these enzymes (Tjäderhane et al. 2013b).

5.11 Conclusion

Since the publication of the first edition of this book in 2015, progress has been made in the understanding of the physiological mechanisms of sensitive teeth. Although care must be exercised in the application of knowledge gained from animal research to human diseases, many insights have been gained. The role of the odontoblasts in dentin sensitivity has moved from "maybe" as we suggested in 2015 to probably "yes". In 2015, we were certain that the hydrodynamic mechanism pointed to a mechanoreceptor in nerves and odontoblasts. Today we are confident that we have identified the receptors and the process by which dentin stimulation is translated into the language of nerve signalling. Other clinically important questions such as the effect of inflammation on pain transduction have been substantiated. The ultimate test of our ideas is translation into improved patient care.

References

Absi EG, Addy M, Adams D. Dentine hypersensitivity. A study of the patency of dentinal tubules in sensitive and non-sensitive cervical dentine. J Clin Periodontol. 1987;14:280–4.

Absi EG, Addy M, Adams D. Dentine hypersensitivity. The development and evaluation of a replica technique to study sensitive and non-sensitive cervical dentine. J Clin Periodontol. 1989;16:190–5.

Addy M. Clinical aspects of dentine hypersensitivity. Proc Finn Dent Soc. 1992;88(Suppl 1):23–30.

Addy M, Mostafa P, Newcombe RG. Dentine hypersensitivity: the distribution of recession, sensitivity and plaque. J Dent. 1987;15(6):242–8.

Ahlquist ML, Franzén OG. Encoding of the subjective intensity of sharp dental pain. Endod Dent Traumatol. 1994;10(4):153–66.

Ahlquist ML, Edwall LG, Franzén OG, Haegerstam GA. Perception of pulpal pain as a function of intradental nerve activity. Pain. 1984;19(4):353–66.

Ahlquist MO, Franzén OG, Coffey J, Pashley D. Dental pain evoked by hydrostatic pressures applied to exposed dentin in man: a test of the hydrodynamic theory of dentin sensitivity. J Endod. 1994;20(3):130–4.

Ahn DK, Doutova EA, McNaughton K, Light AR, Närhi M, Maixner W. Functional properties of tooth pulp neurons responding to thermal stimulation. J Dent Res. 2012;91(4):401–6.

Ajcharanukul OW, Chidchuangchai WP, Charoenlarp PN, Vongsavan N, Matthews B. Sensory transduction in human teeth with inflamed pulps. J Dent Res. 2011;90(5):678–82.

Allard B, Magloire H, Couble ML, Maurin JC, Bleicher F. Voltage-gated sodium channels confer excitability to human odontoblasts: possible role in tooth pain transmission. J Biol Chem. 2006;281(39):29002–10.

Aminoshariae A, Kulild JC. Current concepts of dentinal hypersensitivity. J Endod. 2021;47:1696–702.

Amir R, Argoff CE, Bennett GJ, Cummins TR, Durieux ME, Gerner P, Gold MS, Porreca F, Strichartz GR. The role of sodium channels in chronic inflammatory and neuropathic pain. J Pain. 2006;7(5 Suppl 3):S1–29.

Anderson DJ, Matthews B. Dentinal and periodontal sensory mechanisms. Front Oral Physiol. 1976;2:38–50.

Anderson DJ, Matthews B, Shelton LE. Variations in the sensitivity to osmotic stimulation of human dentine. Arch Oral Biol. 1967;12(1):43–7.

Andrew D, Matthews B. Displacement of the contents of dentinal tubules and sensory transduction in intradental nerves of the cat. J Physiol. 2000;529(Pt 3):791–802.

Andrew D, Matthews B. Properties of single nerve fibres that evoke blood flow changes in cat dental pulp. J Physiol. 2002;542(Pt 3):921–8.

Armstrong CM, Hille B. Voltage-gated ion channels and electrical excitability. Neuron. 1998;20(3):371–80.

Bekes K, Hirsch C. What is known about the influence of dentine hypersensitivity on oral health-related quality of life? Clin Oral Investig. 2013;17(Suppl 1):S45–51.

Bernal L, Sotelo-Hitschfeld P, König C, Sinica V, Wyatt A, Winter Z, Hein A, Touska F, Reinhardt S, Tragl A, Kusuda R, Wartenberg P, Sclaroff A, Pfeifer JD, Ectors F, Dahl A, Freichel M, Vlachova V, Brauchi S, Roza C, Boehm U, Clapham DE, Lennerz JK, Zimmermann K. Odontoblast TRPC5 channels signal cold pain in teeth. Sci Adv. 2021;7:eabf5567.

Bletsa A, Berggreen E, Fristad I, Tenstad O, Wiig H. Cytokine signalling in rat pulp interstitial fluid and transcapillary fluid exchange during lipopolysaccharide-induced acute inflammation. J Physiol. 2006;573(Pt 1):225–36.

Bletsa A, Fristad I, Berggreen E. Sensory pulpal nerve fibres and trigeminal ganglion neurons express IL-1RI: a potential mechanism for development of inflammatory hyperalgesia. Int Endod J. 2009;42(11):978–86.

Boskey AL, Maresca M, Doty S, Sabsay B, Veis A. Concentration-dependent effects of dentin phosphophoryn in the regulation of in vitro hydroxyapatite formation and growth. Bone Miner. 1990;11(1):55–65.

Bowles WR, Withrow JC, Lepinski AM, Hargreaves KM. Tissue levels of immunoreactive substance P are increased in patients with irreversible pulpitis. J Endod. 2003;29(4):265–7.

Brännström M. The elicitation of pain in human dentine and pulp by chemical stimuli. Arch Oral Biol. 1962;7:59–62.

Brännström M. Dentin sensitivity and aspiration of odontoblasts. J Am Dent Assoc. 1963;66:366–70.

Brännström M. The surface of sensitive dentine. An experimental study using replication. Odontol Revy. 1965;16(4):293–9.

Brännström M. Sensitivity of dentine. Oral Surg Oral Med Oral Pathol. 1966;21(4):517–26.

Brännström M. The effect of dentin desiccation and aspirated odontoblasts on the pulp. J Prosthet Dent. 1968;20(2):165–71.

Brännström M. The hydrodynamic theory of dentinal pain: sensation in preparations, caries, and the dentinal crack syndrome. J Endod. 1986;12(10):453–7.

Brännström M. Etiology of dentin hypersensitivity. Proc Finn Dent Soc. 1992;88(Suppl 1):7–13.

Brännström M, Linden LA, Astrom A. The hydrodynamics of the dental tubule and of pulp fluid. A discussion of its significance in relation to dentinal sensitivity. Caries Res. 1967;1(4):310–7.

Buzalaf MA, Kato MT, Hannas AR. The role of matrix metalloproteinases in dental erosion. Adv Dent Res. 2012;24(2):72–6.

Byers MR. Dental sensory receptors. Int Rev Neurobiol. 1984;25:39–94.

Byers MR. Dynamic plasticity of dental sensory nerve structure and cytochemistry. Arch Oral Biol. 1994;39(Suppl):13S–21S.

Byers MR, Närhi MV. Dental injury models: experimental tools for understanding neuroinflammatory interactions and polymodal nociceptor functions. Crit Rev Oral Biol Med. 1999;10(1):4–39.

Byers MR, Sugaya A. Odontoblast processes in dentin revealed by fluorescent Di-I. J Histochem Cytochem. 1995;43(2):159–68.

Byers MR, Westenbroek RE. Odontoblasts in developing, mature and ageing rat teeth have multiple phenotypes that variably express all nine voltage-gated sodium channels. Arch Oral Biol. 2011;56(11):1199–220.

Byers MR, Neuhaus SJ, Gehrig JD. Dental sensory receptor structure in human teeth. Pain. 1982;13(3):221–35.

Byers MR, Närhi MV, Dong WK. Sensory innervation of pulp and dentin in adult dog teeth as demonstrated by autoradiography. Anat Rec. 1987;218:207–15.

Byers MR, Wheeler EF, Bothwell M. Altered expression of NGF and P75 NGF-receptor by fibroblasts of injured teeth precedes sensory nerve sprouting. Growth Factors. 1992;6(1):41–52.

Camps J, Pashley D. Reliability of the dye penetration studies. J Endod. 2003;29(9):592–4. https://doi.org/10.1097/00004770-200309000-00012. PMID: 14503834

Camps J, Salomon JP, Meerbeek BV, Tay F, Pashley D. Dentin deformation after scratching with clinically-relevant forces. Arch Oral Biol. 2003;48(7):527–34.

Carrilho MR, Tay FR, Sword J, Donnelly AM, Agee A, Nishitani Y, Sadek ET, Carvalho RM, Pashley DH. Dentine sealing provided by smear layer/smear plugs vs. adhesive resins/resin tags. Eur J Oral Sci. 2007;115(4):321–9.

Catania KC. The sense of touch in the star-nosed mole: from mechanoreceptors to the brain. Philos Trans R Soc Lond Ser B Biol Sci. 2011;366(1581):3016–25.

Charoenlarp PS, Wanachantararak S, Vongsavan N, Matthews B. Pain and the rate of dentinal fluid flow produced by hydrostatic pressure stimulation of exposed dentine in man. Arch Oral Biol. 2007;52(7):625–31. https://doi.org/10.1016/j.archoralbio.2006.12.014.

Chattipakorn SC, Sigurdsson A, Light AR, Närhi M, Maixner W. Trigeminal c-Fos expression and behavioral responses to pulpal inflammation in ferrets. Pain. 2002;99(1–2):61–9.

Chattipakorn SN, Chattipakorn N, Light AR, Närhi M, Maixner W. Comparison of Fos expression within the ferret's spinal trigeminal nuclear complex evoked by electrical or noxious-thermal pulpal stimulation. J Pain. 2005;6(9):569–80.

Chaussain-Miller C, Fioretti F, Goldberg M, Menashi S. The role of matrix metalloproteinases (MMPs) in human caries. J Dent Res. 2006;85(1):22–32.

Chen C, Huang X, Zhu W, Ding C, Huang P, Li R. TRPA1 triggers hyperalgesia and inflammation after tooth bleaching. Sci Rep. 2021;11(1):17418.

Chidchuangchai W, Vongsavan N, Matthews B. Sensory transduction mechanisms responsible for pain caused by cold stimulation of dentine in man. Arch Oral Biol. 2007;52(2):154–60.

Cho YS, Han HM, Jeong SY, Kim TH, Choi SY, Kim YS, Bae YC. Expression of piezo1 in the trigeminal neurons and in the axons that innervate the dental pulp. Front Cell Neurosci. 2022;16:945948.

Chung MK, Lee J, Duraes G, Ro JY. Lipopolysaccharide-induced pulpitis up-regulates TRPV1 in trigeminal ganglia. J Dent Res. 2011;90(9):1103–7.

Chung MK, Jue SS, Dong X. Projection of non-peptidergic afferents to mouse tooth pulp. J Dent Res. 2012;91(8):777–82.

Chung G, Jung SJ, Oh SB. Cellular and molecular mechanisms of dental nociception. J Dent Res. 2013;92(11):948–55.

Ciucchi B, Bouillaguet S, Holz J, Pashley D. Dentinal fluid dynamics in human teeth, in vivo. J Endod. 1995;21(4):191–4.

Cook SP, McCleskey EW. Cell damage excites nociceptors through release of cytosolic ATP. Pain. 2002;95(1–2):41–7.

Cooper PR, McLachlan JL, Simon S, Graham LW, Smith AJ. Mediators of inflammation and regeneration. Adv Dent Res. 2011;23(3):290–5.

Cowin SC. The significance of bone microstructure in mechanotransduction. J Biomech. 2007;40(Suppl 1):S105–9.

Davidson RM. Neural form of voltage-dependent sodium current in human cultured dental pulp cells. Arch Oral Biol. 1994;39(7):613–20.

Delmas P, Coste B. Mechano-gated ion channels in sensory systems. Cell. 2013;155(2):278–84.

Diogenes A, Ferraz CC, Akopian AN, Henry MA, Hargreaves KM. LPS sensitizes TRPV1 via activation of TLR4 in trigeminal sensory neurons. J Dent Res. 2011;90(6):759–64.

Eckert SP, Taddese A, McCleskey EW. Isolation and culture of rat sensory neurons having distinct sensory modalities. J Neurosci Methods. 1997;77(2):183–90.

El Karim IA, Linden GJ, Curtis TM, About I, McGahon MK, Irwin CR, Lundy FT. Human odontoblasts express functional thermo-sensitive TRP channels: implications for dentin sensitivity. Pain. 2011;152(10):2211–23.

Emrick JJ, von Buchholtz LJ, Ryba NJP. Transcriptomic classification of neurons innervating teeth. J Dent Res. 2020;99(13):1478–85. https://doi.org/10.1177/0022034520941837.

Fehrenbacher JC, Sun XX, Locke EE, Henry MA, Hargreaves KM. Capsaicin-evoked iCGRP release from human dental pulp: a model system for the study of peripheral neuropeptide secretion in normal healthy tissue. Pain. 2009;144(3):253–61.

Fogel HM, Marshall FJ, Pashley DH. Effects of distance from the pulp and thickness on the hydraulic conductance of human radicular dentin. J Dent Res. 1988;67(11):1381–5.

Fors U, Ahlquist ML, Skagerwall R, Edwall LG, Haegerstam GA. Relation between intradental nerve activity and estimated pain in man—a mathematical model. Pain. 1984;18(4):397–408.

Fouad A. Molecular mediators of inflammation, Chap. 11. In: Hargreaves KM, Goodis HE, Tay FR, editors. Seltzer and Bender's Dental Pulp. 2nd ed. Chicago, IL: Quintessence Publishing Co. Inc.; 2012. p. 241–75.

Fried K, Sessle BJ, Devor M. The paradox of pain from tooth pulp: low-threshold algoneurons? Pain. 2011;152(12):2685–9.

Fujita T, Kamisaki Y, Yonehara N. Nitric oxide-induced increase in excitatory amino acid levels in the trigeminal nucleus caudalis of the rat with tactile hypersensitivity evoked by the loose-ligation of the inferior alveolar nerves. J Neurochem. 2004;91(3):558–67.

Fuss Z, Trowbridge H, Bender IB, Rickoff B, Sorin S. Assessment of reliability of electrical and thermal pulp testing agents. J Endod. 1986;12(7):301–5.

Gillam DG, Orchardson R, Närhi MVO, Kontturi-Närhi V. Present and future methods for the evaluation of pain associated with dentine hypersensitivity. In: Addy M, Embery G, Edgar WM, Orchardson R, editors. Tooth wear and sensitivity. London: Martin Dunitz; 2000. p. 283–97.

Gillespie PG, Walker RG. Molecular basis of mechanosensory transduction. Nature. 2001;413(6852):194–202.

Gold MS, Flake MN. Inflammation-mediated hyperexcitability of sensory neurons. Neurosignals. 2005;14(4):147–57.

Goldberg M, Farges JC, Lacerda-Pinheiro S, Six N, Jegat N, Decup F, Septier D, Carrouel F, Durand S, Chaussain-Miller C, Denbesten P, Veis A, Poliard A. Inflammatory and immunological aspects of dental pulp repair. Pharmacol Res. 2008;58(2):137–47.

Goodis HE, Bowles WR, Hargreaves KM. Prostaglandin E2 enhances bradykinin-evoked iCGRP release in bovine dental pulp. J Dent Res. 2000;79(8):1604–7.

Goodis HE, Poon A, Hargreaves KM. Tissue pH and temperature regulate pulpal nociceptors. J Dent Res. 2006;85(11):1046–9.

Guyton AC, Hall JE. Textbook of medical physiology. 10th ed. Philadelphia: W.B. Saunders Company; 2000.

Gysi A. An attempt to explain the sensitiveness of dentine. Br J Dent Sci. 1900;43:865–8.

Hahn CL, Liewehr FR. Update on the adaptive immune responses of the dental pulp. J Endod. 2007;33(7):773–81.

Hahn CL, Overton B. The effects of immunoglobulins on the convective permeability of human dentine in vitro. Arch Oral Biol. 1997;42(12):835–43.

Hahn CL, Falkler WA Jr, Minah GE. Correlation between thermal sensitivity and microorganisms isolated from deep carious dentin. J Endod. 1993;19(1):26–30.

Hargreaves KM, Keiser K. Local anesthetic failure in endodontics: mechanisms and management. Endod Top. 2002;1(1):26–39.
Hargreaves KM, Ruparel S. Role of oxidized lipids and TRP channels in orofacial pain and inflammation. J Dent Res. 2016;95(10):1117–23.
Henry MA, Hargreaves KM. Peripheral mechanisms of odontogenic pain. Dent Clin N Am. 2007;51(1):19–44.
Henry MA, Luo S, Foley BD, Rzasa RS, Johnson LR, Levinson SR. Sodium channel expression and localization at demyelinated sites in painful human dental pulp. Pain. 2009;10(7):750–8.
Henry MA, Luo S, Levinson SR. Unmyelinated nerve fibers in the human dental pulp express markers for myelinated fibers and show sodium channel accumulations. BMC Neurosci. 2012;13:29.
Hermanstyne TO, Markowitz K, Fan L, Gold MS. Mechanotransducers in rat pulpal afferents. J Dent Res. 2008;87(9):834–8.
Heyeraas KJ, Berggreen E. Interstitial fluid pressure in normal and inflamed pulp. Crit Rev Oral Biol Med. 1999;10(3):328–36.
Heyeraas KJ, Kim S, Raab WH, Byers MR, Liu M. Effect of electrical tooth stimulation on blood flow, interstitial fluid pressure and substance P and CGRP-immunoreactive nerve fibers in the low compliant cat dental pulp. Microvasc Res. 1994;47(3):329–43.
Hirafuji M, Ogura Y. 5-Hydroxytryptamine stimulates the release of prostacyclin but not thromboxane A2 from isolated rat dental pulp. Eur J Pharmacol. 1987;136(3):433–6.
Hirvonen TJ, Närhi MV, Hakumäki MO. The excitability of dog pulp nerves in relation to the condition of dentine surface. J Endod. 1984;10(7):294–8.
Horst OV, Tompkins KA, Coats SR, Braham PH, Darveau RP, Dale BA. TGF-beta1 inhibits TLR-mediated odontoblast responses to oral bacteria. J Dent Res. 2009;88(4):333–8.
Ichikawa H, Kim HJ, Shuprisha A, Shikano T, Tsumura M, Shibukawa Y, Tazaki M. Voltage-dependent sodium channels and calcium-activated potassium channels in human odontoblasts in vitro. J Endod. 2012;38(10):1355–62.
Ikeda H, Tokita Y, Suda H. Capsaicin-sensitive a delta fibers in cat tooth pulp. J Dent Res. 1997;76(7):1341–9.
Izumi T, Kobayashi I, Okamura K, Sakai H. Immunohistochemical study on the immunocompetent cells of the pulp in human non-carious and carious teeth. Arch Oral Biol. 1995;40(7):609–14.
Jeske NA, Patwardhan AM, Gamper N, Price TJ, Akopian AN, Hargreaves KM. Cannabinoid WIN 55,212-2 regulates TRPV1 phosphorylation in sensory neurons. J Biol Chem. 2006;281(43):32879–90.
Jontell M, Okiji T, Dahlgren U, Bergenholtz G. Immune defense mechanisms of the dental pulp. Crit Rev Oral Biol Med. 1998;9(2):179–200.
Jyväsjärvi E, Kniffki KD. Cold stimulation of teeth: a comparison between the responses of cat intradental a delta and C fibres and human sensation. J Physiol. 1987;391:193–207.
Jyväsjärvi E, Kniffki KD. Studies on the presence and functional properties of afferent C-fibers in the cat's dental pulp. Proc Finn Dent Soc. 1992;88(Suppl 1):533–42.
Kang S, Jang JH, Price MP, Gautam M, Benson CJ, Gong H, Welsh MJ, Brennan TJ. Simultaneous disruption of mouse ASIC1a, ASIC2 and ASIC3 genes enhances cutaneous mechanosensitivity. PLoS One. 2012;7(4):e35225.
Kerezoudis NP, Olgart L, Edwall L. Evans blue extravasation in rat dental pulp and oral tissues induced by electrical stimulation of the inferior alveolar nerve. Arch O.ral Biol. 1993;38(10):893–901.
Kerns DG, Scheidt MJ, Pashley DH, Horner JA, Strong SL, Van Dyke TE. Dentinal tubule occlusion and root hypersensitivity. J Periodontol. 1991;62(7):421–8.
Kim S. Neurovascular interactions in the dental pulp in health and inflammation. J Endod. 1990;16(2):48–53.
Kim J, Arola DD, Gu L, Kim YK, Mai S, Liu Y, Pashley DH, Tay FR. Functional biomimetic analogs help remineralize apatite-depleted demineralized resin-infiltrated dentin via a bottom-up approach. Acta Biomater. 2010;6(7):2740–50.
Kim HY, Chung G, Jo HJ, Kim YS, Bae YC, Jung SJ, Kim JS, Oh SB. Characterization of dental nociceptive neurons. J Dent Res. 2011;90(6):771–6.
Kontturi-Nahri V, Närhi M. Testing sensitive dentine in man. Int Endod J. 1993;26(1):4.
Kress M. Nociceptor sensitization by Proinflammatory cytokines and chemokines. Open Pain J. 2010;3:97–107.
Kubo K, Shibukawa Y, Shintani M, Suzuki T, Ichinohe T, Kaneko Y. Cortical representation area of human dental pulp. J Dent Res. 2008;87(4):358–62.
Lai J, Porreca F, Hunter JC, Gold MS. Voltage-gated sodium channels and hyperalgesia. Annu Rev Pharmacol Toxicol. 2004;44:371–97.
Law AS, Baumgardner KR, Meller ST, Gebhart GF. Localization and changes in NADPH-diaphorase reactivity and nitric oxide synthetase immunoreactivity in rat pulp following tooth preparation. J Dent Res. 1999;78(10):1585–95.
Lee K, Lee BM, Park CK, Kim YH, Chung G. Ion channels involved in tooth pain. Int J Mol Sci. 2019;20(9):2266.
Lee PR, Lee JY, Kim HB, Lee JH, Oh SB. TRPM8 mediates hyperosmotic stimuli-induced nociception in dental afferents. J Dent Res. 2020;99(1):107–14.
Lilja J, Nordenvall KJ, Branstrom M. Dentin sensitivity, odontoblasts and nerves under desiccated or infected experimental cavities. A clinical, light microscopic and ultrastructural investigation. Swed Dent J. 1982;6(3):93–103.
Lin Y, Ren J, McGrath C. Mechanosensitive Piezo1 and Piezo2 ion channels in craniofacial development and dentistry: recent advances and prospects. Front Physiol. 2022;13:1039714.
Love RM. The effect of tissue molecules on bacterial invasion of dentine. Oral Microbiol Immunol. 2002;17(1):32–7.

Love RM, McMillan MD, Park Y, Jenkinson HF. Coinvasion of dentinal tubules by Porphyromonas gingivalis and Streptococcus gordonii depends upon binding specificity of streptococcal antigen I/II adhesin. Infect Immun. 2000;68(3):1359–65.

Loyd DR, Henry MA, Hargreaves KM. Serotonergic neuromodulation of peripheral nociceptors. Semin Cell Dev Biol. 2013;24(1):51–7.

Lundy T, Stanley HR. Correlation of pulpal histopathology and clinical symptoms in human teeth subjected to experimental irritation. Oral Surg Oral Med Oral Pathol. 1969;27(2):187–201.

Luo S, Perry GM, Levinson SR, Henry MA. Pulpitis increases the proportion of atypical nodes of Ranvier in human dental pulp axons without a change in Nav1.6 sodium channel expression. Neuroscience. 2010;169(4):1881–7.

Magloire H, Maurin JC, Couble ML, Shibukawa Y, Tsumura M, Thivichon-Prince B, Bleicher F. Topical review. Dental pain and odontoblasts: facts and hypotheses. J Orofac Pain. 2010;24(4):335–49.

Markowitz K. The original desensitizers: Strontium and potassium salts. J Clin Dent. 2009;20:145–51.

Markowitz K. Pretty painful: why does tooth bleaching hurt? Med Hypotheses. 2010;74(5):835–40.

Markowitz K. A new treatment alternative for sensitive teeth: A desensitizing oral rinse. J Dent. 2013;41(Suppl 1):S1–S11.

Markowitz K, Pashley DH. Discovering new treatments for sensitive teeth: the long path from biology to therapy. J Oral Rehabil. 2008;35(4):300–15.

Matsunaga M, Kimura M, Ouchi T, Nakamura T, Ohyama S, Ando M, Nomura S, Azuma T, Ichinohe T, Shibukawa Y. Mechanical stimulation-induced calcium signaling by Piezo1 channel activation in human odontoblast reduces dentin mineralization. Front Physiol. 2021;212:704518.

Matthews B, Vongsavan N. Interactions between neural and hydrodynamic mechanisms in dentine and pulp. Arch Oral Biol. 1994;39(Suppl):87S–95S.

Matthews WG, Showman CD, Pashley DH. Air blast-induced evaporative water loss from human dentine, *in vitro*. Arch Oral Biol. 1993;38:517–0523.

McGrath PA, Gracely RH, Dubner R, Heft MW. Non-pain and pain sensations evoked by tooth pulp stimulation. Pain. 1983;15(4):377–88.

McKemy DD. How cold is it? TRPM8 and TRPA1 in the molecular logic of cold sensation. Mol Pain. 2005;1(1):16.

Meier ML, Brugger M, Ettlin DA, Luechinger R, Barlow A, Jancke L, Lutz K. Brain activation induced by dentine hypersensitivity pain—an fMRI study. J Clin Periodontol. 2012;39(5):441–7.

Merchant VA, Livingston MJ, Pashley DH. Dentin permeation: comparison of diffusion with filtration. J Dent Res. 1977;56(10):1161–4.

Michelich V, Pashley DH, Whitford GM. Dentin permeability: a comparison of functional versus anatomical tubular radii. J Dent Res. 1978;57(11–12):1019–24.

Michelich VJ, Schuster GS, Pashley DH. Bacterial penetration of human dentin in vitro. J Dent Res. 1980;59(8):1398–403.

Mjör IA. Pulp-dentin biology in restorative dentistry. Part 5: clinical management and tissue changes associated with wear and trauma. Quintessence Int. 2001;32(10):771–88.

Mjör IA, Nordahl I. The density and branching of dentinal tubules in human teeth. Arch Oral Biol. 1996;41(5):401–12.

Närhi MV. The characteristics of intradental sensory units and their responses to stimulation. J Dent Res. 1985;64 Spec No:564–71.

Närhi MV, Hirvonen TJ, Hakumäki MO. Responses of intradental nerve fibres to stimulation of dentine and pulp. Acta Physiol Scand. 1982a;115(2):173–8.

Närhi M, Jyväsjärvi E, Hirvonen T, Huopaniemi T. Activation of heat-sensitive nerve fibres in the dental pulp of the cat. Pain. 1982b;14(4):317–26.

Närhi M, Virtanen A, Hirvonen T, Huopaniemi T. Comparison of electrical thresholds of intradental nerves and jaw-opening reflex in the cat. Acta Physiol Scand. 1983;119(4):399–403.

Närhi M, Hirvonen T, Huopaniemi T. The function of intradental nerves in relation to the sensations induced by dental stimulation. Acupunct Electrother Res. 1984;9(2):107–13.

Närhi M, Jyväsjärvi E, Virtanen A, Huopaniemi T, Ngassapa D, Hirvonen T. Role of intradental A- and C-type nerve fibres in dental pain mechanisms. Proc Finn Dent Soc. 1992a;88(Suppl 1):507–16.

Närhi M, Kontturi-Närhi V, Hirvonen T, Ngassapa D. Neurophysiological mechanisms of dentin hypersensitivity. Proc Finn Dent Soc. 1992b;88(Suppl 1):15–22.

Ngassapa D, Närhi M, Hirvonen T. Effect of serotonin (5-HT) and calcitonin gene-related peptide (CGRP) on the function of intradental nerves in the dog. Proc Finn Dent Soc. 1992;88(Suppl 1):143–8.

Nishiyama A, Sato M, Kimura M, Katakura A, Tazaki M, Shibukawa Y. Intercellular signal communication among odontoblasts and trigeminal ganglion neurons via glutamate. Cell Calcium. 2016;60(5):341–55.

Nissan R, Segal H, Pashley D, Stevens R, Trowbridge H. Ability of bacterial endotoxin to diffuse through human dentin. J Endod. 1995;21(2):62–4.

Nweeia MT, Eichmiller FC, Hauschka PV, Donahue GA, Orr JR, Ferguson SH, Watt CA, Mead JG, Potter CW, Dietz R, Giuseppetti AA, Black SR, Trachtenberg AJ, Kuo WP. Sensory ability in the narwhal tooth organ system. Anat Rec (Hoboken). 2014;297(4):599–617.

Ohyama S, Ouchi T, Kimura M, Kurashima R, Yasumatsu K, Nishida D, Hitomi S, Ubaidus S, Kuroda H, Ito S, Takano M, Ono K, Mizoguchi T, Katakura A, Shibukawa Y. Piezo1-pannexin-1-P2X3 axis in odontoblasts and neurons mediates sensory transduction in dentinal sensitivity. Front Physiol. 2022;13:891759.

Okiji T, Morita I, Suda H, Murota S. Pathophysiological roles of arachidonic acid metabolites in rat dental pulp. Proc Finn Dent Soc. 1992;88(Suppl 1):433–8.

Olgart L. Neural control of pulpal blood flow. Crit Rev Oral Biol Med. 1996;7(2):159–71.

Olgart L, Gazelius B, Sundstrom F. Intradental nerve activity and jaw-opening reflex in response to mechanical deformation of cat teeth. Acta Physiol Scand. 1988;133(3):399–406.

Olgart L, Edwall L, Gazelius B. Involvement of afferent nerves in pulpal blood-flow reactions in response to clinical and experimental procedures in the cat. Arch Oral Biol. 1991;36(8):575–81.

Orchardson R, Gillam DG. Managing dentin hypersensitivity. J Am Dent Assoc. 2006;137(7):990–998; quiz 1028-1029.

Pan M, Naftel JP, Wheeler EF. Effects of deprivation of neonatal nerve growth factor on the expression of neurotrophin receptors and brain-derived neurotrophic factor by dental pulp afferents of the adult rat. Arch Oral Biol. 2000;45(5):387–99.

Pan Y, Wheeler EF, Bernanke JM, Yang H, Naftel JP. A model experimental system for monitoring changes in sensory neuron phenotype evoked by tooth injury. J Neurosci Methods. 2003;126(1):99–109.

Panopoulos P. Factors influencing the occurrence of pain in carious teeth. Proc Finn Dent Soc. 1992;88(Suppl 1):155–60.

Parirokh M, Abbott PV. Present status and future directions-mechanisms and management of local anaesthetic failures. Int Endod J. 2022;55(Suppl 4):951–94. https://doi.org/10.1111/iej.13697. Epub 2022 Feb 23. PMID: 35119117

Park SJ, Chiang CY, Hu JW, Sessle BJ. Neuroplasticity induced by tooth pulp stimulation in trigeminal subnucleus oralis involves NMDA receptor mechanisms. J Neurophysiol. 2001;85(5):1836–46.

Park CK, Kim MS, Fang Z, Li HY, Jung SJ, Choi SY, Lee SJ, Park K, Kim JS, Oh SB. Functional expression of thermo-transient receptor potential channels in dental primary afferent neurons: implication for tooth pain. J Biol Chem. 2006;281(25):17304–11.

Pashley DH. Smear layer: physiological considerations. Oper Dent Suppl. 1984;3:13–29.

Pashley DH. Dentin permeability, dentin sensitivity, and treatment through tubule occlusion. J Endod. 1986;12(10):465–74.

Pashley DH. Mechanistic analysis of fluid distribution across the pulpodentin complex. J Endod. 1992a;18(2):72–5.

Pashley DH. Smear layer: overview of structure and function. Proc Finn Dent Soc. 1992b;88(Suppl 1):215–24.

Pashley DH. How can sensitive dentine become hypersensitive and can it be reversed? J Dent. 2013;41(Suppl 4):S49–55.

Pashley DH, Matthews WG. The effects of outward forced convective flow on inward diffusion in human dentine in vitro. Arch Oral Biol. 1993;38(7):577–82.

Pashley DH, Whitford GM. Permeability of human dentine in vitro interpreted from reflection coefficients. Arch Oral Biol. 1980;25(2):141–4.

Pashley DH, Livingston MJ, Greenhill JD. Regional resistances to fluid flow in human dentine in vitro. Arch Oral Biol. 1978;23(9):807–10.

Pashley DH, Livingston MJ, Whitford GM. The effect of molecular size on reflection coefficients in human dentine. Arch Oral Biol. 1979;24(6):455–60.

Pashley DH, Michelich V, Kehl T. Dentin permeability: effects of smear layer removal. J Prosthet Dent. 1981;46(5):531–7.

Pashley DH, Galloway SE, Stewart F. Effects of fibrinogen in vivo on dentine permeability in the dog. Arch Oral Biol. 1984;29(9):725–8.

Pashley DH, Andringa HJ, Derkson GD, Derkson ME, Kalathoor SR. Regional variability in the permeability of human dentine. Arch Oral Biol. 1987;32(7):519–23.

Pashley DH, Matthews WG, Zhang Y, Johnson M. Fluid shifts across human dentine in vitro in response to hydrodynamic stimuli. Arch Oral Biol. 1996;41(11):1065–72.

Pashley DH, Agee K, Zhang Y, Smith A, Tavss EA, Gambogi RJ. The effects of outward forced convective flow on inward diffusion of potassium across human dentin. Am J Dent. 2002;15(4):256–61.

Pertl C, Liu MT, Markowitz K, Kim S. Effects of capsaicin on KCl-induced blood flow and sensory nerve activity changes in the tooth pulp. Pain. 1993;52(3):351–8.

Pocket Dentistry. The physiological basis of dentin hypersensitivity. https://pocketdentistry.com. Accessed 7 July 2024.

Quan N, Avitsur R, Stark JL, He L, Shah M, Caligiuri M, Padgett DA, Marucha PT, Sheridan JF. Social stress increases the susceptibility to endotoxic shock. J Neuroimmunol. 2001;115(1–2):36–45.

Reeder OW Jr, Walton RE, Livingston MJ, Pashley DH. Dentin permeability: determinants of hydraulic conductance. J Dent Res. 1978;57(2):187–93.

Renton T, Yiangou Y, Plumpton C, Tate S, Bountra C, Anand P. Sodium channel Nav1.8 immunoreactivity in painful human dental pulp. BMC Oral Health. 2005;5(1):5.

Rodd HD, Boissonade FM. Innervation of human tooth pulp in relation to caries and dentition type. J Dent Res. 2001;80(1):389–93.

Sato M, Ogura K, Kimura M, Nishi K, Ando M, Tazaki M, Shibukawa Y. Activation of mechanosensitive transient receptor potential/piezo channels in odontoblasts generates action potentials in Cocultured Isolectin B_4-negative medium-sized trigeminal ganglion neurons. J Endod. 2018;44(6):984–991.e2. https://doi.org/10.1016/j.joen.2018.02.020. Epub 2018 Apr 27. PMID: 29709295

Sessle BJ. Acute and chronic craniofacial pain: brainstem mechanisms of nociceptive transmission and neuroplasticity, and their clinical correlates. Crit Rev Oral Biol Med. 2000;11(1):57–91.

Sessle BJ, Greenwood LF. Inputs to trigeminal brain stem neurons from facial, oral, tooth pulp and pharyngolaryngeal tissues: I. Responses to innocuous and noxious stimuli. Brain Res. 1976;117(2):211–26.

Shibukawa Y, Sato M, Kimura M, Sobhan U, Shimada M, Nishiyama A, Kawaguchi A, Soya M, Kuroda

H, Katakura A, Ichinohe T, Tazaki M. Odontoblasts as sensory receptors: transient receptor potential channels, pannexin-1, and ionotropic ATP receptors mediate intercellular odontoblast-neuron signal transduction. Pflugers Arch. 2015;467(4):843–63. https://doi.org/10.1007/s00424-014-1551-x.

Sixou JL. How to make a link between oral health-related quality of life and dentin hypersensitivity in the dental office? Clin Oral Investig. 2013;17(Suppl 1):S41–4.

Smith AJ, Scheven BA, Takahashi Y, Ferracane JL, Shelton RM, Cooper PR. Dentine as a bioactive extracellular matrix. Arch Oral Biol. 2012;57(2):109–21.

Sommer C. Serotonin in pain and analgesia: actions in the periphery. Mol Neurobiol. 2004;30(2):117–25.

Suge T, Kawasaki A, Ishikawa K, Matsuo T, Ebisu S. Effects of plaque control on the patency of dentinal tubules: an in vivo study in beagle dogs. J Periodontol. 2006;77(3):454–9.

Sun XF, Qiao WW, Meng LY, Bian Z. PIEZO1 ion channels mediate Mechanotransduction in odontoblasts. J Endod. 2022;48(6):749–58. https://doi.org/10.1016/j.joen.2022.02.005. Epub 2022 Feb 25. PMID: 35219748

Tammaro S, Wennstrom JL, Bergenholtz G. Root-dentin sensitivity following non-surgical periodontal treatment. J Clin Periodontol. 2000;27(9):690–7.

Tay FR, Pashley DH. Biomimetic remineralization of resin-bonded acid-etched dentin. J Dent Res. 2009;88(8):719–24.

Taylor PE, Byers MR, Redd PE. Sprouting of CGRP nerve fibers in response to dentin injury in rat molars. Brain Res. 1988;461(2):371–6.

Tjäderhane L, Nascimento FD, Breschi L, Mazzoni A, Tersariol IL, Geraldeli S, Tezvergil-Mutluay A, Carrilho MR, Carvalho RM, Tay FR, Pashley DH. Optimizing dentin bond durability: control of collagen degradation by matrix metalloproteinases and cysteine cathepsins. Dent Mater. 2013a;29(1):116–35.

Tjäderhane L, Nascimento FD, Breschi L, Mazzoni A, Tersariol IL, Geraldeli S, Tezvergil-Mutluay A, Carrilho M, Carvalho RM, Tay FR, Pashley DH. Strategies to prevent hydrolytic degradation of the hybrid layer-a review. Dent Mater. 2013b;29(10):999–1011. https://doi.org/10.1016/j.dental.2013.07.016. Epub 2013 Aug 14.

Tsumura M, Sobhan U, Sato M, Shimada M, Nishiyama A, Kawaguchi A, Soya M, Kuroda H, Tazaki M, Shibukawa Y. Functional expression of TRPM8 and TRPA1 channels in rat odontoblasts. PLoS One. 2013;8(12):e82233.

Tsunozaki M, Bautista DM. Mammalian somatosensory mechanotransduction. Curr Opin Neurobiol. 2009;19(4):362–9.

Utreras E, Prochazkova M, Terse A, Gross J, Keller J, Iadarola MJ, Kulkarni AB. TGF-beta1 sensitizes TRPV1 through Cdk5 signaling in odontoblast-like cells. Mol Pain. 2013;9:24.

Veerayutthwilai O, Byers MR, Pham TT, Darveau RP, Dale BA. Differential regulation of immune responses by odontoblasts. Oral Microbiol Immunol. 2007;22(1):5–13.

Veis A. Mineral-matrix interactions in bone and dentin. J Bone Miner Res. 1993;8(Suppl 2):S493–7.

Verworn M. Irritability a physiological analysis of the general effect of stimuli in living substance. New Haven: Yale University Mrs. Hepsa Ely Silliman Memorial Lectures Yale University Press; 1913.

Virtanen AS, Huopaniemi T, Närhi MV, Pertovaara A, Wallgren K. The effect of temporal parameters on subjective sensations evoked by electrical tooth stimulation. Pain. 1987;30(3):361–71.

Vongsavan N, Matthews B. Fluid flow through cat dentine in vivo. Arch Oral Biol. 1992;37(3):175–85.

Vongsavan N, Matthews B. The relationship between the discharge of intradental nerves and the rate of fluid flow through dentine in the cat. Arch Oral Biol. 2007;52(7):640–7. https://doi.org/10.1016/j.archoralbio.2006.12.019.

Vongsavan N, Matthews RW, Matthews B. The permeability of human dentine in vitro and in vivo. Arch Oral Biol. 2000;45(11):931–5.

Wadachi R, Hargreaves KM. Trigeminal nociceptors express TLR-4 and CD14: a mechanism for pain due to infection. J Dent Res. 2006;85(1):49–53.

Wallace JA, Bissada NF. Pulpal and root sensitivity rated to periodontal therapy. Oral Surg Oral Med Oral Pathol. 1990;69(6):743–7.

Warfvinge J, Dahlen G, Bergenholtz G. Dental pulp response to bacterial cell wall material. J Dent Res. 1985;64(8):1046–50.

Won J, Vang H, Lee PR, Kim YH, Kim HW, Kang Y, Oh SB. Piezo2 expression in mechanosensitive dental primary afferent neurons. J Dent Res. 2017 Jul;96(8):931–7.

Xu X, Guo Y, Liu P, Zhang H, Wang Y, Li Z, Mei Y, Niu L, Liu R. Piezo mediates the mechanosensation and injury-repair of pulpo-dentinal complex. Int Dent J. 2024;74:71–80.

Yoshiyama M, Masada J, Uchida A, Ishida H. Scanning electron microscopic characterization of sensitive vs. insensitive human radicular dentin. J Dent Res. 1989;68:1498–502.

Yumoto H, Hirao K, Hosokawa Y, Kuramoto H, Takegawa D, Nakanishi T, Matsuo T. The roles of odontoblasts in dental pulp innate immunity. Jpn Dent Sci Rev. 2018;54(3):105–17.

Treatments for Tooth Sensitivity: Nerve Inactivation and Tubule Occlusion—How Do Potassium and Strontium Salts Treat Sensitivity?

6

Kenneth Markowitz and David G. Gillam

6.1 Dedication

We dedicate this chapter to our collaborator, mentor, and friend, Dr. David H. Pashley. During his long career, David has made outstanding contributions to several areas of dental research, including tooth sensitivity and adhesive dentistry. His interests and ability in combining a wide range of biological thinking into dental problem-solving literally changed the way we approach patient care all over the world. His talent for organizing and explaining complex material has had a lasting impact on our writing and teaching. To David, science was incomplete unless it was communicated and acted upon. His influence and citations permeate this book.

When David started his career, biological concepts were an excepted part of many dental disciplines such as periodontics. Restorative dentistry was the last bastion of a mechanical view of dentistry. Along with other investigators, David championed the view that the dentin–pulp complex is a living tissue, which has important properties that must be considered in clinical procedures. The principles learned have had a long and widespread influence on several fields of study and industries. His laboratory in Augusta Georgia always hosted scientists from around the world.

David combined an intense intellect with a warm personal nature. He is always willing to give advice, read a manuscript, and serve the scientific community in many capacities.

K. Markowitz (✉)
Rutgers School of Dental Medicine, Rutgers the State University of New Jersey, Newark, NJ, USA
e-mail: markowkj@sdm.rutgers.edu

D. G. Gillam
Centre for Oral Bioengineering, Institute of Dentistry, Barts and the London School of Medicine and Dentistry, Queen Mary University of London, London, UK
e-mail: d.g.gillam@qmul.ac.uk

6.2 The Challenge of Treating Tooth Sensitivity

Tooth sensitivity is a common dental condition for which there have been many remedies proposed over the years (Emling 1982; Rosenthal 1990; Markowitz 2009). Since the turn of the previous century, the importance of the dentinal tubules in tooth sensitivity has been recognized (Gysi 1900). Many early attempts at treatments for tooth sensitivity either attempted to occlude the dentinal tubules by using harsh chemical treatments to coagulate the poorly understood "protoplasmic" contents of the dentinal tubules or use the anesthetic compounds known at the time such as cocaine derivatives (potent topical and local anesthetics) to inactivate the neuronal elements in the tooth (Rosenthal 1990).

Gysi in 1900 described experiments, performed on human subjects, where attempts at anesthetizing the dentin with cocaine failed

D. G. Gillam (ed.), *Dentine Hypersensitivity*, https://doi.org/10.1007/978-3-031-74321-4_6

unless electric current was used to drive the drug, along with a dye allowing depth of dentin visualization, into the deep areas of dentin. Gysi also recognized that many topical anesthetic preparations induced pain due to their osmotic effect. These observations led Gysi to explain dentin sensitivity by what latter became known as the hydrodynamic hypothesis. Recent studies have confirmed that local anesthetics applied to dentin cavities fail to render the dentin insensitive unless applied in high concentrations and with pressure or iontophoresis to induce inward movement of the anesthetic molecules (Thongkukiatkun et al. 2015). These experiments highlight the difficulties in developing effective tooth sensitivity treatments. Today, progress has been made in understanding the underlying cellular basis and mechanisms of the condition.

In this chapter, we will highlight the historic development of two useful approaches to tooth sensitivity treatment homecare products, namely potassium and strontium salts. Although we will not attempt to review the numerous clinical trials that have been performed since this book's previous edition, we will examine support for various classes of desensitizing treatment by higher levels of evidence. We will also describe biological considerations that should be useful for future work.

6.3 How Can Sensitivity Treatments Work?

In the treatment of most diseases, drugs block or disrupt the events associated with the development or symptoms of the disease being treated. The physiologic process responsible for tooth sensitivity (Chap. 5) involves stimuli activating intradental nerves, resulting in action potential generation. Odontoblasts have been shown to participate in this process. The ability of stimuli to cause fluid shifts in the dentin tubules is an important way of activating both odontoblasts and nerves. Several stimuli such as hot and cold may also activate these cells directly (independently of tubule fluid movements) as well. As stated in works that applied the hydrodynamic hypothesis to tooth sensitivity therapy research (Markowitz and Pashley 2008), materials that reduce dentin permeability or, alternatively, target the activation or conduction of the intradental nerves should reduce tooth sensitivity pain. Advances in the physiological basis of the nerve activation process should provide new and better therapeutic opportunities. Although oversimplified and neglecting many aspects of the pain experience, targeting the initial, peripheral mechanisms of pain generation is something a consumer product can do.

6.4 Desensitization Treatments Targeting Dentin Permeability

The reduction of dentin permeability via tubule occlusion is an important strategy for treating sensitive teeth (Pashley 1986; Cummins 2009). Reducing dentin permeability acts to not only attenuate stimulus-evoked dentin fluid flow but also to prevent the activation of the intradental nerves and odontoblasts by directly acting physical stimuli and by reducing the inward diffusion of irritating chemical agents (Hirvonen et al. 1984; Rifai et al. 2004; Chidchuangchai et al. 2007). This is still true in view of the recent observations clarifying the role of odontoblasts in dentin sensitivity reviewed in Chap. 5.

In vitro studies measuring the impact of treatments on the dentin's permeability and microscopic appearance are used to screen the ability of materials and products to reduce dentin fluid flow (see Chap. 7). Treatments that are effective in vitro and otherwise acceptable are candidates for more focused research activities including clinical trials. Due to the steep relationship between tubule radius and flow (flow $\propto r^4$), it is expected that dentin may be desensitized by treatments that induce partial tubule occlusion, reducing the stimulus-evoked flow to values that fail to activate a sufficient nerve response needed to result in conscious pain sensation. Several clinically tested desensitizing treatments cause high reductions in flow when tested in vitro (Pashley et al. 1978a, b). Other desensitizing agents that have been shown to be effective in clinical trials appear to cause modest (<90%) reductions in dentin permeability when tested in vitro (Patel et al. 2011) (Fig. 6.1). For some of these treatments, repeated applications are required to achieve near total occlusion (Sharma et al. 2013). Stannous fluoride has been introduced into several desensitizing products. This fluoride source gradually produces tubule occlusion and may offer the dentin surface protection from acid erosion (Hines et al. 2019).

In assessing the impact of perspective treatments on dentin permeability, it is important to determine whether the dentin flow evoked by pain-producing stimuli is reduced by the treatments (Markowitz and Pashley 2008). In most experiments where dentin permeability is examined and the effect of potential desensitizing agents is assessed, flow driven by a trans-dentine pressure gradient is measured (Pashley et al. 1978a, b). Air blasts directed to the dentin surface evaporate fluid at the tubule orifice, displacing the tubule fluid in an outward direction. Unlike pressure-driven flow, the movement of evaporated water from the dentin surface is less affected by tubule occlusion (Matthews et al. 1993). Occluding the tubules with a porous material such as the smear layer reduces the effective tubule radius (Fig. 6.1) and reduces pressure-driven convective flow but may have a modest effect on the fluid displacement caused by air blasts. As observed in Fig. 6.2, smear layer formation severely depresses convective flow but has more modest effects on air-blast driven flow. Oxalate compounds (Pashley 1986) occlude dentinal tubules to a greater extent than the smear layer, resulting in near complete blockage of pressure-driven flow and high levels of air-current driven flow reduction. These results indicate that a high level of tubule occlusion may be needed to halt fluid displacements induced by air blasts and other pain-producing stimuli. As a practical matter, it may be easier to make dentin sensitive by increasing dentin permeability than to desensitize dentin by reducing dentin permeability.

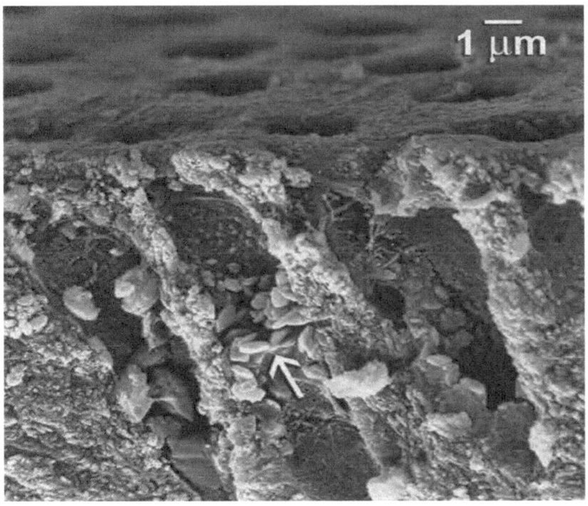

Fig. 6.1 SEM of fracture edge of acid-etched dentin treated with 1.4 wt% potassium oxalate, pH 4.2 experimental desensitizing mouthrinse. Because acid-etching removes all apatite crystallites from the surface of dentin and from peritubular dentin, potassium oxalate cannot react with any calcium ions until it diffuses down into the tubule about 10 μm. There it can etch Ca^{++} from mineralized peritubular dentin, filling the tubule orifice with calcium oxalate crystals of various sizes that block fluid shifts. (From Pashley DH, unpublished micrograph)

The dentin–pulp complex has the capacity for repair (Smith et al. 2012). However, as is evident from clinical observation, individuals with dentin that is exposed to the oral environment do not necessarily experience DH. Several natural mechanisms are known to reduce dentin permeability (Daculsi et al. 1987). In animals with continuously erupting teeth, dentin is exposed, and the tubules mineralize rapidly. Continuously erupting teeth like rat incisors or horse molars wear rapidly. In these teeth, dentin exposure is followed by rapid dentin formation and tubule occlusion (Dimuzio and Veis 1978). In humans, age, chronic exposure to the oral environment, and being subjacent to caries are accompanied by physiological occlusion of dentin tubules (Daculsi et al. 1987; Tagami et al. 1992).

Tertiary and peritubular dentin formation are pulpal processes that reduce dentin permeability and DH (Lundy and Stanley 1969; Senawongse et al. 2008). Growth factors that stimulate tertiary dentin formation are left in the mineralized dentin during development. These growth factors may become exposed and subsequently released by tooth wear, erosion initiated by dietary acids and dentin etching (Smith et al. 2012). These biological and physiochemical processes are

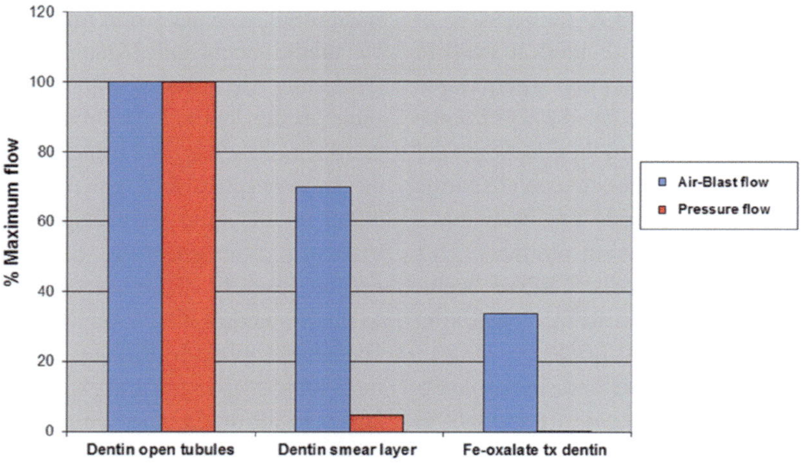

Fig. 6.2 Effects of treatment on fluid flux across dentin disks driven by evaporation of water via air blasts or by pressure-induced fluid flow. On the far left, dentin tubules were opened by acid-etching. In this condition, both pressure and evaporative flow are at their maximal. In the middle section, fluid flux was measured across smear layer-covered dentin. On the far right, acid-etched dentin with open tubules was treated with ferric oxalate to occlude the tubules with calcium oxalate and ferric phosphate crystals. Following the application of ferric oxalate, pressure-driven flow is zero. Creation of porous plugs, for example, smear layers or calcium oxalate crystals has a greater impact on convective flow than flow induced by air blasts. These results indicate that dentin fluid fluxes induced by natural stimuli may be difficult to eliminate unless the tubules are sealed. (Data from Matthews et al. (1993) and Markowitz K, unpublished)

processes by which exposed dentin may become naturally desensitized.

Demineralized dentin matrix retaining acidic proteins has been reported to be capable of remineralization (Clarkson et al. 1991; Bertassoni et al. 2011). This observation has been capitalized on by investigators developing biomimetic analogs of the acidic proteins that would anchor to the appropriate portion of the collagen fibers to facilitate mineral formation in a pattern that replicates the dentin's original structure and restores its physical properties (Tjäderhane et al. 2023). This approach has important applications to the repair of dentin damaged by caries and dietary acid exposure.

Mineralization of the dentin surface can also be achieved by applying materials that adhere to the dentin and interact with saliva to precipitate mineral that can serve as a protective barrier (Markowitz and Pashley 2008; Cummins 2009, see also Orchardson and Gillam 2006). Bioactive glass is an example of a mineralization-promoting material that has been incorporated into dental products (Wang et al. 2010; Wang et al. 2011; Lynch et al. 2012). The formation of a mineral-rich surface layer that extends into the dentin tubules should, in addition to providing desensitization, also improve the resistance of the dentin to acid erosion and mechanical wear (Wang et al. 2010; Seong et al. 2013). Several agents that promote the reduction of DH by facilitating the formation of surface mineral also act to prevent or arrest the development of caries (Reynolds 2008; Cummins 2013) (see Chaps. 7, 9, and 10).

Dentin exposure triggers protective host responses that may subsequently reduce dentin permeability. When the dentin in live animals is left exposed, the permeability is reduced in a matter of hours. In contrast, dentin permeability remained high in animals treated with a type of snake venom that caused the depletion of fibrinogen, a soluble blood-clotting factor that is converted into fibrin, a principal insoluble component of blood clots. That experiment demonstrated that a process related to blood coagulation takes place in the dentin fluid and leads to a reduction in dentin permeability (Pashley et al. 1984). Antibodies reaching the dentin fluid from the pulp have also been demonstrated to reduce dentin permeability in vitro (Hahn and Overton

1997). Large macromolecules like those produced in the pulp during defensive reactions move in a peripheral direction through the dentin tubules, transported by outward dentin fluid flow. In the narrower peripheral portion of the tubules, these molecules bind to the tubule walls, reducing dentin permeability. This mechanism protects the pulp from the ingress of bacterial products and would be expected to lead to a decline in DH with time.

6.5 Strontium Salts

Strontium (Sr) salts are delivered as active agents in dentifrices to treat sensitive teeth (Hughes et al. 2010; Olley et al. 2012; Seong et al. 2013; West et al. 2013). Application of strontium-containing dentifrices to dentin in vitro caused partial tubule occlusion, and as discussed below, shares with other divalent cation solutions some ability to reduce intradental nerve excitability. Strontium shares many biological features of calcium including its ability to be incorporated into bone and some capacity to suppress caries development. This "heritage" prompted the formulation of 10% $SrCl_2$ as an active agent in toothpastes for sensitive teeth in the early 1960s (Markowitz 2009). In contrast to $SrCl_2$, strontium acetate has greater compatibility with fluoride sources in dentifrices. In addition to problems with fluoride compatibility, $SrCl_2$ proved to be a demanding active to formulate owing to the tendency of Sr^{++} to bind many of the common anionic detergents and abrasive particles used in dentifrices (Markowitz 2009). The incorporation of 10% $SrCl_2$ into dentifrices also imparts a strong "medicinal" flavor to the dentifrice that can be a benefit as it signals an expectation of effectiveness in the minds of consumers.

Using an in situ methodology where subjects wore acrylic intraoral devices with dentin chips exposed on the buccal surface, brushing with an 8% strontium acetate toothpaste resulted in progressive build-up of tubule occlusion over time (Claydon et al. 2009). Exposure of intact and demineralized dentin surfaces with strontium acetate solutions and gels results in tubule occlusion and some improvement in the mechanical properties of the surface (Saeki et al. 2016). Although some effects such as the ability to localize Sr on the surface and within the tubules were reduced by water washing, these results support the concept that strontium-containing dentifrices act by reducing dentin permeability. Applications of Sr-containing biomaterials and glasses materials including novel polymer complexes (Xu et al. 2024) demonstrate that future applications of strontium to tooth sensitivity are likely.

6.6 Desensitization Treatments Targeting the Intradental Nerves

In sensitive teeth, stimuli either activate or reach the intradental nerves by way of the dentin tubules. These tubules can also act as a route of administration for therapeutic agents intended to treat sensitive teeth. Drugs delivered topically to the tooth surface may potentially diffuse through dentin to reach the intradental nerves and other targets located in the deep dentin and pulp (Ciarlone and Pashley 1992). Potassium nitrate (KNO_3) was introduced into clinical use as a desensitizing agent based on empirical observations (Hodosh 1974). Several clinical studies indicate that KNO_3 and other potassium salts reduce sensitivity symptoms over a period of approximately 2 weeks when applied by twice daily brushing (Orchardson and Gillam 2000) (see Chap. 8). Potassium salts have also been used to treat pain caused by tooth whitening procedures (Lima et al. 2024). These salts have little effect on dentin permeability when tested in vitro (Greenhill and Pashley 1981), suggesting that they alleviate DH symptoms by interfering with the activation of the intradental nerves.

When potassium salt solutions are applied to deep dentin cavities or placed on isolated nerves in concentrations far exceeding their physiological level, they have a profound action on nerve excitability (Orchardson 1978; Markowitz et al. 1991; Peacock and Orchardson 1999). When first applied to deep dentin cavities, or when applied to shallow cavities under positive pressure to drive the solution through the dentin, potassium salts briefly excite the intradental nerves (Markowitz et al. 1991; Wanachantararak et al. 2011). With elevated potassium ion concentration, the intradental nerves become more sensitive to inward flow than they are when exposed to the normal ionic environment (Wanachantararak et al. 2011). Following the initial excitation induced by solutions containing high potassium ion concentrations, the intradental nerves stop firing and their responses to a variety of stimuli are depressed (Markowitz and Kim 1992). In animals, the normally vigorous nerve response evoked by outward dentin flow during the application of negative pressure is inhibited by the positive pressure application of high potassium ion-containing solutions (Wanachantararak et al. 2011). Since KNO_3 was the first potassium salt investigated clinically, other potassium and nitrate compounds were tested in the animal model. These tests were conducted to determine whether the potassium or nitrate ions were the effective entity in KNO_3. $NaNO_3$ and $LiNO_3$ were found to lack the depressant effect of KNO_3 on intradental nerve activity. In contrast, other potassium salts, such as K chloride, K citrate, and K bicarbonate all share the ability to suppress intradental nerve excitation in a concentration-dependent fashion (Markowitz and Kim 1992). These experiments demonstrate that potassium ions have a desensitizing action, and today, a variety of potassium salts are commercially available in desensitizing products.

When solutions containing high potassium ion concentration are applied using positive pressure to test cavities in human teeth, pain is initially evoked (Ajcharanukul et al. 2007). This pain response corresponded to the nerve excitation observed in the animal experiments. When the dentin floor of these test cavities was probed or air blasted after pressure application of a potassium solution, the pain responses were reduced compared to those measured prior to potassium solution application. Solutions containing elevated sodium ion concentration did not share this desensitizing effect. In contrast, when these potassium ion-containing solutions were applied to human dentin cavities without positive pressure, there was no pain. Furthermore, the pain inhibiting action of potassium salts was modest and of short duration when these solutions were applied to human dentin cavities under atmospheric pressure (Noparatkailas et al. 2009). These results indicate that without the assistance of inward pressure, the penetration of potassium ions to the intradental nerve endings by diffusion is limited.

These experiments imply that although potassium salts can inhibit pain induced by clinically relevant stimuli, this effect may be limited when these agents are applied to the dentin surface of sensitive teeth in clinical use. In a published clinical study designed to test an arginine-calcium carbonate-based toothpaste, a commercially available potassium salt-containing dentifrice was used as a positive control. The potassium salt-based product performed better than the fluoride toothpaste negative control but had an efficacy that was inferior to the arginine compound-containing product (Docimo et al. 2009). Although this and many other clinical studies support the use of potassium salts as a desensitizing agent (Orchardson and Gillam 2000), evidence demonstrating potassium salt's efficacy is considered weak by several authors (Poulsen et al. 2006; Karim and Gillam 2013) (Table 6.1, see also Chap. 8).

Dentin's outward fluid flow acts to oppose and reduce the inward diffusion of solutes such as potassium ions through dentin (Stead et al. 1996; Vongsavan et al. 2000). This aspect of dentin physiology accounts for the difficulty clinicians encounter when attempting to anesthetize teeth by placing local anesthetic solutions on exposed dentin (Rirattanapong et al. 2013). When applied to the dentin surface of sensitive teeth, little of the 500 mmol/l potassium ion concentration found in potassium salt-containing dentifrices diffuses into the innervated inner dentin. The concept that limited transdentinal diffusion hinders the clinical effectiveness of potassium salts as desensitizing agents was based in part on a computer model of potassium diffusion through dentin that considers anatomic and physiological parameters (Stead et al. 1996; Padwal et al. 2022).

Table 6.1 Selected reviews on the effectiveness of strontium- and potassium-based products. Third column quotes the authors conclusion based on the evidence in the paper

Authors	Study type	Author's conclusions
Orchardson and Gillam (2000)	Review	"Although there is evidence that toothpastes containing K^+ are more effective than minus-active preparations in reducing DH, the K-containing preparations are not always superior to controls such as Na MFP. It is postulated that potassium ions released from toothpastes diffuse along the dentinal tubules to inactivate intradental nerves. However, this principle has never been confirmed in intact human teeth. The mechanism of the desensitizing effects of potassium-containing toothpastes remains uncertain at present"
Poulsen et al. (2006)	Cochrane report	"The evidence generated by this review is based on a small number of individuals. Furthermore, the effect varies with the methods applied for assessing the sensitivity. Thus, no clear evidence is available for the support of potassium-containing toothpastes for DH"
Karim and Gillam (2013)	Review	"The results from the present paper would appear to support the conclusions of previous investigators that there is only minimal evidence for the efficacy of both strontium- and potassium-based toothpastes in relieving symptoms of DH"
Bae et al. (2015)	Systematic review and meta-analysis	"The study reports that there is sufficient evidence to support the use of potassium, stannous fluoride, potassium and stannous fluoride, calcium sodium phosphosilicate (CSP), and arginine-containing desensitizing toothpastes for dentin hypersensitivity, but not the use of strontium-containing desensitizing toothpaste"
Hu et al. (2018)	Systematic review and meta-analysis	"Result supports the premise that toothpastes containing potassium, stannous fluoride, potassium and strontium, potassium and stannous fluoride, calcium sodium phosphosilicate (CSP), arginine, and nano-hydroxyapatite relieve the symptoms of DH but does not advise the use of toothpastes that contain strontium and amorphous calcium phosphate. Furthermore, high-quality studies are needed to confirm our results"
Martins et al. (2020)	Network meta-analysis	"CSP was most beneficial for all three stimuli with high to moderate certainty. SnF_2 alone and potassium combined with SnF_2 or hydroxyapatite were beneficial for tactile and air stimulus with high to moderate certainty. Arginine was beneficial for air stimulus, and strontium and potassium were beneficial for tactile stimulus, with moderate certainty"

(continued)

The short-term (measured in minutes) actions of potassium salts on the excitability of the intradental nerves that are observed when these agents are placed in dentin cavities can be explained by the role that extracellular potassium ion concentration has in determining the nerve cell's resting membrane potential (Markowitz and Kim 1992; Markowitz and Pashley 2008). Increasing extracellular potassium ion concentration depolarizes the cell; if the depolarized membrane potential exceeds the action potential threshold, the nerve will fire action potentials (Hodgkin and Huxley 1952; Hodgkin and Horowicz 1959). This excitation is recorded in physiological experiments and resulted in pain when potassium solutions are applied to human dentin under pressure (Markowitz et al. 1991; Ajcharanukul et al. 2007; Wanachantararak et al. 2011).

If high potassium ion concentrations remain, the nerve's action potential threshold adjusts to the depolarization. The maintained depolarization caused the cell's action potential channels to become inactivated and closed (Hodgkin and Huxley 1952). When this occurs, excitation ceases and the nerve cell becomes silent and unresponsive to other stimuli, as was observed in the human and animal experiments described above. In experiments where isolated nerve fibers were exposed to potassium ion-containing solutions, raising the extracellular K^+ to 10 mmol/l resulted in inhibition of nerve responses (Orchardson 1978; Peacock and Orchardson 1999). These effects are dependent on the extracellular potassium ion concentration and reverse rapidly when the ionic gradients return to physiological levels. It is not clear if these physiological actions of potassium salts on nerve excitability contribute to the clinical effectiveness of potassium salts as desensitizing agents (Markowitz and Pashley 2008; Wanachantararak et al. 2011).

6.7 Possible Links Between Potassium and Tubule Occlusion: Other Ions

In experiments that measured the diffusion of potassium ions or other solutes under conditions where there was an opposing transdentinal pressure gradient generating flow, partial tubule occlusion enhanced diffusion of solutes across dentin (Pashley and Matthews 1993; Pashley et al. 2002). Although both convective flow and diffusion are reduced by partial tubule occlusion, occlusion has a greater impact on flow, since flow is $\propto r^4$ (Eq. 5.2 in Chap. 5) as opposed to diffusion which is $\propto r^2$. Hence partial tubule occlusion in dentin with outward flow greatly reduces the opposing action of flow and has a modest blocking effect on diffusion. The net effect being an enhancement of diffusion.

Partial tubule occlusion has been examined as a potential method of enhancing dentifrice-derived potassium ion delivery to the inner dentin (Pashley et al. 2002). There is limited clinical evidence supporting the idea of using partial tubule occlusion as a means of enhancing the effectiveness of potassium-based dentifrices (Schiff et al. 2000; Sowinski et al. 2001). In a pilot clinical trial examining the combination of potassium salts with a polymer that reduces dentin permeability, use of the combination dentifrice exerted slightly greater desensitizing effect; however, this was not statistically significant (Parkinson et al. 2017). Tubule-occluding materials can also release potassium ions. Potassium-releasing bioactive glasses (BAGs) have also been developed and subsequently may offer improved relief for DS in toothpaste formulations (Tiskaya et al. 2021).

The ionic composition of dentin fluid in intact teeth is not known. When the dentinal tubules are exposed and patent, there is an outward flow of dentin fluid that can be observed with sensitive tooth impression techniques (Kerdvongbundit et al. 2004). Since the flowing fluid in exposed sensitive tubules gets replaced by extracellular fluid derived from blood, it is reasoned to be like extracellular fluid elsewhere in the body being high in sodium and low in potassium. The application of oxalate to permeable dentin surfaces causes an immediate drop in dentin permeability when tested in vitro. In contrast, oxalate application to dentin surfaces in human teeth exhibiting sensitivity symptoms reduced pain over a period of approximately half an hour. This was observed using a variety of dentin stimuli including cold, a stimulus that the authors believed would still cause pain after tubule occlusion. The authors hypothesized that occluding the dentin tubules causes a change in the composition of the dentin tubule fluid in addition to reducing stimulus-induced dentin flow (Chinajitphan et al. 2021). Following tubule occlusion, the ionic concentration of the dentin fluid would shift to concentrations found in intact teeth. The odontoblasts are the likely source of the dentin fluid in intact teeth. If the dentin fluid has a potassium concentration exceeding typical extracellular fluid, this may maintain the action potential gates of the intradental nerves in an inactivated configuration-suppressing excitability.

The ionic environment of the dentin may also influence dentin formation. The odontoblasts secrete highly acidic proteins that use phosphate groups to complex calcium and trigger dentin mineralization (Boskey et al. 1990). Using ion imaging, K^+ is observed to be the counter ion secreted along with these highly anionic proteins (Wiesmann et al. 1998). This observation raises the possibility that by transiently raising potassium ion concentrations, potassium ion delivering products restore the healthy ionic environment and facilitate the resolution of sensitivity.

Solutions containing divalent cations, e.g., calcium, magnesium, or strontium, also reduce the excitability of the intradental nerves. Thus, strontium salts can be thought of having a dual desensitizing action on both dentin permeability and nerve excitability. Application of solutions containing these cations blocked the vigorous excitatory response to potassium salt application (Markowitz et al. 1991). Elevated levels of divalent cations in the extracellular environment also reduced neuronal excitability (Markowitz and Kim 1992). In medicine, divalent cation solutions are used to curb neuronal and cardiac hyperexcitability (Karumanchi and Lindheimer 2008).

6.8 Pharmacological Approaches to Tooth Sensitivity Treatment

Pharmacological agents that bind to receptors or have other specific targets are effective at far lower concentrations (have greater potency) and have longer durations of action compared to the effects of potassium ions on intradental nerve activity which is dependent on maintaining high concentrations of potassium in the deep portions of the dentin. For example, the low concentrations of eugenol (0.1 mmol/l) that leach into the dentin fluid from zinc oxide-eugenol fillings have both analgesic and anti-inflammatory effects on the dental pulp (Kozam 1977; Hume 1984; Markowitz et al. 1992). Eugenol has both excitatory and inhibitory actions on nerve cells and interacts with a variety of neuronal receptors (Park et al. 2006; Klein et al. 2014). These studies determining the mechanism of action for eugenol, an old drug, lead us to conclude that more effective targeted treatment of DH and other forms of dental pain is achievable.

One innovative approach is to use the heat/capsaicin receptor (TRPV1) ion channel as a pathway to allow a highly effective but normally impermeant cationic local anesthetic drug to cross cell membranes and block nociceptor activation. This treatment would be accomplished by the simultaneous administration of capsaicin and the cationic local anesthetic. Since many nociceptors (unfortunately not including the neurons responding to dentin stimulation (Närhi et al. 1992a, b)) possess TRPV1 receptors, this approach would selectively target pain without the loss of non-pain sensation (Kim et al. 2010).

Identification of the receptors used by intradental nerves and odontoblast in transducing stimulation into nerve signals can provide targets for future research. As described in Chap. 5, piezo channels are important in mechanical force transduction in both odontoblasts and the intradental nerve endings. There are several drugs that act as antagonists to piezo including gadolinium (Ga^{3+} salts) (Savadipour et al. 2023). In addition, drugs that target the GABA and ATP ion channels associated with release of excitatory transmitters from odontoblasts or agents that block the actions of these transmitters on intradental nerves are attractive targets for pharmacological research (Nishiyama et al. 2016). The drawback for a receptor-targeted pharmacological approach would be safety concerns arising from the drug's unwanted actions on other tissues as well as the likely high cost.

Inflammation and inflammatory mediators sensitize the intradental nerves to pain-evoking dentin stimuli (Ngassapa et al. 1992; Olgart 1996; Byers and Närhi 1999; Ajcharanukul et al. 2011). In acute inflammation triggered by tissue injury, prostaglandins sensitize nociceptors and enhance the actions of other mediators (Goodis et al. 2000). These cell membrane lipid-derived mediators contribute to the alterations in neuronal VGNa channels observed in inflammation (Rush and Waxman 2004).

Inhibition of prostaglandin synthesis counteracts some of the effects that acute injury has on intradental nerve function. Systemic administration of non-steroidal anti-inflammatory drugs (NSAIDs) prevented the activation of the intradental nerves by heat stimulation (Ahlberg 1978). Following tooth injury, systemic administration of NSAIDs reduces pulpal inflammatory mediator production (Chidiac et al. 2009) and prevents central neuroplastic changes that are indicative of enhanced pain perception (Worsley et al. 2008).

Currently, the role of inflammation in DH involving teeth lacking caries or other forms of pathology is not clear. Pulpal blood flow measurements using a laser Doppler flow meter showed that there was no significant blood flow difference between sensitive and non-sensitive teeth and that desensitization with oxalate failed to change the blood flow (Chinajitphan et al. 2021). These results indicate that sensitive teeth do not exhibit vascular manifestations of inflammation. As described above, the pulps of teeth with exposed patent dentin tubules are susceptible to bacterial insults from overlying plaque. The role of systemic and local anti-inflammatory therapy in the treatment of DH is therefore an open area for investigation (Pashley 2013).

6.9 An Ecological Overview

It is evident that the goal of all DH treatments is to return the dentin and pulp to a state of health. Starting with the work of Martin Addy and associates (Addy 1990, 1992), the link between tooth wear and sensitivity became clear (Markowitz and Pashley 2008). Hence in a manner not unlike the etiology of caries, the oral environment is critical to the origin and resolution of tooth sensitivity. Like caries, tooth wear and sensitivity are caused by loss of tooth mineral. Behavioral factors such as oral hygiene practices and diet help determine the oral environmental condition along with the saliva. Control of the etiological factors damaging the dentin and making it sensitive is the first step and an indispensable part of any treatment strategy (Chap. 8).

One way of conceptualizing a desensitizing agent that works with the oral environment would be a material that catalyzes and directs the formation of mineral on the dentin surface (Fig. 6.3). Based on studies of the smear layer, David Pashley recognized the importance of the dentin's capacity to heal as key to both sensitivity treatment and restorative dentistry (Pashley 1984). For example, agents such as the amino acid arginine are metabolized by oral bacteria into alkaline compounds. This favors mineral formation and has been reported as having both anti-caries and desensitizing properties (Cummins and Marsh 2018). As mentioned above, the application of the bioactive glasses such as NovaMin and BioMin F (toothpaste) will react with the Ca, phosphate, and fluoride ions in saliva and deposit a crystalline hydroxyl-carbonate apatite (HCA) or a protective fluorapatite layer, respectively, on the tooth surface. Both products have been shown to be effective in the treatment of DH and the remineralization of lost mineral from enamel (Chaps. 7, 9, and 10). The translation of in vitro results to the clinical arena is complex. Ideally, in vitro testing of agents which encourage mineral formation on the dentin surface would involve incubation of the dentin surface in sterile saliva or by use of an in situ approach. As will be discussed in other chapters in this book, the clinical evaluation of tooth sensitivity treatments is complex and presents unique difficulties in interpreting the outcomes from these studies to the consumer's real-life experience in terms of quality of life (QoL) (Bekes and Hirsch 2013) (see Chaps. 3 and 8).

6.10 Critical Evidence

The evaluation of the evidence for the effectiveness of both strontium- and potassium-based products has been extensively covered over the last 20 years, either in terms of reviews, Cochrane reports, systematic reviews, and meta-analysis. The conclusions from these reviews can be somewhat confusing, for example, an earlier Cochrane report (Poulsen et al. 2006) as well as a previous topical review by Orchardson and Gillam (2000) indicated that there was limited evidence for the effectiveness of potassium-based products, whereas more recent reviews reported more

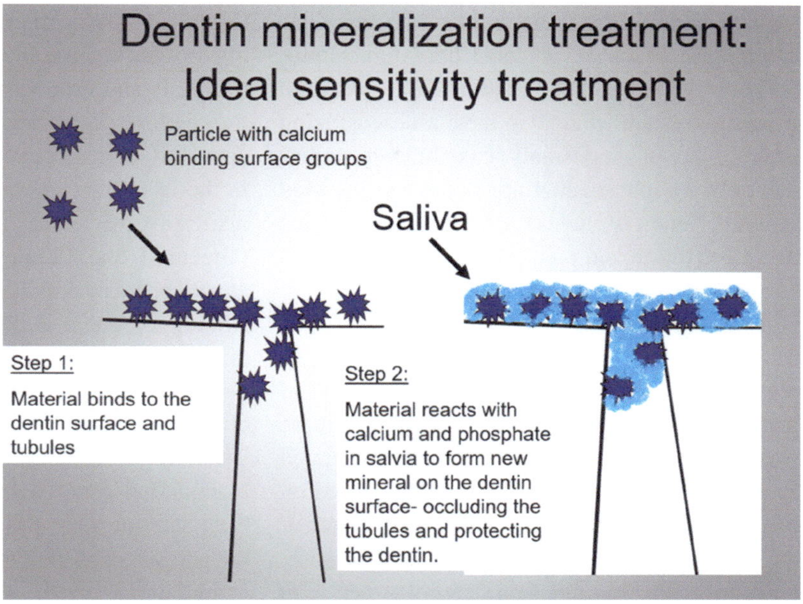

Fig. 6.3 Characteristics of an ideal tooth desensitizer that would work with the oral environment. A particle or polymer having affinity for both the dentin surface and the ability to guide precipitation of mineral from saliva. Treatment with such an agent would make dentin less sensitive and protect the surface from further acid and abrasive damage

favorably on the effectiveness of potassium salts (Bae et al. 2015; Hu et al. 2018; Martins et al. 2020). Similarly, although strontium products have been available in the dental market as a toothpaste in various forms since the early 1950s (Markowitz 2009), the conclusion from the published literature is again somewhat confusing; the earlier historical studies were favorable in terms of effectiveness, but various published reviews have been somewhat negative (Cummins 2011, 2013; Karim and Gillam 2013; Bae et al. 2015; Hu et al. 2018). However, Martins et al. (2020) indicated some relief when using a tactile stimulus (see Table 6.1). According to Karim and Gillam (2013), however, there are problems in analyzing data from the published studies in the literature when evaluating the efficacy of both strontium- and potassium-based toothpastes in that there are variations in the study design, duration, product ingredients, assessment protocols, and inclusion/exclusion criteria which can create difficulties when making direct comparisons between products. For example, both Poulsen et al. (2006) and Karim and Gillam (2013) only included studies that were of a six-week duration and matching ingredients, whereas other views included both short- and long-term studies that were less restricted in including studies in their review (Bae et al. 2015; Hu et al. 2018; Martins et al. 2020).

A further problem when evaluating the effectiveness of desensitizing products is the strong placebo effect reported in clinical studies, although this is in a similar range to that reported in medicine (Karim and Gillam 2013). Most clinical trials of consumer dental products are manufacturer-sponsored. Since many trials were conducted prior to the practice of journals requiring preregistration and disclosure of studies, there is the risk of publication bias in the reporting of clinical trial results.

Evaluating the effectiveness of oxalate-based desensitizing treatments is of particular interest since these constituted a direct clinical application of the hydrodynamic hypothesis when introduced by David Pashley in the 1970s (Pashley 1984, 2013). As initially described by Pashley, high concentration oxalates are used in professionally applied products since oxalate is toxic. In the USA, a topically applied oxalate strip was also available. Oxalates are usually used as monohydrogen monopotassium (acidic), dipotassium (basic), or ferric salts. When applied to dentin, a calcium oxalate precipitate forms on the surface occluding the tubules. Acidic oxalate compounds readily free calcium from the dentin surface forming more precipitate than the basic compounds (Pashley, personal communication). It should be noted that potassium ions delivered by some oxalates may also have a desensitizing action. Animal and small-scale human studies demonstrate that oxalate application to exposed sensitive dentin occludes the tubules and prevents nerve activation and pain evoked by stimuli such as air blasts and probing (Närhi et al. 1992a, b).

Despite the demonstration of oxalate's efficacy, its effectiveness in larger clinical trials remains to be proven. In a systemic review of professionally applied oxalate compounds, there was no benefit for most compounds examined except for 3% monohydrogen monopotassium oxalate. For this compound, although several of the examined studies showed benefit, the summary estimate was not significantly superior to control (Cunha-Cruz et al. 2011).

An oxalate containing mouthwash has been developed and tested in vitro (Fig. 6.1) (Markowitz 2013; Pashley 2013; Eliades et al. 2013) as well as evaluated clinically (Sharma et al. 2013). In a clinical trial, the oxalate mouthwash was observed to reduce sensitivity particularly following 4 weeks of use (Lynch et al. 2018). The oxalate experience, however, highlights the difficulty of translating technologies from the lab into clinical use.

6.11 Direction for Future Clinical and Laboratory Research. Applying Evidence-Based Practice to Tooth Sensitivity Research and Development

One of the problems in research generally is the validation of the results from in vitro, in situ, or animal studies. There is a danger of extrapolating these results into the clinical environment. Invariably what promises to be an exciting new ingredient or product fails to materialize in either the lab or in the clinical environment which not only produces frustration and disappointment to researchers but may also have financial implications in terms of any future development. It is important to acknowledge that most of the historical laboratory studies in DH were in part trying to identify the mechanism of action of the materials and products under test. For example, the action of potassium ions in toothpastes appeared to be successful in clinical practice, but in the laboratory, it was evident that the mechanism involved was not by tubular occlusion (Greenhill and Pashley 1981). Furthermore, it should be recognized that when evaluating desensitizing products currently on the market, the product formulations may not be the same as the original products that were evaluated as being clinically effective. For example, the original strontium chloride did not have fluoride in the formulation (due to interaction between strontium and fluoride within the toothpaste tube) and the abrasive was diatomaceous earth. Subsequent formulations used a silica-based toothpaste (Gillam et al. 1992). The strontium source was also subsequently changed in certain products, to strontium acetate to accommodate fluoride in the toothpaste formulation (Karim and Gillam 2013). Potassium-based toothpastes (and mouthrinses) originally contained the nitrate salt. Later, the product selection was expanded to include chloride and citrate compounds depending on the commercial market. More recently, stannous fluoride (SnF_2) and hydroxyapatite-based products have become popular (Martins et al. 2020).

The problems of assessing and evaluating the efficacy of the various desensitizing toothpaste have been detailed elsewhere (Gillam et al. 2000), but it is evident that the assessment tools and stimuli used to evaluate the effectiveness in clinical studies do not relate to the types of stimuli and daily experiences of the consumer in day-to-day living. Perhaps this is an area for future research. The direction of future laboratory and clinical research has been addressed in Chaps. 7, 9, and 10.

6.12 Conclusion

Desensitizing toothpastes containing potassium, strontium salts, as well as other agents are considered "first-line" therapies for sensitive teeth along with behavioral changes aimed at controlling the etiological factors. Professional interventions as will be described in other chapters in this book can be reserved for cases that fail to respond to homecare agents. Practice-based clinical studies indicate that professionally applied materials that seal the dentin tubules are considerably more effective that potassium salt dentifrices (Veitz-Keenan et al. 2013). Aside from their widespread use and effectiveness, research on agents such as potassium and strontium salts has led to the development of laboratory and clinical research methods that can be applied to other types of treatments. As more is learned concerning the biological basis of dentin sensitivity and new materials become available (Wu et al. 2023), we are hopeful for the future.

References

Addy M. Etiology and clinical implications of dentine hypersensitivity. Dent Clin N Am. 1990;4(3):503–14.

Addy M. Clinical aspects of dentine hypersensitivity. Proc Finn Dent Soc. 1992;88(Suppl 1):23–30.

Ahlberg KF. Dose-dependent inhibition of sensory nerve activity in the feline dental pulp by anti-inflammatory drugs. Acta Physiol Scand. 1978;102(4):434–40.

Ajcharanukul O, Kraivaphan P, Wanachantararak S, Vongsavan N, Matthews B. Effects of potassium ions on dentine sensitivity in man. Arch Oral Biol. 2007;52(7):632–9.

Ajcharanukul O, Chidchuangchai W, Charoenlarp P, Vongsavan N, Matthews B. Sensory transduction in human teeth with inflamed pulps. J Dent Res. 2011;90(5):678–82.

Bae JH, Kim YK, Myung SK. Desensitizing toothpaste versus placebo for dentin hypersensitivity: a systematic review and meta-analysis. J Clin Periodontol. 2015;42:131–41.

Bekes K, Hirsch C. What is known about the influence of dentine hypersensitivity on oral health-related quality of life? Clin Oral Investig. 2013;17(Suppl 1):S45–51.

Bertassoni LE, Habelitz S, Marshall SJ, Marshall GW. Mechanical recovery of dentin following remineralization in vitro—an indentation study. J Biomech. 2011;44(1):176–81.

Boskey AL, Maresca M, Doty S, Sabsay B, Veis A. Concentration-dependent effects of dentin phosphophoryn in the regulation of in vitro hydroxyapatite formation and growth. Bone Miner. 1990;11(1):55–65.

Byers MR, Närhi MV. Dental injury models: experimental tools for understanding neuroinflammatory interactions and polymodal nociceptor functions. Crit Rev Oral Biol Med. 1999;10(1):4–39.

Chidchuangchai W, Vongsavan N, Matthews B. Sensory transduction mechanisms responsible for pain caused by cold stimulation of dentine in man. Arch Oral Biol. 2007;52:154–60.

Chidiac JJ, Al-Asmar B, Rifai K, Jabbur SJ, Saade NE. Inflammatory mediators released following application of irritants on the rat injured incisors. The effect of treatment with anti-inflammatory drugs. Cytokine. 2009;46(2):194–200.

Chinajitphan N, Ajcharanukul O, Kijsamanmith K, Vongsavan N, Matthews B. Time-course of the effect of potassium oxalate in the treatment of hypersensitive dentine in man. Arch Oral Biol. 2021;126:105109.

Ciarlone AE, Pashley DH. Medication of the dental pulp: a review and proposals. Endod Dent Traumatol. 1992;8(1):1–5.

Clarkson BH, Feagin FF, McCurdy SP, Sheetz JH, Speirs R. Effects of phosphoprotein moieties on the remineralization of human root caries. Caries Res. 1991;25(3):166–73.

Claydon NC, Addy M, MacDonald EL, West NX, Maggio B, Barlow A, Parkinson C, Butler A. Development of an in situ methodology for the clinical evaluation of dentine hypersensitivity occlusion ingredients. J Clin Dent. 2009;20:158–66.

Cummins D. Dentin hypersensitivity: from diagnosis to a breakthrough therapy for everyday sensitivity relief. J Clin Dent. 2009;20(1):1–9.

Cummins D. Advances in the clinical management of dentin hypersensitivity: a review of recent evidence for the efficacy of dentifrices in providing instant and lasting relief. J Clin Dent. 2011;22(4):100–7. PMID: 22403985.

Cummins D. The development and validation of a new technology, based upon 1.5% arginine, an insoluble calcium compound and fluoride, for everyday use in the prevention and treatment of dental caries. J Dent. 2013;41 Suppl 2:S1–11.

Cummins D, Marsh PD. Changing the paradigm of daily prevention to achieve whole mouth health in the 21st century. J Clin Dent. 2018;29 Spec No A:A1–9.

Cunha-Cruz J, Stout JR, Heaton LJ, Wataha JC, Northwest PRECEDENT. Dentin hypersensitivity and oxalates: a systematic review. J Dent Res. 2011;90:304–10.

Daculsi G, LeGeros RZ, Jean A, Kerebel B. Possible physico-chemical processes in human dentin caries. J Dent Res. 1987;66(8):1356–9.

Dimuzio MT, Veis A. The biosynthesis of phosphophoryns and dentin collagen in the continuously erupting rat incisor. J Biol Chem. 1978;253(19):6845–52.

Docimo R, Montesani L, Maturo P, Costacurta M, Bartolino M, DeVizio W, Zhang YP, Cummins D, Dibart S, Mateo LR. Comparing the efficacy in reducing dentin hypersensitivity of a new toothpaste containing 8.0% arginine, calcium carbonate, and 1450 ppm fluoride to a commercial sensitive toothpaste containing 2% potassium ion: an eight-week clinical study in Rome, Italy. J Clin Dent. 2009;20(1):17–22.

Eliades G, Mantzourani M, Labella R, Mutti B, Sharma D. Interactions of dentine desensitisers with human dentine: morphology and composition. J Dent. 2013;41(Suppl 4):S28–39. https://doi.org/10.1016/S0300-5712(13)70004-6. PMID: 23929642.

Emling RC. Historical overview of causes and treatment of dental hypersensitivity. Compend Contin Educ Dent. 1982;2:S92–4.

Gillam DG, Newman HN, Davies EH, Bulman JS. Clinical efficacy of a low abrasive dentifrice for the relief of cervical dentinal hypersensitivity. J Clin Periodontol. 1992;19(3):197–201.

Gillam DG, Orchardson R, Närhi MVO, Kontturi-Närhi V. Present and future methods for the evaluation of pain associated with dentine hypersensitivity. In: Addy M, Embery G, Edgar WM, Orchardson R, editors. Tooth wear and sensitivity. London: Martin Dunitz Ltd; 2000. p. 283–97.

Goodis HE, Bowles WR, Hargreaves KM. Prostaglandin E2 enhances bradykinin-evoked iCGRP release in bovine dental pulp. J Dent Res. 2000;79:1604–7.

Greenhill JD, Pashley DH. The effects of desensitizing agents on the hydraulic conductance of human dentin in vitro. J Dent Res. 1981;60(3):686–98.

Gysi A. An attempt to explain the sensitiveness of dentine. Br J Dent Sci. 1900;43:865–8.

Hahn CL, Overton B. The effects of immunoglobulins on the convective permeability of human dentine in vitro. Arch Oral Biol. 1997;42:835–43.

Hines D, Xu S, Stranick M, Lavender S, Pilch S, Zhang YP, Sullivan R, Montesani L, Montesani L, Mateo LR, Williams M. Effect of a stannous fluoride toothpaste on dentinal hypersensitivity: in vitro and clinical evaluation. J Am Dent Assoc. 2019;150(4S):S47–59.

Hirvonen TJ, Närhi MV, Hakumäki MO. The excitability of dog pulp nerves in relation to the condition of dentine surface. J Endod. 1984;10(7):294–8.

Hodgkin AL, Horowicz P. The influence of potassium and chloride ions on the membrane potential of single muscle fibres. J Physiol. 1959;148:127–60.

Hodgkin AL, Huxley AF. The dual effect of membrane potential on sodium conductance in the giant axon of Loligo. J Physiol. 1952;116(4):497–506.

Hodosh M. A superior desensitizer—potassium nitrate. J Am Dent Assoc. 1974;88(4):831–2.

Hu ML, Zheng G, Zhang YD, Yan X, Li XC, Lin H. Effect of desensitizing toothpastes on dentine hypersensitivity: a systematic review and meta-analysis. J Dent. 2018;75:12–21.

Hughes N, Mason S, Jeffery P, Welton H, Tobin M, O'Shea C, Browne M. A comparative clinical study investigating the efficacy of a test dentifrice containing 8% strontium acetate and 1040 ppm sodium fluoride versus a marketed control dentifrice containing 8% arginine, calcium carbonate, and 1450 ppm sodium monofluorophosphate in reducing dentinal hypersensitivity. J Clin Dent. 2010;21(2):49–55.

Hume WR. An analysis of the release and the diffusion through dentin of eugenol from zinc oxide-eugenol mixtures. J Dent Res. 1984;63(6):881–4.

Karim BF, Gillam DG. The efficacy of strontium and potassium toothpastes in treating dentine hypersensitivity: a systematic review. Int J Dent. 2013;2013:573258.

Karumanchi SA, Lindheimer MD. Advances in the understanding of eclampsia. Curr Hypertens Rep. 2008;10:305–12.

Kerdvongbundit V, Thiradilok S, Vongsavan N, Matthews B. The use of the replica technique to record fluid emerging from exposed dentine. Arch Oral Biol. 2004;49:613–9.

Kim HY, Kim K, Li HY, Chung G, Park CK, Kim JS, Jung SJ, Lee MK, Ahn DK, Hwang SJ, Kang Y, Binshtok AM, Bean BP, Woolf CJ, Oh SB. Selectively targeting pain in the trigeminal system. Pain. 2010;150(1):29–40.

Klein AH, Joe CL, Davoodi A, Takechi K, Carstens MI, Carstens E. Eugenol and carvacrol excite first- and second-order trigeminal neurons and enhance their heat-evoked responses. Neuroscience. 2014;271:45–55.

Kozam G. The effect of eugenol on nerve transmission. Oral Surg Oral Med Oral Pathol. 1977;44:799–805.

Lima NLB, Sette-de-Souza PH, Siqueira AHC, Costa SGA, Alves PVM, Silvestre FA, Meneses NE, Santiago SL, Peixoto RF. Preemptive use of ibuprofen and desensitizer decreases immediate tooth sensitivity after in-office bleaching: a triple-blind, randomized, placebo-controlled clinical trial. J Am Dent Assoc. 2024;155:304–11.

Lundy T, Stanley HR. Correlation of pulpal histopathology and clinical symptoms in human teeth subjected to experimental irritation. Oral Surg Oral Med Oral Pathol. 1969;27:187–201.

Lynch E, Brauer DS, Karpukhina N, Gillam DG, Hill RG. Multi-component bioactive glasses of varying fluoride content for treating dentin hypersensitivity. Dent Mater. 2012;28(2):168–78.

Lynch MC, Perfekt R, McGuire JA, Milleman J, Gallob J, Amini P, Milleman K. Potassium oxalate mouthrinse reduces dentinal hypersensitivity: a randomized controlled clinical study. J Am Dent Assoc. 2018;149:608–18.

Markowitz K. The original desensitizers: strontium and potassium salts. J Clin Dent. 2009;20:145–51.

Markowitz K. A new treatment alternative for sensitive teeth: a desensitizing oral rinse. J Dent. 2013;41(Suppl 1):S1–S11.

Markowitz K, Kim S. The role of selected cations in the desensitization of intradental nerves. Proc Finn Dent Soc. 1992;88(Suppl 1):39–54.

Markowitz K, Pashley DH. Discovering new treatments for sensitive teeth: the long path from biology to therapy. J Oral Rehabil. 2008;35(4):300–15.

Markowitz K, Bilotto G, Kim S. Decreasing intradental nerve activity in the cat with potassium and divalent cations. Arch Oral Biol. 1991;36(1):1–7.

Markowitz K, Moynihan M, Liu M, Kim S. Biologic properties of eugenol and zinc oxide-eugenol. A clinically oriented review. Oral Surg Oral Med Oral Pathol. 1992;73(6):729–37.

Martins CC, Firmino RT, Riva JJ, Ge L, Carrasco-Labra A, Brignardello-Petersen R, Colunga-Lozano LE, Granville-Garcia AF, Costa FO, Yepes-Nuñez JJ, Zhang Y, Schünemann HJ. Desensitizing toothpastes for dentin hypersensitivity: a network meta-analysis. J Dent Res. 2020;99:514–22.

Matthews WG, Showman CD, Pashley DH. Air blast-induced evaporative water loss from human dentine, in vitro. Arch Oral Biol. 1993;38:517–23.

Närhi M, Jyväsjärvi E, Virtanen A, Huopaniemi T, Ngassapa D, Hirvonen T. Role of intradental A- and C-type nerve fibres in dental pain mechanisms. Proc Finn Dent Soc. 1992a;88(Suppl 1):507–16.

Närhi M, Kontturi-Närhi V, Hirvonen T, Ngassapa D. Neurophysiological mechanisms of dentin hypersensitivity. Proc Finn Dent Soc. 1992b;88 Suppl 1:15–22.

Ngassapa D, Närhi M, Hirvonen T. Effect of serotonin (5-HT) and calcitonin gene-related peptide (CGRP) on the function of intradental nerves in the dog. Proc Finn Dent Soc. 1992;88(Suppl 1):143–8.

Nishiyama A, Sato M, Kimura M, Katakura A, Tazaki M, Shibukawa Y. Intercellular signal communication among odontoblasts and trigeminal ganglion neurons via glutamate. Cell Calcium. 2016;60:341–55.

Noparatkailas S, Wanachantararak S, Vongsavan N, Matthews B. The effect of applying potassium chloride solutions at atmospheric pressure on the sensitivity of dentine in man. Arch Oral Biol. 2009;54(1):50–4.

Olgart L. Neural control of pulpal blood flow. Crit Rev Oral Biol Med. 1996;7:159–71.

Olley RC, Pilecki P, Hughes N, Jeffery P, Austin RS, Moazzez R, Bartlett D. An in-situ study investigating dentine tubule occlusion of dentifrices following acid challenge. J Dent. 2012;40(7):585–93.

Orchardson R. An electrophysiological investigation of the sensitivity of intradental nerves in the cat to changes in the ionic composition of extracellular fluid. Arch Oral Biol. 1978;23(6):471–5.

Orchardson R, Gillam DG. The efficacy of potassium salts as agents for treating dentin hypersensitivity. J Orofac Pain. 2000;14(1):9–19.

Orchardson R, Gillam DG. Managing dentin hypersensitivity. J Am Dent Assoc. 2006;137(7):990-998; quiz 1028-1029.

Padwal MS, Gillam D, Davis G. Measurement of potassium ion diffusion through dentine using ISE. J Dent Maxillofac Res. 2022;5(2):1–9.

Park CK, Li HY, Yeon KY, Jung SJ, Choi SY, Lee SJ, Lee S, Park K, Kim JS, Oh SB. Eugenol inhibits sodium currents in dental afferent neurons. J Dent Res. 2006;85(10):900–4.

Parkinson C, Constantin P, Goyal C, Hall C. An exploratory clinical trial to evaluate the efficacy of an experimental dentifrice formulation in the relief of dentine hypersensitivity. J Dent. 2017;56:39–44.

Pashley DH. Smear layer: physiological considerations. Oper Dent Suppl. 1984;3:13–29.

Pashley DH. Dentin permeability, dentin sensitivity, and treatment through tubule occlusion. J Endod. 1986;12(10):465–74.

Pashley DH. How can sensitive dentine become hypersensitive, and can it be reversed? J Dent. 2013;41(Suppl 4):S49–55.

Pashley DH, Matthews WG. The effects of outward forced convective flow on inward diffusion in human dentine in vitro. Arch Oral Biol. 1993;38(7):577–82.

Pashley DH, Livingston MJ, Greenhill JD. Regional resistances to fluid flow in human dentine in vitro. Arch Oral Biol. 1978a;23(9):807–10.

Pashley DH, Livingston MJ, Reeder OW, Horner J. Effects of the degree of tubule occlusion on the permeability of human dentine in vitro. Arch Oral Biol. 1978b;23(12):1127–33.

Pashley DH, Galloway SE, Stewart F. Effects of fibrinogen in vivo on dentine permeability in the dog. Arch Oral Biol. 1984;29:725–8.

Pashley DH, Agee K, Zhang Y, Smith A, Tavss EA, Gambogi RJ. The effects of outward forced convective flow on inward diffusion of potassium across human dentin. Am J Dent. 2002;15(4):256–61.

Patel R, Chopra S, Vandeven M, Cummins D. Comparison of the effects on dentin permeability of two commercially available sensitivity relief dentifrices. J Clin Dent. 2011;22(4):108–12.

Peacock JM, Orchardson R. Action potential conduction block of nerves in vitro by potassium citrate, potassium tartrate and potassium oxalate. J Clin Periodontol. 1999;26(1):33–7.

Poulsen S, Errboe M, Hovgaard O, Worthington HW. Potassium nitrate toothpaste for dentine hypersensitivity. Cochrane Database Syst Rev. 2006;3:CD001476.

Reynolds EC. Calcium phosphate-based remineralization systems: scientific evidence? Aust Dent J. 2008;53(3):268–73.

Rifai K, Chidiac JJ, Hawwa N, Baliki M, Jabbur SJ, Saade NE. Occlusion of dentinal tubules and selective block of pulp innervation prevent the nociceptive behaviour induced in rats by intradental application of irritants. Arch Oral Biol. 2004;49(6):457–68.

Rirattanapong P, Vongsavan K, Kraivaphan P, Vongsavan N, Matthews B. Effect of the topical application of 50% lignocaine hydrochloride on the sensitivity of dentine in man. Arch Oral Biol. 2013;58(10):1549–55.

Rosenthal MW. Historic review of the management of tooth hypersensitivity. Dent Clin N Am. 1990;34:403–27.

Rush AM, Waxman SG. PGE2 increases the tetrodotoxin-resistant Nav1.9 sodium current in mouse DRG neurons via G-proteins. Brain Res. 2004;1023:264–71.

Saeki K, Marshall GW, Gansky SA, Parkinson CR, Marshall SJ. Strontium effects on root dentin tubule occlusion and nanomechanical properties. Dent Mater. 2016;32(2):240–51.

Savadipour A, Palmer D, Ely EV, Collins KH, Garcia-Castorena JM, Harissa Z, Kim YS, Oestrich A, Qu

F, Rashidi N, Guilak F. The role of PIEZO ion channels in the musculoskeletal system. Am J Physiol Cell Physiol. 2023;324:C728–40.

Schiff T, Zhang YP, DeVizio W, Stewart B, Chaknis P, Petrone ME, Volpe AR, Proskin HM. A randomized clinical trial of the desensitizing efficacy of three dentifrices. Compend Contin Educ Dent Suppl. 2000;27:4–10. quiz 28

Senawongse P, Otsuki M, Tagami J, Mjör IA. Morphological characterization and permeability of attrited human dentine. Arch Oral Biol. 2008;53:14–9.

Seong J, Macdonald E, Newcombe RG, Davies M, Jones SB, Johnson S, West NX. In situ randomised trial to investigate the occluding properties of two desensitising toothpastes on dentine after subsequent acid challenge. Clin Oral Investig. 2013;17(1):195–203.

Sharma D, McGuire JA, Amini P. Randomized trial of the clinical efficacy of a potassium oxalate-containing mouthrinse in rapid relief of dentin sensitivity. J Clin Dent. 2013;24(2):62–7.

Smith AJ, Scheven BA, Takahashi Y, Ferracane JL, Shelton RM, Cooper PR. Dentine as a bioactive extracellular matrix. Arch Oral Biol. 2012;57:109–21.

Sowinski J, Ayad F, Petrone M, DeVizio W, Volpe A, Ellwood R, Davies R. Comparative investigations of the desensitising efficacy of a new dentifrice. J Clin Periodontol. 2001;28(11):1032–6.

Stead WJ, Orchardson R, Warren PB. A mathematical model of potassium ion diffusion in dentinal tubules. Arch Oral Biol. 1996;41(7):679–87.

Tagami J, Hosoda H, Burrow MF, Nakajima M. Effect of aging and caries on dentin permeability. Proc Finn Dent Soc. 1992;88(Suppl 1):149–54.

Thongkukiatkun W, Vongsavan K, Kraivaphan P, Rirattanapong P, Vongsavan N, Matthews B. Effects of the iontophoresis of lignocaine with epinephrine into exposed dentine on the sensitivity of the dentine in man. Arch Oral Biol. 2015;60:1098–103.

Tiskaya M, Gillam D, Shahid S, Hill R. A potassium based fluorine containing bioactive glass for use as a desensitizing toothpaste. Molecules. 2021;17(26):4327.

Tjäderhane L, Nascimento FD, Breschi L, Mazzoni A, Tersariol IL, Geraldeli S, Tezvergil-Mutluay A, Carrilho MR, Carvalho RM, Tay FR, Pashley DH. Optimizing dentin bond durability: control of collagen degradation by matrix metalloproteinases and cysteine cathepsins. Dent Mater. 2023;29:116–35.

Veitz-Keenan A, Barna JA, Strober B, Matthews AG, Collie D, Vena D, Curro FA, Thompson VP. Treatments for hypersensitive noncarious cervical lesions: a Practitioners Engaged in Applied Research and Learning (PEARL) network randomized clinical effectiveness study. J Am Dent Assoc. 2013;144:495–506.

Vongsavan N, Matthews RW, Matthews B. The permeability of human dentine in vitro and in vivo. Arch Oral Biol. 2000;45:931–5.

Wanachantararak S, Vongsavan N, Matthews B. Electrophysiological observations on the effects of potassium ions on the response of intradental nerves to dentinal tubular flow in the cat. Arch Oral Biol. 2011;56(3):294–305.

Wang Z, Sa Y, Sauro S, Chen H, Xing W, Ma X, Jiang T, Wang Y. Effect of desensitising toothpastes on dentinal tubule occlusion: a dentine permeability measurement and SEM in vitro study. J Dent. 2010;38(5):400–10.

Wang Z, Jiang T, Sauro S, Pashley DH, Toledano M, Osorio R, Liang S, Xing W, Sa Y, Wang Y. The dentine remineralization activity of a desensitizing bioactive glass-containing toothpaste: an in vitro study. Aust Dent J. 2011;56(4):372–81.

West N, Newcombe RG, Hughes N, Mason S, Maggio B, Sufi F, Claydon N. A 3-day randomised clinical study investigating the efficacy of two toothpastes, designed to occlude dentine tubules, for the treatment of dentine hypersensitivity. J Dent. 2013;41(2):187–94.

Wiesmann HP, Plate U, Zierold K, Höhling HJ. Potassium is involved in apatite biomineralization. J Dent Res. 1998;77:1654–7.

Worsley MA, Clayton NM, Bountra C, Boissonade FM. The effects of ibuprofen and the neurokinin-1 receptor antagonist GR205171A on Fos expression in the ferret trigeminal nucleus following tooth pulp stimulation. Eur J Pain. 2008;12(3):385–94.

Wu W, Chi H, Zhang Q, Zheng C, Hu N, Wu Y, Liu J. Self-propelled bioglass janus nanomotors for dentin hypersensitivity treatment. Nanoscale. 2023;15:19681–90.

Xu Y, Pan X, Shen D, Sun Y, Liu W, Lin Y, Fu B, Zhang L. In-depth occlusion of dentine tubules via the application of (poly-L-aspartic acid) strontium and phosphate/fluoride to treat dentine hypersensitivity. Int J Biol Macromol. 2024;254(Pt 3):127780.

7 Treatment Modalities and Procedures

Victor Mosquim, Linda Wang, Giovanna Speranza Zabeu, Luciana Fávaro Francisconi-dos-Rios, David G. Gillam, and Ana Carolina Magalhães

7.1 Brief Overview of the Chapter

There is evidence that patients might not know that dentine hypersensitivity (DH) is a preventable and treatable condition and might not seek professional assistance (Gillam et al. 2013; Exarchou et al. 2019; Mosquim et al. 2023). Therefore, it is essential for the clinician to identify possible aetiological factors for the disease and educate the patients regarding hygiene, dietary, and parafunctional deleterious habits that have been associated with DH development and/or aggravation over time (Canadian Advisory Board on Dentin Hypersensitivity 2003; Gillam et al. 2013) (see also Chaps. 4 and 8).

It is important to highlight that, without a definite diagnosis of DH, the clinician cannot successfully treat the condition. As previously defined, DH is essentially a diagnosis of exclusion, and this will clearly take the clinician some time to record the necessary information during the screening process and subsequent clinical examination (Canadian Advisory Board on Dentin Hypersensitivity 2003). Following these steps is important because a treatment based on the prescription of products and procedures without the removal of the aetiological and causal factors that originated the problem in the first place will likely fail. Once the clinician is confident that the correct diagnosis of DH has been made, then the treatment of the condition can be undertaken (see also Chap. 8).

Nonetheless, the clinician who treats patients suffering from DH is often faced with a variety of products from different companies claiming to be effective against the symptoms of DH. According to Orchardson and Gillam (2006), the treatment of DH has been traditionally based on products or procedures (in-office and over-the-counter (OTC)) that may either block the tubules on the exposed dentine surface or desensitize the nerves in the pulp. However, there is still considerable

V. Mosquim (✉) · L. Wang
Department of Operative Dentistry, Endodontics and Dental Materials, Bauru School of Dentistry, University of São Paulo, Bauru, SP, Brazil
e-mail: victor.mosquim@usp.br

G. S. Zabeu
Department of Operative Dentistry, Endodontics and Dental Materials, Bauru School of Dentistry, University of São Paulo, Bauru, SP, Brazil

School of Dentistry, Centro Universitário Sagrado Coração – UNISAGRADO, Bauru, SP, Brazil

L. F. Francisconi-dos-Rios
Department of Operative Dentistry, School of Dentistry, University of São Paulo, São Paulo, SP, Brazil

D. G. Gillam
Centre for Oral Bioengineering, Institute of Dentistry, Barts and the London School of Medicine and Dentistry, Queen Mary University of London, London, UK
e-mail: d.g.gillam@qmul.ac.uk

A. C. Magalhães
Department of Biological Sciences, Bauru School of Dentistry, University of São Paulo, Bauru, SP, Brazil

D. G. Gillam (ed.), *Dentine Hypersensitivity*, https://doi.org/10.1007/978-3-031-74321-4_7

confusion on the mechanism of action of different products and procedures, whether they can provide long-lasting desensitizing effects, and if an ideal treatment (i.e., gold-standard) exists for this condition (Gillam et al. 2002a; Orchardson and Gillam 2006; Cunha-Cruz et al. 2010; Gillam et al. 2013; Exarchou et al. 2019; Zeola et al. 2020; Mosquim et al. 2024, 2023) (see also Chaps. 5 and 6). Therefore, the aim of this chapter is to review the scientific evidence behind the various approaches recommended for the treatment of DH, including recently introduced products, along with recommendations for the future development of desensitizing strategies.

7.2 Classification of Desensitizing Agents

To be both effective and acceptable to the patient and clinician, an ideal product for DH should have specific criteria, such as fast action, sustained efficacy, easy application, not dangerous to the pulp, not cause pain, and not stain the teeth. To this day, a product that fulfils all these requirements is still not available, but knowing the characteristics of the patient as well as the mode of action of the products might help the clinician in the decision-making process of what desensitizing agent to use.

There have been several previous classifications published in the literature, some relatively simple, others more complex in nature. For instance, there is a simple classification of products into in-office and OTC products (Orchardson and Gillam 2006), but there is also a classification for in-office products, dividing them into those that (1) do not polymerise (varnishes/precipitants/primers containing glutaraldehyde and HEMA), (2) undergo setting or polymerisation reactions (varnishes, conventional glass ionomer cements, or resin-modified glass ionomers/compomers, adhesive resin primers, adhesive resin bonding systems) or whether these agents are used in conjunction with (3) mouthguards, (4) iontophoresis combined with fluoride pastes or solutions, or (5) lasers (Pashley 2000). However, clinicians appear uncertain not only about the most successful way to treat DH but also express a level of dissatisfaction with the various products and techniques available (Cunha-Cruz et al. 2010). For this reason, the classification that gained most popularity is based on the mechanism of action of the desensitizing products (Miglani et al. 2010).

As addressed in Chap. 5, the most accepted theory to justify DH is the hydrodynamic theory, which assumes that the abrupt movement of the fluid within the dentinal tubules can stimulate the nerve cells within the dentinal tubules or in the pulp, which leads to the onset of pain. Based on that, there are basically two mechanisms to prevent this pain from being generated: (1) preventing the nerve cells from being stimulated (neural action) and (2) blocking the flow of fluid by occluding the patent dentinal tubules, which can be either by protein precipitation, mineral deposition onto dentine, or simply by mechanically covering the dentine with a restoration or periodontal tissue (see also Chaps. 5 and 6). It is important to note that an agent can also accommodate both mechanisms (for example, potassium oxalate-containing products). The division of agents and products into this classification is presented in Table 7.1.

7.3 Current Therapies for Dentine Hypersensitivity (DH)

As discussed throughout this chapter, most studies on desensitizing agents focus on the materials that work through tubule occlusion. This occurs because the efficiency of these materials can be somehow estimated in vitro and in situ by measuring the dentine permeability and by analysing the deposits formed onto the dentine surface and the degree of penetration into the dentinal tubule under a microscope (e.g., scanning electron microscope-SEM, confocal laser scanning microscopy-CLSM, etc.), whereas those agents with a nerve desensitization effect may require other study designs to determine their mode of action. There are, however, problems with the application of both in-office and OTC products that work through tubule occlu-

Table 7.1 Classification of dentine desensitizers according to their mechanism of action

Mechanism of action		Desensitizing agents
Nerve desensitization		Potassium salts (chloride, citrate, nitrate, oxalate) Low-power lasers (photobiomodulation)
Tubule occlusion	Protein precipitation	Glutaraldehyde + HEMA[a], silver diamine fluoride (SDF), silver nitrate, zinc chloride, strontium chloride hexahydrate
	Mineral deposition	Aluminium compounds (oxalate, lactate) Amorphous calcium phosphate (ACP) Arginine and calcium carbonate Calcium hydroxide Calcium phosphate Calcium sodium phosphosilicate (CSPS) Ferric oxalate Fluoride salts (amine, stannous, sodium, MFP[a]) Fluoro calcium phosphosilicate (FCSPS) High-power lasers (CO_2[a]; Er,Cr:YSGG[a]; erbium-YAG[a]; GaAlAs[a]; Nd-YAG[a]) Potassium oxalate Silver diamine fluoride (SDF) Strontium chloride Tricalcium phosphate (TCP)
	Covering the dentine surface	Periodontal surgery Bonding agents and other polymeric materials Tooth restoration (with GICs[a], RMGICs[a], or bonding agents + resin composite)

Adapted from Miglani et al. (2010)

[a]*CO_2* Carbon dioxide, *Er,Cr:YSGG* Erbium, chromium:yttrium–scandium–gallium–garnet, *Erbium-YAG* Erbium–yttrium–aluminium–garnet, *GaAlAs* Gallium–aluminium–arsenide, *GIC* Glass ionomer cement, *HEMA* 2-hydroxyethyl methacrylate, *MFP* Sodium monofluorophosphate, *Nd-YAG* Neodymium-doped yttrium–aluminium–garnet, *RMGIC* Resin-modified glass ionomer cement

sion, as the tubular occlusion promoted by mineral deposition is not permanent and can be removed over time, especially following an acid challenge. Nonetheless, the occlusion promoted by the application of a polymeric material appears to be more acid-resistant, but could cause other problems over time, such as staining. Furthermore, compounds such as resin or toothpaste products that precipitate into the dentine tubule may only provide a chemical–physical blockage rather than induce the initiation of new dentine, which could have a much more efficient desensitizing effect.

Therefore, it is evident that the application of desensitizing agents on the dentine is not necessarily a permanent definitive treatment for DH, and it is necessary to not only treat the symptoms of DH but also continuously prevent any symptoms from developing or aggravating DH. The treatment of DH should be conducted by taking into account the extent, location, and severity of the condition, as well as by removing or at least controlling the aetiological or predisposing factors by counselling the patient with regard to dietary intake (e.g., excessive consumption of acidic drinks), toothbrushing techniques, and also by monitoring the patient (Orchardson and Gillam 2006; Gillam et al. 2013; Grover et al. 2022).

Gillam et al. (2013) discussed the importance of not using a single treatment philosophy to treat all patients suffering from DH but recommended different strategies based on the aetiology and predisposing factors detected in the patient. More recently, the Indian Society of Periodontology (ICS) published a useful guide and a flowchart to help the clinicians properly diagnose DH as well as recommendations on how to conduct the active treatment of DH associating in-office and OTC products (Grover et al. 2022). Both documents are clear on stating that more conservative treatments should be conducted before more invasive procedures, and that, without these mentioned actions, the solely application of desensitizing products will most likely fail to treat the painful condition.

7.4 In-Office (Professionally Applied) Versus Over-the-Counter (OTC) Products

After a successful diagnosis of DH and treatment of the aetiological factors associated with its development, patients with moderate to intense pain in a few teeth might benefit from a localized professional in-office application of a desensitizing agent. Due to its higher cost, this approach is normally conducted after several unsuccessful attempts to resolve the patient's pain with OTC products. Nonetheless, one major benefit from in-office procedures is that it might present an immediate desensitizing effect, whereas OTC products might take 2–4 weeks to relief the symptoms of DH (Lynch et al. 2012). There are, however, a vast array of desensitizing products currently available which may make the choice of the most appropriate product both confusing and difficult for the clinician (Cunha-Cruz et al. 2010).

Nonetheless, individuals with mild to moderate local or generalized DH may seek products aiming to resolve the pain arising from DH without going to see a clinician. In the study of Mosquim et al. (2023), 21.2% and 30.1% of the participants reported never and rarely scheduling an appointment with a dentist after experiencing and episode of DH, respectively. According to Mantzourani and Sharma (2013), there are three main reasons that contribute to this behaviour: (1) the need of a fast and urgent relief, (2) the easy availability of OTC products (also known as home-care products) in pharmacies and markets, and (3) their low cost, as this does not include the expenses of professional appointments.

Normally, OTC products are generally based on formulations with the same active ingredients as in-office products, yet the concentration of the active ingredients in OTC products is considerably lower than those used professionally. These OTC products are available most commonly in the form of toothpastes or mouthrinses that are sold without prescription, but their indications of use are limited, so patients should be advised to see a clinician if the symptoms last longer than 2–4 weeks. Also, it is likely that the clinician recommends the patient to associate an OTC product with an in-office procedure when the pain from DH is generalized and/or mild to moderate in severity (Miglani et al. 2010; Orchardson and Gillam 2006; Karim and Gillam 2013; Talioti et al. 2014; França et al. 2015). Examples of OTC products with different desensitizing ingredients are provided in Table 7.2, but it is worth mentioning that occluding agents that work by protein precipitation are available solely in professional in-office products.

7.5 In-Office Fluoride Application (Gels, Varnishes, and Resins)

High concentrated-fluoride gels, varnishes, and resins have been recommended for in-office treatment for DH (Orchardson and Gillam 2006; Cummins 2010; Trushkowsky and Oquendo 2011), promoting instant and relative long-term relief for 3–6 months (Al-Sabbagh et al. 2009; Pradeep et al. 2012; Petersson 2013; Glockner 2013; Schmidlin and Sahrmann 2013). The combined use of fluoride with iontophoresis has also been reported in the literature (Aparna et al. 2010; da Rosa et al. 2013; Das et al. 2023). The mechanism of this technique has been based on three different hypotheses: (1) reparative dentine formation; (2) paraesthesia by modifying the pain conduction mechanism; and (3) helps to transfer fluoride ions deep into dentine, which appears to prolong the effect of the desensitizing agent (da Rosa et al. 2013; Das et al. 2023). This effect has been proved in some clinical studies (Aparna et al. 2010; Das et al. 2023), but more long-term evidence still appears to be necessary.

The mode of action of conventional fluorides, such as NaF, is by precipitation of CaF_2 globules that can occlude the dentinal tubule (Table 7.1). The formation of this layer is influenced by the F concentration, pH of the agent, and the frequency of application; however, it is generally not resis-

Table 7.2 Examples of OTC toothpastes available for the treatment of DH

Mechanism of action	Active ingredient	Commercial name[a]
Nerve desensitization	Potassium chloride	Sensodyne F Total Care
	Potassium citrate	Colgate Sensitive Multi Protection
	Potassium nitrate	Sensodyne Pronamel Mineral Boost; Sensodyne Complete Protection+; Sensodyne Nourish
Tubule occlusion by mineral deposition	Arginine and calcium carbonate	Colgate Sensitive Instant Relief; Colgate Sensitive Pro-Relief; Elmex Sensitive Professional
	Calcium sodium phosphosilicate (CSPS)	Sensodyne Repair and Protect Deep Repair
	Amine fluoride	Elmex Erosion Protection (now Elmex Opti-namel); Elmex Sensitive Professional
	Stannous fluoride	Sensodyne Sensitivity and Gum; Sensodyne Rapid Relief; Crest Complete Sensitivity
	Stannous chloride	Elmex Erosion Protection (now Elmex Opti-namel)
	Fluoro calcium phosphosilicate (FCSPS)	BioMin F
	Tricalcium phosphate (TCP)[b]	3 M Clinpro 5000; Colgate Prevident 5000

[a]Commercial name and composition may vary between countries
[b]Prescription strength fluoride content

tant to the frequent acid challenges in the oral environment, resulting in the need for reapplication (Cummins 2010; Calabria et al. 2014; Francisconi-Dos-Rios et al. 2021; Mosquim et al. 2022b). The mechanism of action is supported by the results of in vitro study showing reduction in dentine permeability values after the fluoride application (Calabria et al. 2014; Francisconi-Dos-Rios et al. 2021; Mosquim et al. 2022b).

Currently, other fluoride compounds containing polyvalent metals (TiF_4, SnF_2) have been tested against erosive tooth wear (ETW) (Lussi and Carvalho 2015), which is a condition that may be associated with DH development (O'Toole and Bartlett 2017) (see also Chap. 4). Despite their preventive effect against ETW being superior to NaF (Lussi and Carvalho 2015), an in vitro study has shown no reduction in dentine permeability following application of a TiF_4 varnish (Calabria et al. 2014), and no published clinical trial has been conducted testing this compound on tooth pain relief so far.

Although currently no systematic review exclusively addressed the role of professionally applied fluoride in DH control (Sharif et al. 2013), there is some evidence reported in the published literature that indicates that professionally applied fluoride, especially varnishes, are effective in relieving pain associated with DH (Orchardson and Gillam 2006; Sharif et al. 2013; Wang et al. 2016) in a way comparable to potassium nitrate (Osmari et al. 2018; Abdollahi and Jalalian 2019).

7.6 Over-the-Counter Fluoride Use (Toothpastes and Mouthrinses)

Toothpastes and mouthrinses containing sodium, stannous, or amine fluoride (NaF, SnF_2, or AmF) or sodium monofluorphosphate (MFP) have been used OTC to alleviate DH (Rösing et al. 2009; Pradeep et al. 2012). Nevertheless, inconsistent data are available on its clinical effectiveness (Orchardson and Gillam 2006; Pradeep et al. 2012).

With respect to calcium fluoride globules formation, they apparently do not contribute effectively to dentinal tubules occlusion (Petersson 2013), probably due to the small amount and size of the precipitated crystals (Calabria et al. 2014; Mosquim et al. 2022b). Considering that a F toothpaste is less concentrated than a F varnish, its effect is likely less evident on tooth pain relief, as reported by Mosquim et al. (2022b), in which a NaF toothpaste was less effective to reduce the dentine permeability and produced much less mineral deposits onto the dentine surface when compared to a NaF varnish. According to Calabria et al. (2014), relatively small number of particles can be observed inside the tubules after F application, whereas in the potassium oxalate sample, numerous dentinal tubules are occluded undersurface. This apparently ineffective action observed in the in vitro study does not, however, correspond to the clinical study results using fluoride formulations and this may be due to the difficulties in completely mimicking the oral environment in the laboratory.

The incorporation of metal ions (e.g., zinc, tin, strontium, and potassium) and abrasive components in toothpaste or mouthrinse formulation (e.g., alumina, silica, calcium carbonate, zinc, etc.) may also have a synergistic effect with the active ingredient on the dentine surface, thereby blocking the dentinal tubules (Petersson 2013). For example, a F toothpaste with 0.454% stannous fluoride (SnF_2) has been reported to be more effective in reducing DH following 4 weeks of daily use when compared to toothpaste with 0.76% MFP (Martins et al. 2020), whereas other studies do not show superiority effect for SnF_2 (Tao et al. 2020). Other desensitizing agents in combination with fluoride (e.g., strontium, 8% arginine, and calcium carbonate) have also been reported to be effective in clinical studies (Orchardson and Gillam 2006). Amine fluorides (Amflor™; Olaflur™, and even Dectaflur™, an organic amine fluoride) have also been reported to reduce DH, although currently there are limited data on its effectiveness (Pradeep et al. 2012).

Most of the cited studies evaluated toothpastes containing 1100–1450 ppm F. Nevertheless, the efficacy of toothpastes with high fluoride concentrations, such as those containing 2800-5000 ppm F (e.g. Duraphat), has not been comprehensively investigated as desensitizers; although highly concentrated products have a recognized anti-caries effect and may be effective on preventing and controlling root caries (Walsh 2010; Castelo et al. 2021).

The use of a fluoridated mouthrinse therapy in controlling DH in association with the regular use of a desensitizing toothpaste may also be recommended (e.g., potassium and amine fluoride) (Yates et al. 2004; Pradeep et al. 2012; Glockner 2013; Petersson 2013), although currently there are limited data on their effectiveness (Petersson 2013). Other fluoridated mouthrinses incorporating the various desensitizing agents mentioned in this chapter may also enhance the effectiveness of fluoride toothpaste and perhaps favour the remineralisation of dentine (Glockner 2013).

Irrespective of the actual active agent, the effectiveness of OTC products is dependent on the individual (patient or consumer) maintaining regular and effective oral hygiene practices by applying the toothpastes and/or mouthrinse on a twice daily basis (Petersson 2013) without exerting over-zealous brushing that could potentialize DH. However, depending on the nature of these OTC products, its active component may take up to 2–4 weeks to achieve relief from DH (Talioti et al. 2014).

One of the problems in evaluating the claims of these desensitizing products in clinical studies is the heterogeneity of the published studies, which makes the results difficult to understand (Karim and Gillam 2013; Talioti et al. 2014). Furthermore, both placebo and non-placebo effects may also impact the results of these studies, although Lin et al. (2013) and Bae et al. (2015), in their systematic reviews, reported that despite these observed effects both *in-office* and OTC products, techniques, and treatment approaches may have a real effect on DH. In addition, the systematic review of Bae et al. (2015) support the use of stannous fluoride with or without potassium-containing toothpastes for DH treatment.

One of the advantages of formulations containing both F^- and Sn^{2+} is their potential to reduce ETW even in the absence of demineralized collagen, whereas NaF is unable to reduce ETW when the demineralized dentine organic layer is lost by enzymatic action (Ganss et al. 2014) (see also Sect. 7.21.1 in this chapter). Chitosan has been incorporated into a commercial fluoride toothpaste containing tin with a positive effect against ETW (Ganss et al. 2014) but was unable to reduce dentine permeability as showed by João-Souza et al. (2019). As recently demonstrated (Pini et al. 2020) in vitro with a toothpaste formulation containing AmF, $SnCl_2$, and chitosan, brushing itself seems to play an important role in the formation of stannous compounds formed on the surface of the tooth. Also, the viscosity (i.e., the molecular weight) of chitosan also seems to be important for the control of ETW. Chitosan that is too fluid might not reduce tissue loss, whilst chitosan that is too thick could create excessive friction, which is undesirable (Pini et al. 2020). Thus, future studies on the use of chitosan for the prevention of ETW should also be conducted, especially in more complex study designs such as in situ models.

To this day, there is currently no published randomized clinical trial testing the effect of F^-, Sn^{2+}, and chitosan toothpaste in the control of DH. Therefore, twice daily application of self-applied fluoride toothpaste containing either tin, potassium with or without tin, or arginine with calcium carbonate can be recommended for the reduction of DH pain. Nonetheless, there is a need for standardized methodology guideline development to improve the conduct, analysis, and reporting of DH in clinical studies (Pollard et al. 2023).

7.7 Potassium Salts in In-Office Products

One of the most investigated agents to treat DH are those containing potassium salts, such as potassium oxalate (Wang et al. 2016; Osmari et al. 2018; Sgreccia et al. 2020, 2022). The mechanism of action of this product is based on the presence of potassium and the formation of calcium oxalate. Potassium ions can prolong the duration of the repolarization stage of the nerve fibre, which is essential for a stimulus to occur (Nanjundasetty and Ashrafulla 2016). A study by Peacock and Orchardson (1995) demonstrated that 8–16 mM concentrations of potassium ions around axons are necessary to sustain the nerve depolarization. However, there has been a degree of controversy because of its proposed mode of action (nerve desensitization) based on an animal model (Markowitz et al. 1991; Schmidlin and Sahrmann 2013; Boneta et al. 2013). Several investigators have, however, challenged this mode of action as indicated above and have suggested that these formulations may instead be through tubule occlusion and attributed to other constituents (e.g., abrasives or even the presence of fluoride salts) than the potassium ion per se (Addy and Mostafa 1989; Gillam et al. 1996; West et al. 1997; Orchardson and Gillam 2000). Conversely, the oxalate is known to react with calcium and precipitate calcium oxalate, which can occlude the patent dentinal tubules and has been shown to resist a subsequent erosive challenge (Calabria et al. 2014; Francisconi-Dos-Rios et al. 2021) (see also Chap. 6).

Formulations are launched in different vehicles to the dental profession (Fig. 7.1) (Sgreccia et al. 2020, 2022) or for OTC use (Orchardson and Gillam 2000; Lynch et al. 2018; Burnett et al. 2018; Anderson et al. 2020; Chapman et al. 2020), including solutions (Lynch et al. 2018; Burnett et al. 2018) and strips (Amini et al. 2016; Lynch et al. 2018; Chapman et al. 2020). Regardless of the vehicle, potassium oxalate shows reliable and long-lasting effect compared with other occluding products. Along the clinical effect, the self-reported quality of life (QoL) has also been investigated, in which the individuals demonstrate satisfaction once treated with potassium oxalate (Sgreccia et al. 2022). Agheli et al.

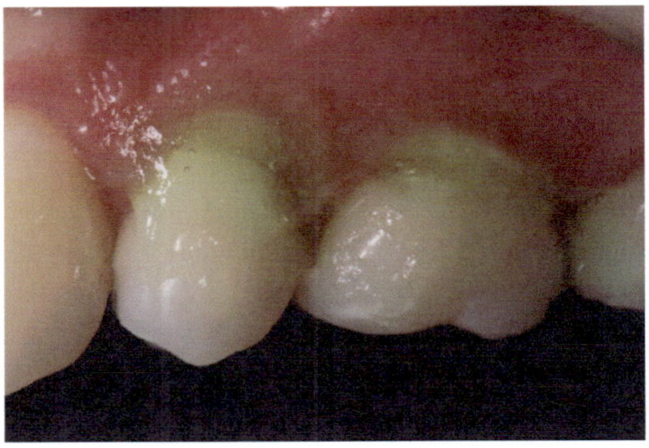

Fig. 7.1 Application of an in-office potassium oxalate gel on sensitive dentine. As recommended by the manufacturer, the product was kept on the exposed dentine for 3 min and removed without rinsing. (Images provided by Dr. Victor Mosquim and Dr. Mariele Vertuan)

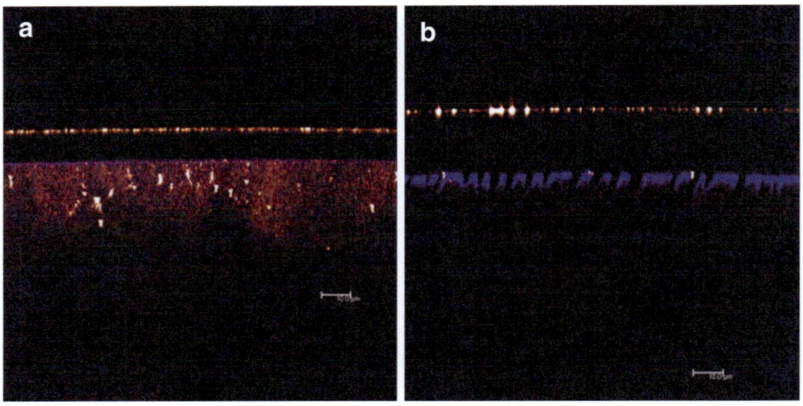

Fig. 7.2 Confocal laser scanning microscopy (CLSM; XZ axis) of mineralized sound dentine (**a**) and after etching with phosphoric acid (**b**). (Images provided by Dr. Linda Wang, Dr. Marcela Pagani Calabria and Dr. Luciana Fávaro Francisconi-dos-Rios)

(2023) reported that increased exposure to DH treatment in dental school curricula and continuing education courses helps students and professionals recognize the importance of accurate diagnosis and treatment of DH. This also increases their willingness to use oxalate and arginine/calcium-based products (Agheli et al. 2023) (Fig. 7.1).

The in vitro testing of desensitizing agents has been conducted traditionally through the observation of the surface and subsurface of the dentine tubules using several techniques, such as SEM and CLSM, and comparing the obtained images before and after treatment (Fig. 7.2a, b). By comparing the images of potassium oxalate-treated dentine before and after an acid challenge (Fig. 7.3a, b), one can observe the greater precipitation of crystals inside the dentinal tubules following an acid challenge, effectively occluding the dentine, which is reflected in lower dentine permeability values (Pereira et al. 2005; Cummins 2010; Calabria et al. 2014; Francisconi-Dos-Rios et al. 2021).

Nevertheless, several investigators have reported that any relief from DH may be transient in nature as the precipitated crystals may be dissolved or removed over time (Al-Sabbagh et al. 2009). Classically, 6% ferric, 30% dipotassium, and 3% monohydrogen monopotassium have been the oxalate formulation associated with potassium to occlude the dentinal tubules and reduce DH (Pashley et al. 2001; Al-Sabbagh et al. 2009; Schmidlin and Sahrmann 2013); yet, according to Al-Sabbagh et al. (2009), oxalate-containing phytocomplexes may also be an alternative to the traditional oxalate preparations. For example, Sauro et al. (2007) reported that these complexes reduced dentine permeability following a single application in an in vitro study. These investigators also postulated that these complexes may protect the smear layer formed by scaling procedures on the root dentine from an acidic challenge (Sauro et al. 2007).

7.8 Potassium-Containing OTC Products

Potassium-containing (nitrate, chlorine, and citrate) toothpastes, mouthrinses, and strips have been reported to be effective in reducing DH compared to placebo controls (Orchardson and Gillam 2000; Markowitz 2009; Bae et al. 2015; Lynch et al. 2018). Of these formulations, 5% potassium nitrate toothpastes formulations have been the most extensively evaluated desensitizing toothpastes (Rösing et al. 2009). Overall, most studies have reported favorable outcomes for potassium-containing toothpastes when compared to controls (Schiff et al. 2009; Orchardson and Gillam 2000; Pradeep and Sharma 2010; Pradeep et al. 2012) and to other desensitizing agents, such as 10% strontium chloride (Orchardson and Gillam 2000), 2% sodium citrate, and 1.4% formaldehyde toothpaste (Orchardson and Gillam 2000).

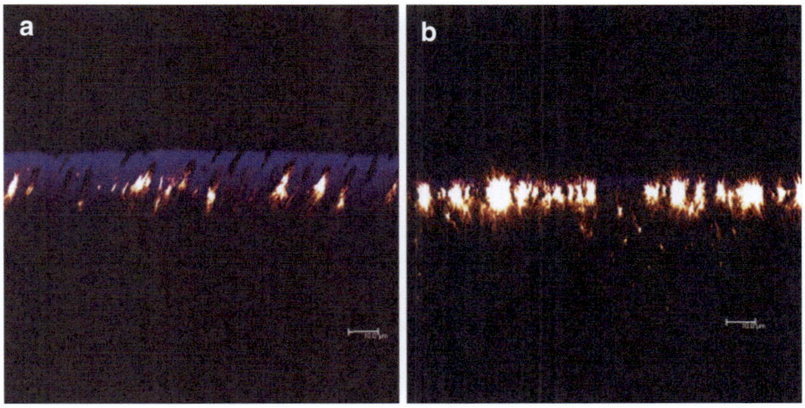

Fig. 7.3 Confocal laser scanning microscopy (CLSM, XZ axis) of dentine treated with 3% potassium oxalate before (**a**) and after (**b**) a citric acid challenge. (Images provided by Dr. Linda Wang, Dr. Marcela Pagani Calabria and Dr. Luciana Fávaro Francisconi-dos-Rios)

However, according to Jackson (2000) and Panagakos et al. (2009), potassium-containing toothpastes are no more effective than regular fluoride toothpastes. Conversely, a systematic review with meta-analysis (Bae et al. 2015) reported that potassium-containing toothpastes were more effective than placebo, and a network meta-analysis also reported that potassium worked better against the symptoms of DH when in combination with stannous fluoride or hydroxyapatite, especially for tactile and air stimuli, with a moderate certainty of the evidence (Martins et al. 2020).

As described above, the focus in most of the earlier desensitizing studies was on toothpaste formulations and relatively few studies have been conducted examining the effectiveness of potassium-containing mouthrinse formulations. Several investigators have reported that these mouthrinse formulations containing potassium nitrate and sodium fluoride (Gillam et al. 1996; Pereira and Chavas 2001), potassium citrate or sodium fluoride (Yates et al. 1998), or a mixture of fluorides (Yates et al. 2004) may reduce DH. Gillam et al. (1996) demonstrated that the 3% potassium nitrate and sodium fluoride mouthrinses significantly reduced DH compared to the sodium fluoride mouthrinse after 2 and 6 weeks of use. Pereira and Chavas (2001) also demonstrated that, after 2 weeks, there were no statistically significant differences between the two groups using tactile and thermal stimuli. At 6 weeks, however, the 3% potassium nitrate and 0.2% sodium fluoride mouthwash demonstrated a significant difference in DH when stimulated by cold air, as compared to the control 0.2% sodium fluoride mouthwash.

More recently, a mouthrinse containing 1.4% potassium oxalate (Listerine Advanced Defence Sensitive, LADS) has been developed (Johnson and Johnson Consumer and Personal Products Worldwide, Skillman and Morris Plains, NJ, USA). There are limited data on its long-term effectiveness on DH with only three published studies (five different randomized clinical trials (RCTs)) (Sharma et al. 2013a, b; Burnett et al. 2018). In two of the studies, the investigators reported that the potassium oxalate mouthrinse significantly reduced DH compared to the negative control groups (Sharma et al. 2013a, b). However, in the study of Burnett et al. (2018), which included three different RCTs, only one of them found that a 1.5% potassium oxalate mouthrinse, and a 2% potassium oxalate + 45 ppm F mouthrinse were superior to the placebo mouthrinse after 4 and 8 weeks. In this publication, the authors discuss the importance of the placebo effect, which has been estimated to be responsible for 20–60% of symptom relief in DH studies. The authors then conclude that, due to the high sensitivity of DH investigations to a placebo effect, further research is necessary to evaluate the effectiveness of this mouthrinse when used as an adjunct to a fluoride-containing toothpaste (Burnett et al. 2018).

Three published in vitro studies used a dentine disc model to demonstrate the mode of action by the oxalate deposit, and the LADS mouthrinse was significantly more effective in tubule occlusion (intratubular penetration was more evident) and in reducing dentine permeability compared to the other tested products (Eliades et al. 2013; Sharma et al. 2013c). Furthermore, according to these investigators, the tubule occlusion associated with LADS was substantially more stable in resisting an acid challenge compared to the other test products. However, these results were not confirmed in the study of Grandizoli et al. (2022).

7.9 Arginine and Calcium Carbonate-Containing Products for In-Office Use

Formulations containing arginine and calcium carbonate have been reported to effectively occlude the dentinal tubules and to provide immediate and lasting relief for DH (Hamlin et al. 2009; Schiff et al. 2009; Pei et al. 2013). According to the manufacturers, arginine is a positively charged amino acid naturally available in saliva. Since dentine is negatively charged, in association with calcium, arginine may play an important role favouring the deposition of an arginine, calcium, and phosphate complex that physically occludes the dentinal tubules and appears to be resistant to normal pulpal pressures (Hamlin et al. 2009; Schiff et al. 2009; Cummins 2010; Pei et al. 2013). Therefore, arginine/calcium carbonate products are currently available as in-office product and as an OTC toothpaste that can be used in association with in-office treatment (Hamlin et al. 2009).

Most of the available clinical trials have proven immediate relief as the main benefit of this agent (Collins et al. 2013; Ayad et al. 2018; Hirsiger et al. 2019). Studies have investigated the use of a professional arginine/calcium carbonate prophylaxis paste compared with a fluoride-free prophylaxis paste. The results demonstrated a significant desensitizing effect of the arginine/calcium carbonate paste, even in patients who had undergone scaling or exhibited gingival recession (Kapferer et al. 2013; Collins et al. 2013; Ayad et al. 2018; Hirsiger et al. 2019).

There is evidence that the deposits generated by arginine/calcium carbonate are effective at occluding the patent dentinal tubules (Cummins 2010). However, there are also some concerns that these formulations are not able to resist an acid challenge (Francisconi-Dos-Rios et al. 2021). Evidence also indicates that arginine/calcium carbonate-containing products are more effective in treating the symptoms of DH derived from air stimuli rather than by tactile stimuli (Collins et al. 2013; Ayad et al. 2018; Bae et al. 2015; Hu et al. 2019; Martins et al. 2020, 2022).

As mentioned previously, the erosive oral condition is one of the main causes of DH (João-Souza et al. 2019; Lopes et al. 2021), thus remineralizing the tooth structure is frequently encouraged to treat this condition. Ding et al. (2023), under this perspective, associated 2.5% sodium trimetaphosphate (STMP) with arginine/calcium carbonate. This combination allowed firstly the remineralization through phosphorylation, resulting in more stable mineral nucleation. Also, this new formation provided a more reliable substrate for the use of bonding agents, which is usually recommended for the conditions that require further restorative treatment.

7.10 Arginine and Calcium Carbonate-Based Toothpastes and Mouthrinses

Current products containing calcium carbonate and arginine are based on Kleinberg's original formulation SensiStat (Kleinberg 2002) and are available in toothpastes (elmex Sensitive Professional, Colgate Sensitive Instant Relief; Colgate Sensitive Pro-Relief, Colgate Total) and, more recently, in the form of a mouthrinse (Colgate Sensitive Pro-Relief mouthwash) (Mello et al. 2013; Hu et al. 2013; Boneta et al. 2013) for the treatment of DH.

Arginine/calcium carbonate-containing toothpastes have also been reported to reduce DH in randomized clinical studies when compared to placebo and other desensitizing products (Petrou et al. 2009; Ayad et al. 2009; Docimo et al. 2009a, b; Que et al. 2010; Fu et al. 2010; Boneta et al. 2013; Hall et al. 2017). Several clinical studies have also reported that arginine/calcium carbonate mouthrinse containing 0.8% arginine, PVM/MA copolymer, pyrophosphates, and 0.05% sodium fluoride in an alcohol-free base mouthrinse was effective compared to control mouthrinses in reducing DH (Hu et al. 2013; Boneta et al. 2013). Several investigators have suggested a role for these products in treating DH (Fu et al. 2010; Que et al. 2010; Sharif et al. 2013), although Sharif et al. (2013) have suggested that more robust and well-designed randomized clinical studies with larger sample sizes should be conducted to determine their clinical efficacy in reducing DH. Ongphichetmetha et al. (2022) and Champaiboon et al. (2024) also stated that the arginine/calcium carbonate toothpaste was an effective desensitizing ingredient in non-surgically treated periodontal patients. Evidence would also suggest that arginine/calcium carbonate-containing products are more effective in treating the symptoms of DH derived from air stimuli (Martins et al. 2020).

More recently, due to the awareness about molar incisor hypomineralization, dental pain is frequently reported by patients with this enamel malformation. In this way, Bekes et al. (2017) demonstrated that the in-office and OTC arginine/calcium carbonate products were efficient to minimize the pain after 8 weeks.

7.11 Calcium Phosphate Compounds

Calcium phosphate has also been reported in in vitro studies to be effective in occluding the dentinal tubules (Francisconi-Dos-Rios et al. 2021), and some studies have reported this material to be more effective than potassium oxalate (Al-Sabbagh et al. 2009), which could provide an effective product to treat DH. Recently, nano-hydroxyapatite (HAp) based agents (for example, Desensibilize NanoP® containing HAp and Clinpro white varnish containing $Ca^{2+}/PO_4^{3-}/F^-$) with both bioactive and biocompatibility potential have been reported to be effective both as a remineralizing and desensitizing agent (Hanning and Hanning 2010; Tschoppe et al. 2011; Calabria et al. 2014; Wang et al. 2016; Francisconi-Dos-Rios et al. 2021; Handa et al. 2023). These agents contain nano-sized particles, which act in a similar manner to dental apatite regarding the morphology, structure, and crystallinity arrangement (Vandiver et al. 2005).

One of the problems, however, is the inability of the HAp layer produced by the application of HAp products to resist an acid challenge in the oral environment overtime. Machado et al. (2022) showed that Clinpro white varnish (a 5% NaF varnish) did not differ from placebo in DH control after 6 months of treatment. This issue has subsequently led investigators to develop innovative bioactive formulations to enhance the remineralizing and tubule occluding properties of the marketed products (Reynolds et al. 2008; Cummins 2010; Nongonierma and Fitzgerald 2012; Pei et al. 2013; Calabria et al. 2014; Wang et al. 2016; Francisconi-Dos-Rios et al. 2021; Mosquim et al. 2022a).

Casein phosphopeptide-amorphous calcium phosphate (CPP-ACP), a milk derivative, has also been reported to be effective in remineralizing enamel and dentine (Reynolds et al. 2008; Agnihotri et al. 2012; Nongonierma and Fitzgerald 2012; Handa et al. 2023). CPP is a bioactive peptide released from casein, which has been shown to enhance bivalent mineral solubility and optimize binding ability to minerals, such as calcium. Amorphous calcium phosphate (ACP) is the precursor of HAp and, in an oral environment in the presence of saliva, is converted to HAp. At the dental surface interface, both calcium and phosphate can precipitate as HAp (Nongonierma and Fitzgerald 2012). It has often been tested to reduce tooth pain following bleaching. With respect to DH treatment, although one study showed that the effectiveness of ACP for DH was no different from the placebo control after approximately 3 months (Al-Sabbagh et al. 2009), a more recent study attested that MI Varnish reduced DH immediately after treatment up to 6 months (Chebel et al. 2018).

Several recent products containing tricalcium phosphate (TCP) have been developed for professional application (3M™ ESPE™, St. Paul, Minneapolis, USA), namely (1) a dental varnish (Clinpro™) containing 5% sodium fluoride with TCP and (2) Vanish™ XT Extended Contact Varnish, which is a light-cured resin-modified glass ionomer cement (RMGIC) based on the patented methacrylate-modified polyalkenoic acid. The indications for their use are based on tooth remineralizing and dentinal tubule occlusion actions (Vanichvatana and Auychai 2013; Asaizumi et al. 2013). Only one clinical trial showed benefit of RMGIC Clinpro™ XT in controlling DH in a 6-month follow-up (Madruga et al. 2017). Nonetheless, to date, most studies on TCP addressed the effect of this component in OTC products, which will be further elaborated in this chapter.

When CPP-ACP is compared to TCP, the former has shown a highest calcium and fluoride release capacity than the TCP varnish (Cochrane et al. 2014), which may indicate better action on DH control despite not appropriately being demonstrated in clinical trials, which highlights the need of further studies comparing these agents not only between them but also to similar products containing F and potassium nitrate.

7.12 Casein Phosphopeptide-Amorphous Calcium Phosphate (CPP-ACP)

Casein phosphopeptide (CPP) (Recaldent™ technology, GC Tooth Mousse) was primarily developed for both anti-caries and remineralisation strategies rather than for the treatment of DH per se (Kowalczyk et al. 2006). Casein phosphopeptide-amorphous calcium phosphate (CPP-ACP) was previously marketed as GC Tooth Mousse (Recaldent™), which was a water based, sugar-free dental topical crème for home-care use. The stabilization of ACP component by the CPP ensured the delivery of both Ca^{2+} and PO_4^{3-} ions onto the enamel surface for remineralisation. Several studies reported that CPP-ACP can effectively remineralize the enamel subsurface lesions (Cai et al. 2003; Lata et al. 2010). The manufacturer indicated that CPP–ACP would be ideal for treating DH on the basis of its remineralizing potential, and a number of in vitro and in vivo studies were conducted demonstrating that calcium phosphate preparations deposit a mineral precipitate onto the dentine surface, blocking dentinal tubules and consequently reducing dentine permeability in the dentine disk model, with potential to be used for treatment of DH (Azarpazhooh and Limeback 2008; Charig et al. 2009; Gandolfi et al. 2010; Walsh 2010). However, it is questionable if the CPP-ACP formulation would demonstrate any long-lasting effect on DH. A systematic review by Talioti et al. (2014) reported that, although the CPP-ACP containing products may provide some benefit in reducing DH, there was insufficient data from the published studies to support any claims of efficacy in reducing DH up to now. More recently, Kijsamanmith et al. (2019) showed that conventional and acid-modified CPP-ACP-containing crème decreased dentine permeability and partially occluded the dentinal tubules, which resisted an acid challenge, for 2 weeks. Clinically, CPP-ACP-containing crèmes are effective in the reduction of DH in an orthodontic patient following debonding (Vatturu et al. 2021), but there is a need for further studies on DH treatment over time.

7.13 Functionalized Tricalcium Phosphate (fTCP)

According to Vanichvatana and Auychai (2013), fTCP is produced by the solid-state ball milling of beta-tricalcium phosphate and sodium lauryl sulphate and has been demonstrated by several investigators to prevent calcium ions from prematurely interacting with ionic fluoride and forming calcium fluoride, thus delivering more fluoride and calcium ions to the enamel surface (Karlinsey et al. 2010; Karlinsey et al. 2012).

fTCP has also been reported to have remineralizing effects in both in vitro and in situ studies (Karlinsey et al. 2009a, b; Mensinkai et al. 2012; Vanichvatana and Auychai 2013). fTCP has been commercially developed and is now available as a 950-ppm fluoride toothpaste (Clinpro Tooth Crème; 3M ESPE, Saint Paul, MN, USA). Asaizumi et al. (2013) also assessed the effect of 0.21 and 1.1% NaF toothpastes containing fTCP on the density of white-spot lesions in vitro, and Mensinkai et al. (2012), in an in situ remineralization study of white-spot lesions, compared a non-fluoride toothpaste with 500 and 1100 ppm F fTCP-containing toothpastes. Both studies showed a good potential of the fTCP toothpaste to be applied for dental caries control. With respect to DH treatment, Jang et al. (2023) demonstrated a significant DH reduction (by a Visual Analogue Scale (VAS) analysis) using an fTCP toothpaste compared to a fluoride-free and to a strontium chloride toothpaste, but there is still a need of further clinical trials to support this result.

7.14 Calcium Sodium Phosphosilicate (Bioactive Glass) in In-Office Products

Calcium sodium phosphosilicate glasses (bioactive glasses) were developed by Professor Larry Hench in the late 1960s, originally called Bioglass 45S5 (Hench 2006). The mechanism of action of this material was previously reported by Hench (2006) and further elaborated by Hill (1996) and is initiated with a rapid exchange of ions from the glass with protons from the solution in which it is immersed, followed by hydrolysis. As this ion exchange occurs, there is migration of Ca^{2+} and PO_4^{3-} to the surface of the glass and formation of an amorphous calcium phosphate (ACP) film, which will further incorporate more Ca^{2+} and PO_4^{3-}, as well as OH^-, CO_3^{2-}, and even F^- from the solution in which it is immersed (e.g., saliva), leading to the crystallization of the film, forming octacalcium phosphate (OCP) and/or different forms of apatite. It is important to note that ACP and OCP are considered precursors of apatite (Brauer et al. 2010; Kovrlija et al. 2021), and it has been shown over the years that these glasses are able to precipitate different forms of apatite (hydroxyapatite, hydroxycarbonate apatite, and even fluorapatite) (Brauer et al. 2010; Tiskaya et al. 2021), depending on their composition and on the composition of the solution in which they are immersed.

Despite also being known as "calcium sodium phosphosilicate", these glasses were shown to be bioactive (i.e., precipitate apatite) even without sodium in their composition (Chen et al. 2017; Sugumaran et al. 2022). Moreover, due to its ability to form apatite, which is the natural mineral component of teeth (both enamel and dentine) and bones, 45S5 has also been used for orthopaedic applications (Hench 2006); however, it was only in the 1990s that it started being used for dental applications under the name of NovaMin (NovaMin Technology Inc., Alachua, FL, USA, now Haleon), especially for the treatment of DH. Based on the Brännström and Åström hydrodynamic theory (Brännström and Åström 1964) explaining the mechanisms involved in DH (see also Chap. 5), the bioactive glasses would be able to precipitate apatite on the tooth surface and help occlude the patent dentinal tubules, thus reducing the permeability of fluids that may lead to the pain sensation (Brauer et al. 2010; Mneimne et al. 2011; Lynch et al. 2012; Tiskaya et al. 2021).

Based on this premise, several studies were developed over the years to investigate the behaviour of these glasses in situations simulating the oral environment (Brauer et al. 2010; Mneimne et al. 2011; Lynch et al. 2012; Tiskaya et al. 2021). These studies evidenced that these glasses were able to increase the local pH (buffering effect), and a higher content of phosphate led to an increase in the amount of apatite being precipitated (Mneimne et al. 2011). Moreover, due to the understanding that fluorapatite (FAp) is more acid-resistant than conventional hydroxyapatite (HAp) and hydroxycarbonate apatite (HCAp) (Tiskaya et al. 2021), fluoride-containing glasses such as Biomin F (Biomin Technologies

Ltd., London, UK) were developed to promote these additional benefits. Also, there is evidence that fluoride-containing bioactive glasses would precipitate apatite more rapidly than fluoride-free glasses because FAp is formed directly, without the formation of ACP and OCP precursors (Tiskaya et al. 2021) (see also Chap. 10).

Due to these characteristics, these calcium sodium phosphosilicate glasses (CSPS) and even fluoride calcium sodium phosphosilicate glasses (FCSPS) have been inserted in *in-office* products for DH such as prophylaxis pastes and varnishes (Zhu et al. 2015). *In-office* prophylaxis pastes containing both arginine/calcium carbonate and bioactive glasses (for example, CSPS) have been reported to provide effective clinical pain relief from DH (Cummins 2010; Hughes et al. 2010; Pradeep and Sharma 2010; Pradeep et al. 2012). In previous in vitro studies, a CSPS-containing prophylaxis paste was able to reduce the permeability of dentine and maintain a lower permeability value even after a 5-day erosive-abrasive challenge (João-Souza et al. 2018; Viana et al. 2022). In the clinical study conducted by Milleman et al. (2012), the prophylaxis paste with CSPS was effective in reducing the DH of patients immediately and after 4 weeks, regardless of the presence of fluoride in the composition of the paste (Milleman et al. 2012). Similarly, in the clinical study conducted by Chałas et al. (2015), DH was also reduced 1 week following a single one-minute application of the prophylaxis paste containing 15% 45S5 glass using a rubber cup on a low-speed handpiece (Chałas et al. 2015). A systematic review with meta-analysis reported that the prophylaxis paste containing 15% CSPS was significantly better than a product with no active ingredient (i.e., negative control), indicating that this *in-office* paste indeed presents a beneficial effect for the control of post-periodontal therapy DH in patients (Zhu et al. 2015). Nonetheless, the authors classified the quality of the evidence as low (Zhu et al. 2015). Also, there is currently insufficient evidence on its clinical efficacy in reducing DH following in-office procedures (Sharif et al. 2013), and most of the studies address the use of CSPS or FCSPS in OTC products.

7.15 Calcium Sodium Phosphosilicate (Bioactive Glass) in OTC Products

As previously described, the process in which CSPS and FCSPS glasses can form apatite starts with ion exchange with water (Hill 1996; Hench 2006); therefore, toothpastes containing a glass formulation need to be anhydrous (water free), and it is for this reason that CSPS and FSCPS are not available in mouthrinses; otherwise, HCA or FAp would form inside the container.

The ability of these glasses to precipitate apatite onto the dentine surface and reduce the lumen of the patent dentinal tubules was reported in several in vitro studies over the years (Dong et al. 2011; João-Souza et al. 2018; Viana et al. 2022), and their clinical efficacy was also compared to other desensitizing products, indicating its use as a desensitizing product with clinically relevant results over time (Du Min et al. 2008; Pradeep and Sharma 2010; Pradeep et al. 2012; Sharif et al. 2013; Petersson 2013; Zhu et al. 2015; Hall et al. 2017; Arantes et al. 2019; Patel et al. 2019). In OTC products, the concentration of glass in the toothpaste ranges from 2.5% to 7.5% (Gillam et al. 2002b; Litkowski and Greenspan 2010), and in a systematic review with meta-analysis (Zhu et al. 2015), CSPS-containing toothpastes provided relief from DH symptoms when compared to products with no active ingredients (i.e., negative control). However, clinical studies evidenced that toothpastes with CSPS provided as much as or even more DH relief than arginine/calcium carbonate toothpastes and potassium nitrate toothpastes (Pradeep and Sharma 2010; Pradeep et al. 2012; Sharif et al. 2013; Hall et al. 2017; Arantes et al. 2019), which are two of the most popular toothpastes used for treating the DH symptoms.

In respect of FCSPS glasses, in the study of Ashwini et al. (2018), the FCSPS-containing toothpaste was more effective than the CSPS-containing toothpaste to reduce DH discomfort, and Patel et al. (2019) demonstrated that a 5% FCSPS toothpaste (Biomin F) was able to reduce DH more efficaciously than an 8% arginine/calcium carbonate toothpaste. Arshad et al. (2021) indicated that arginine/calcium carbonate-based toothpaste and a strontium acetate-based toothpaste may provide a faster desensitizing effect than a 5% FCSPS-based toothpaste, which, in turn, appears to be the best option for the treatment of the DH symptoms in the long-term (Arshad et al. 2021; Petrović et al. 2023). This statement was also supported by a recent systematic review (Petrović et al. 2023). However, despite demonstrating promising results, there are still limited clinical studies on the use of FCSPS glasses for DH (Petrović et al. 2023), and there is lack of homogeneity in the methodology and study designs of the available studies, which makes the analysis of these results difficult (Talioti et al. 2014; Petrović et al. 2023).

7.16 Strontium-Containing Products

Strontium-containing desensitizing agents have been widely investigated over the years (Markowitz 2009; Magno et al. 2015; Bae et al. 2015; Hu et al. 2018; Martins et al. 2020, 2022), and the original strontium acetate-based toothpaste was reformulated as Sensodyne Rapid Relief containing 8% strontium acetate in a silica base and 1040 ppm sodium fluoride. Based on in vitro studies, the main mode of action of strontium formulations (historically in the form of strontium chloride and more recently as strontium acetate) was considered to be one of tubular occlusion by the precipitation of metallic compounds that are more acid-resistant to an acid challenge than arginine-based products (Hughes et al. 2010; Mason et al. 2010; Olley et al. 2012; Seong et al. 2013; Martins et al. 2020, 2022). Also, there is a discussion that strontium can also desensitize nerve cells, similarly to potassium-containing agents (Martins et al. 2020, 2022). However, the actual effect attributed to strontium in clinical studies has yet to be defined and its efficacy has been considered controversial by some authors (Rösing et al. 2009; Cummins 2010; Karim and Gillam 2013; Hu et al. 2018; Martins et al. 2020).

The two in vivo studies by Hughes et al. (2010) and Mason et al. (2010) reported that the formulated strontium acetate toothpaste was effective in reducing DH compared to a control fluoride toothpaste (Mason et al. 2010) and to a marketed control dentifrice containing 8% arginine, calcium carbonate, and 1450 ppm sodium monofluorophosphate (Hughes et al. 2010). However, although in a review on strontium toothpastes conducted by Jackson (2000), there was a lack of significant improvement in the participant's symptoms from DH when compared with negative control toothpastes, a more recent network meta-analysis reported that strontium appears to be effective for DH arising from tactile stimuli with a moderate level of certainty and a very low level of certainty for DH arising from cold stimuli (Martins et al. 2020).

In a 16-week cross-over design study comparing Colgate Sensitive Pro-Relief (also marketed as elmex Sensitive Professional, containing arginine/calcium carbonate) and Sensodyne Rapid Relief (containing strontium acetate), it was reported that following 8 weeks of brushing with Colgate Sensitive Pro-Relief provided a significant reduction in mean DH values compared to the Sensodyne Rapid Relief toothpaste. A further observation from this study was that the Colgate Sensitive Pro-Relief subjects achieved significantly improved reductions in DH following the cross-over from the initial use of brushing with the Sensodyne Rapid Relief toothpaste. However, those subjects who initially brushed with the Colgate Sensitive Pro-Relief toothpaste did not benefit from the cross-over to the Sensodyne Rapid Relief (Schiff et al. 2009).

In other two studies (Bae et al. 2015; Hu et al. 2018), strontium-containing toothpastes appear to be effective against DH if it was associated with potassium, but its effect alone was very limited. For an evaporative stimulus, toothpastes containing arginine/calcium carbonate were significantly superior to those containing strontium acetate in clinical studies (Magno et al. 2015). In a systematic review with network meta-analysis, the level of certainty supporting the use of strontium salts over fluoride was considered low, and the authors pointed out that strontium salts appear to be effective in controlling the DH symptoms only if the stimulus was tactile, with a moderate level of certainty (Martins et al. 2020).

7.17 Dentine Bonding Agents/Adhesives and Adhesive Restorations

Adhesive systems have proven to be valuable tools in the reduction of DH, providing effective solutions for patients experiencing discomfort. The use of adhesive systems for DH involves various techniques and materials designed to reduce pain and reinforce the integrity of compromised structure (Abuzinadah and Alhaddad 2021).

In adhesion evolution, previous adhesive systems relied on the application of phosphoric acid to facilitate the interlocking of the resin material with the dental surface. However, the necessity for acidic dentine conditioning prior to the adhesive application may be detrimental to the integrity of the pulp. The advent of self-etching and universal or multi-mode agents has revitalized the interest in employing adhesive systems as dentine desensitizers. This was attributed to their ease of application and less aggressiveness to the dentine–pulp complex when compared to traditional etch-and-rinse systems (Pei et al. 2013; Abuzinadah and Alhaddad 2021). These systems, incorporating 10-methacryloyloxydecyl dihydrogen phosphate (10-MDP) and/or other functional monomers, establish a chemical bond with calcium from the apatite, leading to the formation of a stable salt (Yoshida et al. 2000; Pei et al. 2013). This introduces an additional chemical bond to enhance the micromechanical bond promoted by conventional systems, presenting an advantageous approach for patients with DH, especially for inducing less postoperative sensitivity (Costa et al. 2017).

One common application of adhesive systems is as a dentine surface sealant, which involves the application of a thin layer of adhesive material directly onto the exposed dentine. The adhesive forms a protective barrier, sealing the dentinal tubules and reducing the transmission of external stimuli that can trigger DH (Wegehaupt et al. 2012a, b; Abuzinadah and Alhaddad 2021). This technique not only provides immediate relief but also helps prevent further enamel erosion (Wegehaupt et al. 2017). Whilst there have been promising results, the enduring effectiveness of adhesive systems as dentine desensitizers remains uncertain. Potential drawbacks are linked to durability and mechanical challenges, as studies on this subject report treatment durability ranging from 3 to 12 months (Wegehaupt et al. 2012a, b; Abuzinadah and Alhaddad 2021). Moreover, the absence of comprehensive clinical studies on this matter exacerbates the uncertainty regarding their long-term efficacy. Another concern with certain products was the absence of a filler material, which could potentially increase susceptibility to wear on the material's surface (Schmidlin and Sahrmann 2013).

Considering postoperative sensitivity and substrate resistance to new insults in the oral environment, the use of glutaraldehyde-based agents, applied either before the use of the adhesive system or incorporated directly into the system itself, has been successfully reported in the treatment of DH (Albar 2022). This product's efficacy relies on the coagulation of proteins within the dentinal tubules, resulting in the creation of a precipitate of serum albumin that seals off these tubules. This phenomenon is commonly linked to 2-hydroxyethyl methacrylate (HEMA), whose polymerization is initiated by the precipitation of serum albumins, thereby aiding in the closure of dentinal tubules (Jiang et al. 2022). Regarding adhesives containing glutaraldehyde and HEMA, numerous researchers have documented its effect on dentine permeability and both immediate and sustained alleviation of pain resulting from DH (Lopes and Aranha 2013; Albar 2022; Mosquim et al. 2022a). Special attention, however, should be paid to the clinical use of HEMA-based products, particularly when applied in proximity or in direct contact with pulpal and epithelial gingival tissues. According to investigators (Chang et al. 2005; de Groot and Rustemeyer 2023, 2024), HEMA not only inhibits cellular growth but may also trigger allergic reactions in both patients and professionals when used in high or low doses

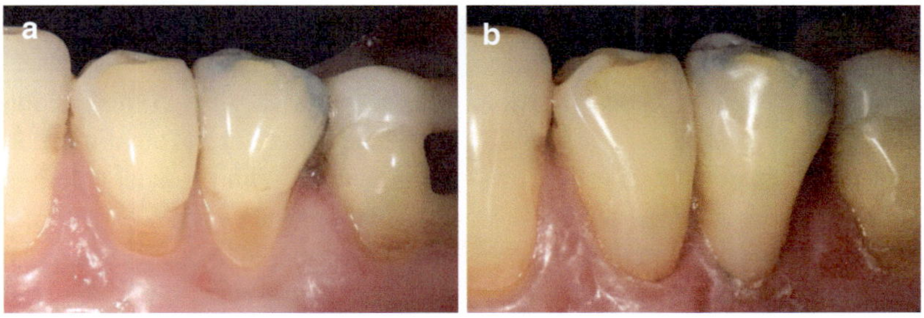

Fig. 7.4 (**a**) initial aspect of the lesions, with enamel loss and exposure of dentine above the cemento-enamel junction (CEJ). (**b**) Final aspect of the restorations with self-etching adhesive. (Case kindly provided by Dr. Karin Cristina da Silva Modena and Dr. Giovanna Speranza Zabeu)

over extended periods, potentially resulting in conditions such as dermatitis.

Whilst a minimally invasive approach is generally preferred when addressing DH with restorative materials (Orchardson and Gillam 2006), clinicians may encounter situations where there is significant loss of dental structure associated with DH. In such cases, restoring the tooth shape becomes necessary to preserve both its aesthetic appearance and functionality.

Of the available restorative materials, resin-modified glass ionomer cements (RMGICs) are highly recommended for areas experiencing indirect mechanical impact. The chemical bonding between the material and substrate is primarily driven by ionic forces, where the carboxylic groups in the material replace phosphate (PO_4^{3-}) ions and form ionic bonds with calcium (Ca^{2+}) ions present in the hydroxyapatite (Yoshida et al. 2000; Fukuda et al. 2003). For decades, glass ionomer-based materials were the main option due to their ability to conciliate both good bonding ability to hypermineralized tissues and ideal elastic modulus (Zabeu et al., 2022; Boing et al. 2018). However, due to the high surface roughness and colour alteration over time (Boing et al. 2018), coupled with the emergence of new resinous materials, the use of ionomeric materials has experienced a decline in their recommendation. Numerous researchers still recommend the use of GICs in conjunction with periodontal procedures, such as root coverage techniques. It has also been reported that the application of GICs may enhance the attachment of periodontal fibres and facilitate the release of fluoride (Francisconi et al. 2009).

Resin materials are often chosen for the restoration of non-carious lesions due to their versatility, aesthetic appeal, and ability to bond effectively to the tooth structure, providing a durable and natural-looking solution (Fig. 7.4a, b). Also, monomeric materials offer more resistance compared to glass ionomers upon toothbrushing forces for abrasion lesions and resist more than GICs during acidic erosive episodes (Peumans et al. 2020). Despite the evolution of restorative materials, the restorative approach in these cases remains challenging, requiring further clinical studies to assess the longevity and marginal integrity of the tooth.

7.18 Laser Technology

Lasers have been thoroughly explored for their potential in treating DH through different mechanisms, rendering their application for this purpose an intriguing and controversial subject (Asnaashari and Moeini 2013; Kong et al. 2020; Pion et al. 2023). The use of lasers in treating DH involves several potential mechanisms, determined by the laser therapy utilized. The impact on the dentine surface during DH treatment varies significantly based on the irradiation parameters (especially wavelength and energy density), the duration of the treatment, and the laser's wavelength, which can vary between low and high intensity (Kong et al. 2020; Pion et al. 2023).

Based on these parameters, different mechanisms can be involved in the laser treatment for DH. These mechanisms include desensitization of nerve cells, dentine sealing, and anti-inflammatory effects (Pion et al. 2023). The low-power laser therapy has been suggested to have anti-inflammatory effects by stimulating cell activity, potentially influencing the inflammatory response, and diminishing the neural response to a hypersensitive stimulus (Kong et al. 2020; Pion et al. 2023). Furthermore, this type of laser can interact with the dental pulp, leading to an increase in odontoblastic activity and, consequently, to formation of a microscopically altered surface layer, which could act as a barrier to external stimuli, reducing the transmission of sensory signals to the nerve cells in the pulp, thereby alleviating pain associated with DH (Sgolastra et al. 2013; Kong et al. 2020).

Alternatively, the most common category of high-power laser for treating DH is the erbium family of lasers, which includes the erbium:yttrium–aluminium–garnet (Er:YAG), erbium, chromium:yttrium–scandium–gallium–garnet (Er,Cr:YSGG), and carbon dioxide (CO_2) laser. These lasers operate in the infrared spectrum, and their wavelengths are well-absorbed by water and hydroxyapatite, the primary mineral component of tooth enamel and dentine (Pion et al. 2023). The Nd:YAG laser, with power density parameters ranging from 0.3 to 2 W, has been reported to reduce discomfort immediately after application (Al-Sabbagh et al. 2009; Lopes and Aranha 2013) and exhibits an additional analgesic effect compared to other high-power lasers (Lin et al. 2013). Despite the limited number of studies, the Er,Cr:YSGG laser, with an output power varying from 0.25 to 0.5 W, has been shown to be effective in reducing DH when compared to placebo (Aranha and Eduardo 2012; Kong et al. 2020).

The GaAlAs diode laser, with a wavelength ranging from 780 nm (low power) to 980 nm (high power), stands as one of the most frequently employed lasers for DH treatment due to its cost-effectiveness and compact design. Despite demonstrating satisfactory results in both in vitro and clinical studies when used in high-power mode (Umberto et al. 2012; Rizzante et al. 2016), low-power utilization of the diode laser has garnered a greater number of promising outcomes in the published literature (Tolentino et al. 2022; Pion et al. 2023). With protocols ranging from 1 to 3 applications with 15 mW to 1 W of power and the combined use of desensitizing agents, the diode laser has demonstrated effectiveness in reducing pain after 3 and 6 months (Bal et al. 2015; Tolentino et al. 2022; Pion et al. 2023).

The long-term effectiveness of lasers compared to the other types of treatment approaches has also been favourably reported (Lopes and Aranha 2013; Tolentino et al. 2022; Pion et al. 2023). Furthermore, according to Pion et al. (2023), high-power lasers showed lower average pain scores after 3 months of treatment compared to low-power lasers on pretreatment pain (baseline); however, no significant differences were observed between the groups. Given the similar outcomes promoted by different types of lasers, low-power options, such as diode lasers, appear to be more cost-effective for clinicians. However, currently there is a lack of cost-effectiveness assessments, and additional long-term studies are required (Pion et al. 2023).

7.19 Combined Treatment of Lasers with Other Treatment Approaches

The combination of techniques, such as integrating laser technology with fluoride varnish or toothpaste, although not being a recommended clinical protocol, has been studied as a strategy in the treatment of DH. The rationale for this approach is the association of the combined effects, which may result in significantly better outcomes (Lin et al. 2013; Lopes and Aranha 2013; Bal et al. 2015; Tolentino et al. 2022). Dentine desensitizers with occlusive properties may be employed in conjunction with low-power lasers to concurrently seal the dentinal tubules and reduce neural stimulation levels. This dual action may, in turn, contribute to the initiation of tertiary dentine formation (Lopes and Aranha 2013; Rizzante et al. 2016).

It is important to note that, despite a considerable number of studies supporting the use of lasers for DH, the effectiveness of laser therapy varies due to heterogeneity among studies, lack of parameter standardization, and the subjectivity and personal experience of both the professional and the patient, making it not a clinically recommended protocol. Therefore, additional research is essential to establish standardized protocols and assess long-term outcomes. In comparison to traditional approaches, laser treatment for DH presents certain drawbacks, such as high cost, complexity of use, and a diminishing effectiveness over time, thereby limiting its clinical utility (Asnaashari and Moeini 2013). Furthermore, the efficacy and mechanism of action of laser therapy for DH remains a subject of considerable controversy and a potential placebo effect must be carefully considered (Sgolastra et al. 2013). As a definitive treatment for DH remains unclear, the combination of laser therapy with topical desensitizing agents may present a promising approach compared to either isolated treatment/technique, but clinical studies are still necessary.

7.20 Periodontal Plastic Surgery (Root Coverage Procedures)

Recession of the marginal tissues (gingival recession) has been reported to be associated with DH because of the exposure of the root surface to the oral environment. Several factors have been associated with gingival recession, such as anatomic characteristics, restorative procedures, habits, smoking, and even with the natural ageing process (Kassab and Cohen 2003; Chambrone and Tatakis 2016; Massaro et al. 2018). According to a recent systematic review, more than three-fourths of the worldwide population appear to present some level of gingival recession (Yadav et al. 2023).

Root coverage procedures associated with root scaling and the covering of the exposed root through surgical periodontal procedures have been reported to reduce or completely resolve DH over time (Orchardson and Gillam 2006; Lin and Gillam 2012; Kotsailidi et al. 2023). Nevertheless, despite promising results of root coverage procedures against the DH symptoms, the clinician should be aware that a thin periodontal biotype is more frequently affected by gingival recession and may tear during both probing and surgical intervention, making the root coverage a more challenging procedure than in a thicker biotype, in which higher mean gain or complete root coverage has been observed (Müller et al. 2000; Hwang and Wang 2006; Kim et al. 2020). Therefore, it is necessary for the clinician to be trained and to consider not only the root coverage aspect but also the resultant aesthetics together with the treatment of DH whilst bearing in mind that the aetiological factors that led to the root exposure must also be addressed (Ahmedbeyli et al. 2014; Cairo et al. 2014; Polack and Mahn 2013; West et al. 2013).

Three different gingival biotypes have been described in the published literature: (1) thin scalloped, (2) thick flat, and (3) thick scalloped (Zweers et al. 2014). Teeth in the thin scalloped category have the characteristics of a thin gingival tissue with a more pronounced contour of the gingival margin, with a greater height of the interproximal papilla and with an underlying thin buccal bone that can present fenestrations. The thick flat biotype category is characterized by thicker bone tissue surrounding the teeth and covered by a thick and smooth contour gingival tissue, which results in a small height of the papilla. The thick scalloped category displays the characteristics of the two other patterns (Zweers et al. 2014).

Moreover, to facilitate both the diagnosis and to assist the clinician on the correction of gingival recession defects, several classifications for gingival recession have been suggested, with the Miller classification system being one of the most widely used (Miller Jr 1985; Pini-Prato et al. 2010; Cairo et al. 2011; Cortellini and Bissada 2018; Pini Prato and Di Gianfilippo 2021) (Table 7.3). However, the Miller classification system disregarded some characteristics that were important to predict the success of the gingival recession treatment, such as the tissue thickness and the possible anomalies on the root surface (e.g., concavities due to the presence of

Table 7.3 Gingival recession classifications and characteristics

Cairo et al. classification	Miller classification	Characteristics
RT1	Class I	Marginal tissue recession that does not extend to the mucogingival junction (MGJ) with no interproximal tissue loss
	Class II	Marginal tissue recession that extends to or beyond the MGJ, with no periodontal attachment loss (bone or soft tissue) in the interdental area
RT2	Class III	Marginal tissue recession that extends to or beyond the MGJ with periodontal attachment loss in the interdental area or malpositioning of teeth
RT3	Class IV	Marginal tissue recession that extends to or beyond the MGJ with severe bone or soft tissue loss in the interdental area, to a level apically to the buccal/labial soft tissue margin and/or severely malpositioned teeth

Modified from Kassab and Cohen (2003)

Table 7.4 The 2018 Classification of Gingival Recession Defects and Gingival Phenotype

Gingival site				Tooth site	
	Recession depth	Gingival thickness	Keratinized tissue width	CEJ (A/B)[a]	Step (+/−)[b]
No recession					
RT1					
RT2					
RT3					

Modified from Cortellini and Bissada (2018)
[a]*CEJ* cemento-enamel junction. In this case, A is marked if CEJ can be detected, and B if it cannot be detected;
[b]in the "step column", + is marked if a cervical step >0.5 mm is present, or—if absent

non-carious cervical lesions, NCCLs) (Pini Prato and Di Gianfilippo 2021).

The classification of Cairo et al. (2011) also considered the interproximal attachment level and combined Miller's classes I and II into recession type (RT) 1, in which the treatment outcomes are favourable. Cases where the interproximal tissue are located at the same level or coronally to the midfacial recession were classified as RT2, whereas those where the interproximal tissue was apical to the midfacial recession were classified as RT3 (Cairo et al. 2011) (Table 7.3). Nonetheless, this classification also disregarded the presence of defects on the root surface (Pini-Prato et al. 2010) and the thickness of the gingival tissue (Zweers et al. 2014).

For this reason, in the 2017 World Workshop, the 2018 Classification of Gingival Recession Defects and Gingival Phenotype was proposed combining both previous classifications and anatomical characteristics (Cortellini and Bissada 2018) (Table 7.4). By using a 4 x 5 matrix, the authors based this classification on three major characteristics: (1) recession: based on the recession depth (in millimetres) and the classification of Cairo et al. (2011) described above; (2) tissue: based on the tissue thickness (Zweers et al. 2014) and the width of keratinized tissue present; and (3) root surface: based on the detectability of the cemento-enamel junction (CEJ) and presence of possible defects, such as NCCLs. This classification enabled the clinician to predict possible outcomes of the surgical procedure based on the type of defect whilst also considering the anatomical features.

Several materials and techniques have been reported in the published literature and these include guided tissue regeneration (GTR), coronally advanced flap and Emdogain (CAF + EMD), connective tissue graft (CTG), and free gingival graft (acellular dermal matrix allograft/mucograft, ADM) (Gillam 2014). Yet, regardless of the surgical procedures, associated techniques, flap design, or materials, the desired outcome for treating gingival recession defects is that the resulting gingival tissue covering the root surface must have the characteristics of a thick keratinized mucosa, enabling biofilm control without any change in the graft's position (e.g., apical direction).

As mentioned above, gingival recession naturally occurs during ageing (Chambrone and Tatakis 2016; Massaro et al. 2018), but it is important to state that, if an associated pathological factor that is aggravating the recession is not removed, untreated recession defects are likely to progress even in patients with good hygiene habits in the long-term (Chambrone and Tatakis 2016). Nonetheless, regardless of the used surgical technique, root coverage surgery has been reported to significantly reduce the frequency and the intensity of stimulated DH with a high and moderate level of evidence (Kotsailidi et al. 2023). Yet, in those cases with good biofilm control, absence of pathological factors that cause gingival recession, and absence of DH symptoms, root coverage surgery might not be necessary.

7.21 Innovations on Tooth Wear Management as Strategies for Treating DH

7.21.1 Protease Inhibitors

Host-derived proteolytic enzymes (also known as proteases), such as matrix metalloproteinases (MMPs) and cysteine cathepsins (CCs) were advocated to contribute to ETW progression since they hydrolyse the demineralized organic matrix (DOM) remaining over the dentine surface when enamel is irreversibly lost (Tjäderhane et al. 2013, 2015). The use of protease inhibitors is thus currently evaluated for the prevention or arrest of the DOM degradation, ETW and, supposedly, DH (see also Chap. 4). Chlorhexidine (CHX) (Magalhães et al. 2009; Kato et al. 2010a; Vertuan et al. 2021), iron sulphate ($FeSO_4$) (Kato et al. 2010b), epigallocatechin gallate (EGCG) (Magalhães et al. 2009; Kato et al. 2010a; Silveira et al. 2014), sodium fluoride (NaF) (Kato et al. 2010a, 2014; Silveira et al. 2014), anacardic acid (Silveira et al. 2014), proanthocyanidin (PA) (Boteon et al. 2017; Vertuan et al. 2021), quercetin (Jiang et al. 2020; Hong et al. 2022), 1,10-phenanthroline, trans-epoxysuccinyl-L-leucylamido-[4-guanidino] butane (E-64), and even combined quercetin and E64 (Yang et al. 2023) have been investigated.

Most MMP inhibitors act because of their ability to chelate metal ions, such as zinc in MMPs active site (Wojtowicz-Praga et al. 1997), and most CCs inhibitors work by binding to CCs' highly reactive thiol group through a thioether covalent bond (Yamamoto et al. 1991). Some protease inhibitors are capable of inhibiting both MMPs and CCs (Scaffa et al. 2012); furthermore, it is also speculated that CCs inhibition can also reduce MMPs activity as the CCs themselves are also believed to activate MMPs (Bafail et al. 2020). Some inhibitors still have a collagen crosslinking effect and could maybe enhance the mechanical properties of demineralized dentine (Epasinghe et al. 2014; Hong et al. 2022).

Several reviews are categorical in stating that the use of protease inhibitors leads to a significantly thicker DOM and to a reduced substance loss in the case of dentine erosive wear (Buzalaf et al. 2012, 2014, 2015; Tjäderhane et al. 2015). Nonetheless, further evidence, and especially that derived from randomized controlled clinical trials, are needed to endorse the use of such inhibitors for tooth wear management (Yang et al. 2023).

Regarding their effect in DH, it has been inferred that some protease inhibitors could also act as traditional desensitizers (Sales-Peres et al. 2011; Calabria et al. 2014), or they could be used in association with these desensitizers (Bhavan Ram et al. 2023). The studies evaluating the role of protease inhibitors on treating DH, or mainly on in vitro dentine permeability, are, however, scarce. Table 7.5 summarizes them, including the pioneers, conducted at a time when researchers were possibly unaware of the role of protease inhibitors on ETW and DH, since the knowledge of the identities and function of collagenolytic enzymes in dentine has accumulated only from the 2000s (Buzalaf et al. 2015).

Table 7.5 Summary of the studies evaluating the role of protease inhibitors on treating DH or mainly on in vitro dentine permeability

Studied substances	Comparisons	Findings	References
0.12% CHX[a] rinse	Placebo rinse 0.2% NaF rinse 0.12% CHX plus 0.2% NaF rinse	CHX and NaF rinses alone significantly reduced DH pain (quantified by applying successively decreasing temperature [20, 15, 10, 5, and 0 °C] intervals of water) to exposed dentin at 4 weeks compared to baseline; sequential CHX plus NaF rinse disclosed a significantly greater reduction compared to placebo, CHX and NaF alone at the 4-week interval	Lawson et al. (1991)
TiF_4 solution	Placebo solution	Eighty percent of the teeth with cervical DH responded (explorer and air blast stimuli) to the treatment with TiF_4 after 1 month and 55–84% thereafter (4, 8, and 12 months), compared to no response in any of the placebo-treated teeth	Charvat et al. (1995)
1% TiF_4 solution 0.5% TiF_4 solution 0.1% TiF_4 solution	NaF solution APF solution Deionized water	Smear layer formation considerably reduced dentinal permeability of extracted mandibular molars dentine discs; fluoride or deionized water application to smeared surfaces did not cause any significant change in hydraulic conductance; after citric acid application, lower permeability values were observed for 1%, 0.5%, and 0.1% TiF_4 and APF groups when compared to the control and NaF groups	Kazemi et al. (1999)
$FeSO_4$ gel (10 mmol/L $FeSO_4$)	1.23% APF gel 3% potassium oxalate gel	$FeSO_4$ gel (applied after 37% phosphoric acid and before 6% citric acid) reduced dentine permeability of human dentine discs similarly to the comparisons; they produced significantly lower reduction in permeability when compared to presence of smear layer	Sales-Peres et al. (2011)
TiF_4 varnish TiF_4 solution (2.45% F)	NaF varnish NaF solution (2.45% F) 3% potassium oxalate gel Placebo varnish (F free) No treatment (control)	All treatments were effective in reducing dentine hydraulic conductance compared with the control immediately after the application; only the potassium oxalate and NaF varnish significantly differed from placebo varnish; same results were found after 6% citric acid challenge; both NaF varnish and potassium oxalate gel reduced the dentine hydraulic conductance similarly to the presence of smear layer. TiF_4 solution and varnish did not differ from the placebo varnish	Calabria et al. (2014)

(continued)

Table 7.5 (continued)

Studied substances	Comparisons	Findings	References
nHAp synthesized from OS	CPP-ACP with 15% PA pretreatment CPP-ACP without 15% PA pretreatment	OS-nHAp and PA/OS-nHAp groups showed significantly superior tubule occlusion, deeper penetration, and lower permeability compared to CPP-ACP; PA pretreatment accentuated mineral deposition on demineralized dentine; citric acid challenge eroded only the surface mineralized layer in both OS-nHAp and PA/OS-nHAp groups, although, the tubular plugs, intratubular precipitates and dentine permeability remained unaffected compared to CPP-ACP	Bhavan Ram et al. (2023)

[a]*APF* Acidulated phosphate fluoride, *CHX* chlorhexidine, *CPP-ACP* Casein phosphopeptide-amorphous calcium phosphate, $FeSO_4$ Iron sulphate, *NaF* Sodium fluoride, *nHAp* Nano-hydroxyapatite, *OS* Oyster shell, *PA* Proanthocyanidin, TiF_4 Titanium tetrafluoride

Despite the results presented above, the authors are currently unaware of any published study that has assessed whether protease inhibitors have a simultaneous effect on reducing ETW and on reducing the dentine hydraulic conductance or on DH pain per se. One suggestion would be to proceed with in situ studies and, when justified, clinical trials. Depending on these results, the use of these protease inhibitors could be included in the management of ETW as a strategy for treating DH.

7.22 Conclusions

Given this wide range of agents and procedures used to treat DH, it would be unreasonable for the clinician to expect that one product would resolve every aspect of the problem or that these treatment strategies would be appropriate for every individual. In general, depending on the desensitizing agent used to treat the problem and on the most painful form of stimulus (e.g., air blast, tactile, or cold), in-office treatments are successful in treating DH in patients with a localized severe problem in one or more teeth. Conversely, OTC products are recommended for mild to moderate pain or generalized DH and they usually demonstrate a reduction in DH over time. The main advantage of using OTC products is that they are easily available and more affordable than *in-office* products. Conversely, longer periods of time are required for the remission of symptoms (2–4 weeks), whilst in-office products might promote instant DH relief (see also Chap. 8).

Despite comparing the outcomes of studies on DH agents being problematic due to their high heterogeneity, reasonable evidence is available to guide the clinician on the decision-making process of choosing the most appropriate agent for each case. Additionally, evidence is also available to help the clinician to effectively diagnose DH, control the aetiological factors associated with the development of the condition, and monitor the patient over time. Nonetheless, it cannot be overstressed that following these steps still is the key condition that needs to be addressed to achieve a successful and long-lasting result.

7.23 Future Trends

Currently, there are two major concerns that need to be addressed in the field of DH:

1. The need for desensitizing agents able to be incorporated into affordable OTC products with fast-acting desensitizing effects that can mineralize the dental tissue as well as precipitate acid-resistant minerals onto the dentine, such as FAp. For this reason, FCSPS glasses maybe the best available agent for the use in DH so far, with promising results. However,

its cost might be limiting for some populations, especially in underdeveloped and developing countries.

2. There is also a need for standardizing the conduction of randomized clinical trials; otherwise, a comparison between studies will be more difficult as the number of studies with different methodologies increases over time.

References

Abdollahi A, Jalalian EJ. Effectiveness of two desensitizer materials, potassium nitrate and fluoride varnish in relieving hypersensitivity after crown preparation. Contemp Dent Pract. 2019;20(4):489–93.

Abuzinadah SH, Alhaddad AJ. A randomized clinical trial of dentin hypersensitivity reduction over one month after a single topical application of comparable materials. Sci Rep. 2021;11(1):6793.

Addy M, Mostafa P. Dentine hypersensitivity. II. Effects produced by the uptake in vitro of toothpastes onto dentine. J Oral Rehabil. 1989;16(1):35–48.

Agheli N, De Faria NG, Maia RR, Siddanna GD, Inglehart MR. Dentists' education, knowledge, and professional behavior concerning the diagnosis and treatment of dentin hypersensitivity: an exploration. J Dent Educ. 2023;87(12):1705–17.

Agnihotri Y, Pragada NP, Patri G, Thajuraj PK. The effect of CPP-ACP on remineralization of artificial caries like lesions: an in vitro study. Indian J Multidiscip Dent. 2012;2(1):366.

Ahmedbeyli C, Ipçi ŞD, Cakar G, Kuru BE, Yılmaz S. Clinical evaluation of coronally advanced flap with or without acellular dermal matrix graft on complete defect coverage for the treatment of multiple gingival recessions with thin tissue biotype. J Clin Periodontol. 2014;41(3):303–10.

Albar NH. Efficacy of GLUMA for the treatment of dentin hypersensitivity compared to lasers: a systematic review. J Contemp Dent Pract. 2022;23(10):1057–65.

Al-Sabbagh M, Brown A, Thomas MV. In-office treatment of dentinal hypersensitivity. Dent Clin N Am. 2009;53(1):47–60.

Amini P, Miner M, Sagel PA, Gerlach RW. Comparative effects of 1.5% oxalate strips versus 5% potassium nitrate dentifrice on dentin hypersensitivity. Compend Contin Educ Dent. 2016;37(1):e21–5.

Anderson CJ, Kugel G, Zou Y, Ferrari M, Gerlach R. A randomized, controlled, two-month pilot trial of stannous fluoride dentifrice versus sodium fluoride dentifrice after oxalate treatment for dentinal hypersensitivity. Clin Oral Investig. 2020;24(11):4043–9.

Aparna S, Setty S, Thakur S. Comparative efficacy of two treatment modalities for dentinal hypersensitivity: a clinical trial. Indian J Dent Res. 2010;21:544–8.

Aranha AC, Eduardo C de P. Effects of Er:YAG and Er,Cr:YSGG lasers on dentine hypersensitivity. Short-term clinical evaluation. Lasers Med Sci. 2012;27(4):813–8.

Arantes DC, Limeira FIR, Yamauti M, Moreira AN, Abreu LG, Magalhães CS. Comparison of clinical efficacy of Pro-Argin and NovaMin toothpastes in relieving dentin hypersensitivity: a systematic review and meta-analysis. Oral Health Prev Dent. 2019;17(5):403–12.

Arshad S, Zaidi SJA, Farooqui WA. Comparative efficacy of BioMin-F, Colgate sensitive pro-relief and Sensodyne rapid action in relieving dentin hypersensitivity: a randomized controlled trial. BMC Oral Health. 2021;21(1):498.

Asaizumi M, Karlinsey RL, Mackey AC, Kato T, Kuga T. In vitro assessments of white-spot lesions treated with NaF plus tricalcium phosphate (TCP) toothpastes using microtomography (micro-CT). J Dent Oral Hyg. 2013;5(7):68–76.

Ashwini S, Swatika K, Kamala DN. Comparative evaluation of desensitizing efficacy of dentifrice containing 5% fluoro calcium phosphosilicate versus 5% calcium sodium phosphosilicate: a randomized controlled clinical trial. Contemp Clin Dent. 2018;9(3):330–6.

Asnaashari M, Moeini M. Effectiveness of lasers in the treatment of dentin hypersensitivity. J Lasers Med Sci. 2013;4(1):1–7.

Ayad F, Ayad N, Delgado E, Zhang YP, DeVizio W, Cummins D, Mateo LR. Comparing the efficacy in providing instant relief of dentin hypersensitivity of a new toothpaste containing 8.0% arginine, calcium carbonate, and 1450 ppm fluoride to a benchmark desensitizing toothpaste containing 2% potassium ion and 1450 ppm fluoride, and to a control toothpaste with 1450 ppm fluoride: a three-day clinical study in Mississauga, Canada. J Clin Dent. 2009;20(4):115–22.

Ayad F, Ayad N, Vazquez J, Zhang YP, Mateo LR, Cummins D. Use of a toothpaste containing 8% arginine and calcium carbonate for immediate and lasting relief of dentin hypersensitivity: a simple and effective in-office procedure. Am J Dent. 2018;31(3):135–40.

Azarpazhooh A, Limeback H. Clinical efficacy of casein derivatives: a systematic review of the literature. J Am Dent Assoc. 2008;139(7):915–24.

Bae JH, Kim YK, Myung SK. Desensitizing toothpaste versus placebo for dentin hypersensitivity: a systematic review and meta-analysis. J Clin Periodontol. 2015;42(2):131–41.

Bafail A, Carrilho MR, Kishen A, Prakki A. Effect of protease inhibitor specificity on dentin matrix properties. J Mech Behav Biomed Mater. 2020;109:103861.

Bal MV, Keskiner İ, Sezer U, Açıkel C, Saygun I. Comparison of low-level laser and arginine-calcium carbonate alone or combination in the treatment of dentin hypersensitivity: a randomized split-mouth clinical study. Photomed Laser Surg. 2015;33(4):200–5.

Bekes K, Heinzelmann K, Lettner S, Schaller HG. Efficacy of desensitizing products containing 8% arginine and calcium carbonate for hypersensitivity relief in

MIH-affected molars: an 8-week clinical study. Clin Oral Investig. 2017;21(7):2311–7.

Bhavan Ram U, Sujatha V, Vidhya S, Jayasree R, Mahalaxmi S. Oyster shell-derived nano-hydroxyapatite and proanthocyanidin pretreatment on dentinal tubule occlusion and permeability before and after acid challenge-an in vitro study. J Mater Sci Mater Med. 2023;34(4):17.

Boing TF, de Geus JL, Wambier LM, Loguercio AD, Reis A, Gomes OMM. Are glass-ionomer cement restorations in cervical lesions more long-lasting than resin-based composite resins? A systematic review and meta-analysis. J Adhes Dent. 2018;20(5):435–52.

Boneta AR, Ramirez K, Naboa J, Mateo LR, Stewart B, Panagokos F, De Vizio W. Efficacy in reducing dentine hypersensitivity of a regimen using a toothpaste containing 8% arginine and calcium carbonate, a mouthwash containing 0.8% arginine, pyrophosphate and PVM/MA copolymer and a toothbrush compared to potassium and negative control regimens: an eight-week randomized clinical trial. J Dent. 2013;41(Suppl 1):S42–9.

Boteon AP, Prakki A, Rabelo Buzalaf MA, Rios D, Honorio HM. Effect of different concentrations and application times of proanthocyanidin gels on dentin erosion. Am J Dent. 2017;30(2):96–100.

Brännström M, Åström A. A study on the mechanism on pain elicited from the dentin. J Dent Res. 1964;43:619–25.

Brauer DS, Karpukhina N, O'Donnell MD, Law RV, Hill RG. Fluoride-containing bioactive glasses: effect of glass design and structure on degradation, pH and apatite formation in simulated body fluid. Acta Biomater. 2010;6:3275–82.

Burnett GR, Gallob JT, Milleman KR, Mason S, Patil A, Budhawant C, Milleman JL. Potassium oxalate oral rinses for long-term relief from dentinal hypersensitivity: three randomised controlled studies. J Dent. 2018;70:23–30.

Buzalaf MA, Kato MT, Hannas AR. The role of matrix metalloproteinases in dental erosion. Adv Dent Res. 2012;24(2):72–6.

Buzalaf MA, Magalhães AC, Wiegand A. Alternatives to fluoride in the prevention and treatment of dental erosion. Monogr Oral Sci. 2014;25:244–52.

Buzalaf MA, Charone S, Tjäderhane L. Role of host-derived proteinases in dentine caries and erosion. Caries Res. 2015;49(Suppl 1):30–7.

Cai F, Shen P, Morgan MV, Reynolds EC. Remineralization of enamel subsurface lesions in-situ by sugar free lozenges containing casein phosphopeptide—amorphous calcium phosphate. Aust Dent J. 2003;48:240–3.

Cairo F, Nieri M, Cincinelli S, Mervelt J, Pagliaro U. The interproximal clinical attachment level to classify gingival recessions and predict root coverage outcomes: an explorative and reliability study. J Clin Periodontol. 2011;38(7):661–6.

Cairo F, Nieri M, Pagliaro U. Efficacy of periodontal plastic surgery procedures in the treatment of localized facial gingival recessions. A systematic review. J Clin Periodontol. 2014;41(Suppl 15):S44–62.

Calabria M, Porfirio R, Fernandes S, Wang L, Buzalaf M, Pereira J, Magalhães A. Comparative in vitro effect of TiF4 to NaF and potassium oxalate on reduction of dentin hydraulic conductance. Oper Dent. 2014;39(4):427–32.

Canadian Advisory Board on Dentin Hypersensitivity. Consensus-based recommendations for the diagnosis and management of dentin hypersensitivity. J Can Dent Assoc. 2003;69(4):221–6.

Castelo R, Attik N, Catirse ABCEB, Pradelle-Plasse N, Tirapelli C, Grosgogeat B. Is there a preferable management for root caries in middle-aged and older adults? A systematic review. Br Dent J. 2021. https://doi.org/10.1038/s41415-021-3003-2.

Chałas R, Wójcik-Chęcińska I, Zamościńska J, Bachanek T. Assessment of pain intensity in patients with dentin hypersensitivity after application of prophylaxis paste based on calcium sodium phosphosilicate formula. Med Sci Monit. 2015;21:2950–5.

Chambrone L, Tatakis DN. Long-term outcomes of untreated buccal gingival recessions: a systematic review and meta-analysis. J Periodontol. 2016;87(7):796–808.

Champaiboon C, Ongphichetmetha N, Lertpimonchai A. Bioactive glass and arginine dentifrices reduce root sensitivity during daily activities following non-surgical periodontal therapy: a randomized controlled trial. J Periodontol. 2024;95(2):135–45. https://doi.org/10.1002/JPER.23-0197.

Chang HH, Guo MK, Kasten FH, Chang MC, Huang GF, Wang YL, Wang RS, Jeng JH. Stimulation of glutathione depletion, ROS production and cell cycle arrest of dental pulp cells and gingival epithelial cells by HEMA. Biomaterials. 2005;26(7):745–53.

Chapman NR, Jones SB, Bahal P, He T, Drake P, Zou Y, West NX. The ability of a potassium oxalate gel strip to occlude human dentine tubules; a novel in vitro: in situ study. J Dent. 2020;100:103437.

Charig AJ, Chapin CA, Major EE, Thong S, Winston AE. Mechanism of action of a desensitizing fluoride toothpaste delivering calcium and phosphate ingredients in the treatment of dental hypersensitivity. Part I: in vitro SEM, EDX, profilometry, and dentin permeability studies. Compend Contin Educ Dent. 2009;30(8) Online access only.

Charvat J, Söremark R, Li J, Vacek J. Titanium tetrafluoride for treatment of hypersensitive dentine. Swed Dent J. 1995;19(1–2):41–6.

Chebel F, Zogheib CM, Baba NZ, Corbani KA. Clinical comparative evaluation of Nd:YAG laser and a new varnish containing casein phosphopeptides-amorphous calcium phosphate for the treatment of dentin hypersensitivity: a prospective study. J Prosthodont. 2018;27(9):860–7.

Chen X, Chen X, Brauer DS, Wilson RM, Law RV, Hill RG, Karpukhina N. Sodium is not essential for high bioactivity of glasses. Int J Appl Glas Sci. 2017;8(4):428–37.

Cochrane NJ, Shen P, Yuan Y, Reynolds EC. Ion release from calcium and fluoride containing dental varnishes. Aust Dent J. 2014;59(1):100–5.

Collins JR, Richardson D, Sotero K, Mateo LR, Mauriz I. Beneficial effects of an arginine-calcium carbonate desensitizing paste for treatment of dentin hypersensitivity. Am J Dent. 2013;26(2):63–7.

Cortellini P, Bissada NF. Mucogingival conditions in the natural dentition: narrative review, case definitions, and diagnostic considerations. J Periodontol. 2018;89(Suppl 1):S204–13.

Costa T, Rezende M, Sakamoto A, Bittencourt B, Dalzochio P, Loguercio AD, Reis A. Influence of adhesive type and placement technique on postoperative sensitivity in posterior composite restorations. Oper Dent. 2017;42(2):143–54.

Cummins D. Recent advances in dentin hypersensitivity: clinically proven treatments for instant and lasting sensitivity relief. Am J Dent. 2010;23 Spec No A:3A–13A.

Cunha-Cruz J, Wataha JC, Zhou L, Manning W, Trantow M, Bettendorf MM, Heaton LJ, Berg J. Treating dentin hypersensitivity: therapeutic choices made by dentists of the northwest PRECEDENT network. J Am Dent Assoc. 2010;141(9):1097–105.

da Rosa WL, Lund RG, Piva E, da Silva AF. The effectiveness of current dentin desensitizing agents used to treat dental hypersensitivity: a systematic review. Quintessence Int. 2013;44(7):535–46.

Das CA, James EP, Jayasree S, Parvathy V, Vidya KG, Varughese A, Rajesh V, Balan P. Effect of iontophoresis on the effectiveness of nano-hydroxyapatite and pro-argin in in-office treatment of dentin hypersensitivity: a split-mouth randomized clinical trial. Cureus. 2023;15(12):e50990.

de Groot AC, Rustemeyer T. 2-hydroxyethyl methacrylate (HEMA): a clinical review of contact allergy and allergic contact dermatitis—part 1. Introduction, epidemiology, case series and case reports. Contact Derm. 2023;89(6):401–33.

de Groot AC, Rustemeyer T. 2-hydroxyethyl methacrylate (HEMA): a clinical review of contact allergy and allergic contact dermatitis. Part 2. Cross- and co-sensitization, other skin reactions to HEMA, position of HEMA among (meth)acrylates, sensitivity as screening agent, presence of HEMA in commercial products and practical information on patch test procedures. Contact Derm. 2024;90(1):1–16.

Ding J, Zhu X, Lin Q, Lin L, Yang Z, Zhu S. Effects of arginine-calcium carbonate pretreatment on the remineralizing and bonding performance of phosphorylated dentin. J Mech Behav Biomed Mater. 2023;140:105718.

Docimo R, Montesani L, Maturo P, Costacurta M, Bartolino M, DeVizio W, Zhang YP, Cummins D, Dibart S, Mateo LR. Comparing the efficacy in reducing dentin hypersensitivity of a new toothpaste containing 8.0% arginine, calcium carbonate, and 1.450 ppm fluoride to a commercial sensitive toothpaste containing 2% potassium ion: an eight-week clinical study in Rome, Italy. J Clin Dent. 2009a;20(1):17–22.

Docimo R, Montesani L, Maturo P, Costacurta M, Bartolino M, Zhang YP, DeVizio W, Delgado E, Cummins D, Dibart S, Mateo LR. Comparing the efficacy in reducing dentin hypersensitivity of a new toothpaste containing 8.0% arginine, calcium carbonate, and 1.450 ppm fluoride to a benchmark commercial desensitizing toothpaste containing 2% potassium ion: an eight-week clinical study in Rome, Italy. J Clin Dent. 2009b;20(4):137–43.

Dong Z, Chang J, Deng Y, Joiner A. Tricalcium silicate induced mineralization for occlusion of dentinal tubules. Aust Dent J. 2011;56(2):175–80.

Du Min Q, Bian Z, Jiang H, Greenspan DC, Burwell AK, Zhong J, Tai BJ. Clinical evaluation of a dentifrice containing calcium sodium phosphosilicate (NovaMin) for the treatment of dentin hypersensitivity. Am J Dent. 2008;21(4):210–4.

Eliades G, Mantzourani M, Labella R, Mutti B, Sharma D. Interactions of dentine desensitisers with human dentine: morphology and composition. J Dent. 2013;41(Suppl 4):S28–39.

Epasinghe DJ, Yiu CK, Burrow MF, Tsoi JK, Tay FR. Effect of flavonoids on the mechanical properties of demineralised dentine. J Dent. 2014;42(9):1178–84.

Exarchou C, Betsani I, Sakellari D, Chatzopoulou D, Gillam D. A survey of dentists in the management of dentine hypersensitivity: a questionnaire-based study. Eur J Dent. 2019;13(3):383–90.

França IL, Sallum EA, Do Vale HF, Casati MZ, Sallum AW, Stewart B. Efficacy of a combined in-office/home-use desensitizing system containing 8% arginine and calcium carbonate in reducing dentin hypersensitivity: an 8-week randomized clinical study. Am J Dent. 2015;28(1):45–50.

Francisconi LF, Graeff MS, Martins L de M, Franco EB, Mondelli RF, Francisconi PA, Pereira JC. The effects of occlusal loading on the margins of cervical restorations. J Am Dent Assoc. 2009;140(10):1275–82.

Francisconi-Dos-Rios LF, Dantas LM, Calabria MP, Pereira JC, Mosquim V, Wang L. Obliterating potential of active products for dentin hypersensitivity treatment under an erosive challenge. J Dent. 2021;112:103745.

Fu Y, Li X, Que K, Wang M, Hu D, Mateo LR, DeVizio W, Zhang YP. Instant dentin hypersensitivity relief of a new desensitizing dentifrice containing 8.0% arginine, a high cleaning calcium carbonate system and 1.450 ppm fluoride: a 3-day clinical study in Chengdu, China. Am J Dent. 2010;23(Spec A):20A–7A.

Fukuda R, Yoshida Y, Nakayama Y, Okazaki M, Inoue S, Sano H, Suzuki K, Shintani H, Van Meerbeek B. Bonding efficacy of polyalkenoic acids to hydroxyapatite, enamel and dentin. Biomaterials. 2003;24(11):1861–7.

Gandolfi MG, Taddei P, Tinti A, Prati C. Apatite-forming ability (bioactivity) of ProRoot MTA. Int Endod J. 2010;43(10):917–29.

Ganss C, Klimek J, Schlueter N. Erosion/abrasion-preventing potential of NaF and F/Sn/chitosan toothpastes in dentine and impact of the organic matrix. Caries Res. 2014;48(2):163–9.
Gillam DG. Treatment approaches for dentin hypersensitivity. In: Taha S, Clarkson BH, editors. Clinician's guide to the diagnosis and management of tooth sensitivity. Berlin/Heidelberg: Springer; 2014. p. 51–80. Chapter 5.
Gillam DG, Bulman JS, Jackson RJ, Newman HN. Efficacy of a potassium nitrate mouthwash in alleviating cervical dentine sensitivity (CDS). J Clin Periodontol. 1996;23(11):993–7.
Gillam DG, Bulman JS, Eijkman MA, Newman HN. Dentists' perceptions of dentine hypersensitivity and knowledge of its treatment. J Oral Rehabil. 2002a;29(3):219–25.
Gillam DG, Tang JY, Mordan NJ, Newman HN. The effects of a novel bioglass dentifrice on dentine sensitivity: a scanning electron microscopy investigation. J Oral Rehabil. 2002b;29(4):305–13. Erratum in: J Oral Rehabil 2003;30(4):446.
Gillam D, Chesters R, Attrill D, Brunton P, Slater M, Strand P, Whelton H, Bartlett D. Dentine hypersensitivity—guidelines for the management of a common oral health problem. Dent Update. 2013;40(7):514–516, 518–20, 523–4.
Glockner K. What are the unmet needs in the dental office/at home to treat dentin hypersensitivity? Clin Oral Investig. 2013;17(Suppl 1):S61–2.
Grandizoli D, Renzo A, Sakae LO, Lopes RM, Zezell DM, Aranha A, Scaramucci T. Assessment of the ability of desensitizing and conventional mouth rinses to promote dentin tubule occlusion. Oper Dent. 2022;47(5):549–61.
Grover V, Kumar A, Jain A, Chatterjee A, Grover HS, Pandit N, Satpathy A, Madhavan Pillai BR, Melath A, Dhruvakumar D, Thakur R, Joshi NV, Deshpande N, Dadlani H, Meenakshi AA, Ashok KP, Reddy KV, Bhasin MT, Salaria SK, Verma A, Gaikwad RP, Darekar H, Amirisetty R, Phadnaik M, Karemore V, Dhulipalla R, Mody D, Rao TS, Chakarpani S, Ranganath V. ISP good clinical practice recommendations for the management of dentin hypersensitivity. J Indian Soc Periodontol. 2022;26(4):307–33.
Hall C, Mason S, Cooke J. Exploratory randomised controlled clinical study to evaluate the comparative efficacy of two occluding toothpastes—a 5% calcium sodium phosphosilicate toothpaste and an 8% arginine/calcium carbonate toothpaste—for the longer-term relief of dentine hypersensitivity. J Dent. 2017;60:36–43.
Hamlin D, Williams KP, Delgado E, Zhang YP, DeVizio W, Mateo LR. Clinical evaluation of the efficacy of a desensitizing paste containing 8% arginine and calcium carbonate for the in-office relief of dentin hypersensitivity associated with dental prophylaxis. Am J Dent. 2009;22(Spec A):16A–20A.
Handa A, Chengappa D, Sharma P, Handa JK. Effectiveness of Clinpro Tooth Crème in comparison with MI Varnish with RECALDENT™ for treatment of white spot lesions: a randomized controlled trial. Clin Oral Investig. 2023;27(4):1473–81.
Hanning M, Hanning C. Nanomaterials in preventive dentistry. Nat Nanotechnol. 2010;5(8):565–9.
Hench LL. The story of bioglass. J Mater Sci Mater Med. 2006;17(11):967–78.
Hill R. An alternative view of the degradation of bioglass. J Mater Sci Lett. 1996;15:1122–5.
Hirsiger C, Schmidlin PR, Michaelis M, Hirsch C, Attin T, Heumann C, Doméjean S, Gernhardt CR. Efficacy of 8% arginine on dentin hypersensitivity: a multicenter clinical trial in 273 patients over 24 weeks. J Dent. 2019;83:1–6.
Hong DW, Chen LB, Lin XJ, Attin T, Yu H. Dual function of quercetin as an MMP inhibitor and crosslinker in preventing dentin erosion and abrasion: an in situ/in vivo study. Dent Mater. 2022;38(12):e297–307.
Hu D, Stewart B, Mello S, Arvanitidou L, Panagakos F, De Vizio W, Zhang YP, Mateo LR, Yin W. Efficacy of a mouthwash containing 0.8% arginine, PVM/MA copolymer, pyrophosphates, and 0.05% sodium fluoride compared to a negative control mouthwash on dentin hypersensitivity reduction. A randomized clinical trial. J Dent. 2013;41(Suppl 1):S26–33.
Hu ML, Zheng G, Zhang YD, Yan X, Li XC, Lin H. Effect of desensitizing toothpastes on dentine hypersensitivity: a systematic review and meta-analysis. J Dent. 2018;75:12–21.
Hu ML, Zheng G, Lin H, Yang M, Zhang YD, Han JM. Network meta-analysis on the effect of desensitizing toothpastes on dentine hypersensitivity. J Dent. 2019;88:103170.
Hughes N, Mason S, Jeffery P, Welton H, Tobin M, O'Shea C, Browne M. A comparative clinical study investigating the efficacy of a test dentifrice containing 8% strontium acetate and 1,040 ppm sodium fluoride versus a marketed control dentifrice containing 8% arginine, calcium carbonate, and 1,450 ppm sodium monofluorophosphate in reducing dentinal hypersensitivity. J Clin Dent. 2010;21(2):49–55.
Hwang D, Wang HL. Flap thickness as a predictor of root coverage: a systematic review. J Periodontol. 2006;77(10):1625–34.
Jackson RJ. Potential treatment modalities for dentine hypersensitivity: home use products. In: Addy M, Edgar WM, Orchardson R, editors. Tooth wear and sensitivity. London: Martin Dunitz; 2000. p. 328–38.
Jang JH, Oh S, Kim HJ, Kim DS. A randomized clinical trial for comparing the efficacy of desensitizing toothpastes on the relief of dentin hypersensitivity. Sci Rep. 2023;13(1):5271.
Jiang N, Hong DW, Attin T, Cheng H, Yu H. Quercetin reduces erosive dentin wear: evidence from laboratory and clinical studies. Dent Mater. 2020;36(11):1430–6.
Jiang R, Xu Y, Wang F, Lin H. Effectiveness and cytotoxicity of two desensitizing agents: a dentin permeability measurement and dentin barrier testing in vitro study. BMC Oral Health. 2022;22(1):391.

João-Souza SH, Machado AC, Lopes RM, Zezell DM, Scaramucci T, Aranha ACC. Effectiveness and acid/tooth brushing resistance of in-office desensitizing treatments-a hydraulic conductance study. Arch Oral Biol. 2018;96:130–6.

João-Souza SH, Scaramucci T, Bühler Borges A, Lussi A, Saads Carvalho T, Corrêa Aranha AC. Influence of desensitizing and anti-erosive toothpastes on dentine permeability: an in vitro study. J Dent. 2019;89:103176.

Kapferer I, Pflug C, Kisielewsky I, Giesinger J, Beier US, Dumfahrt H. Instant dentin hypersensitivity relief of a single topical application of an in-office desensitizing paste containing 8% arginine and calcium carbonate: a split-mouth, randomized-controlled study. Acta Odontol Scand. 2013;71(3–4):994–9.

Karim BF, Gillam DG. The efficacy of strontium and potassium toothpastes in treating dentine hypersensitivity: a systematic review. Int J Dent. 2013;2013:573258.

Karlinsey RL, Mackey AC, Stookey GK. In vitro remineralization efficacy of NaF systems containing unique forms of calcium. Am J Dent. 2009a;22(3):185–8.

Karlinsey RL, Mackey AC, Stookey GK, Pfarrer AM. In vitro assessments of experimental NaF dentifrices containing a prospective calcium phosphate technology. Am J Dent. 2009b;22(3):180–4.

Karlinsey RL, Mackey AC, Walker ER, Frederick KE. Surfactant-modified beta-TCP: structure, properties, and in vitro remineralization of subsurface enamel lesions. J Mater Sci Mater Med. 2010;21(7):2009–20.

Karlinsey RL, Mackey AC, Schwandt CS. Effects on dentin treated with eluted multi-mineral varnish in vitro. Open Dent J. 2012;6:157–63.

Kassab MM, Cohen RE. The etiology and prevalence of gingival recession. J Am Dent Assoc. 2003;134(2):220–5.

Kato MT, Leite AL, Hannas AR, Buzalaf MA. Gels containing MMP inhibitors prevent dental erosion in situ. J Dent Res. 2010a;89(5):468–72.

Kato MT, Leite AL, Hannas AR, Oliveira RC, Pereira JC, Tjäderhane L, Buzalaf MA. Effect of iron on matrix metalloproteinase inhibition and on the prevention of dentine erosion. Caries Res. 2010b;44(3):309–16.

Kato MT, Bolanho A, Zarella BL, Salo T, Tjäderhane L, Buzalaf MA. Sodium fluoride inhibits MMP-2 and MMP-9. J Dent Res. 2014;93(1):74–7.

Kazemi RB, Sen BH, Spångberg LS. Permeability changes of dentine treated with titanium tetrafluoride. J Dent. 1999;27(7):531–8.

Kijsamanmith K, Banomyong D, Burrow MF, Kanchanasantikul P, Wipawiwat S, Srikam S, Laojarungphesatchakorn S. Effect of conventional and acid-modified casein phosphopeptide-amorphous calcium phosphate crèmes on dentin permeability before and after acid challenge. Oper Dent. 2019;44(5):530–5.

Kim DM, Bassir SH, Nguyen TT. Effect of gingival phenotype on the maintenance of periodontal health: an American Academy of Periodontology best evidence review. J Periodontol. 2020;91(3):311–38.

Kleinberg I. SensiStat. A new saliva-based composition for simple and effective treatment of dentinal sensitivity pain. Dent Today. 2002;21(12):42–7.

Kong Y, Lei Y, Li S, Zhang Y, Han J, Hu M. Network meta-analysis of the desensitizing effects of lasers in patients with dentine hypersensitivity. Clin Oral Investig. 2020;24(6):1917–28.

Kotsailidi EA, Michelogiannakis D, Barmak AB, Madianos P, Caton JG, Tsigarida A. Root coverage surgery for dentin hypersensitivity reduction: a systematic review and meta-analysis of randomized controlled trials. Quintessence Int. 2023;54(6):484–97.

Kovrlija I, Locs J, Loca D. Octacalcium phosphate: innovative vehicle for the local biologically active substance delivery in bone regeneration. Acta Biomater. 2021;135:27–47.

Kowalczyk A, Botuliński B, Jaworska M, Kierklo A, Pawińska M, Dabrowska E. Evaluation of the product based on Recaldent technology in the treatment of dentin hypersensitivity. Adv Med Sci. 2006;51(Suppl 1):40–2.

Lata S, Varghese NO, Varughese JM. Remineralization potential of fluoride and amorphous calcium phosphate-casein phosphopeptide on enamel lesions: an in vitro comparative evaluation. J Conserv Dent. 2010;13(1):42–6.

Lawson K, Gross KB, Overman PR, Anderson D. Effectiveness of chlorhexidine and sodium fluoride in reducing dentin hypersensitivity. J Dent Hyg. 1991;65(7):340–4.

Lin YH, Gillam DG. The prevalence of root sensitivity following periodontal therapy: a systematic review. Int J Dent. 2012;2012:407023.

Lin PY, Cheng YW, Chu CY, Chien KL, Lin CP, Tu YK. In-office treatment for dentin hypersensitivity: a systematic review and network meta-analysis. J Clin Periodontol. 2013;40(1):53–64.

Litkowski L, Greenspan DC. A clinical study of the effect of calcium sodium phosphosilicate on dentin hypersensitivity—proof of principle. J Clin Dent. 2010;21(3):77–81.

Lopes AO, Aranha AC. Comparative evaluation of the effects of Nd:YAG laser and a desensitizer agent on the treatment of dentin hypersensitivity: a clinical study. Photomed Laser Surg. 2013;31(3):132–8.

Lopes RM, Scaramucci T, Walker CL, Feitosa SA, Aranha ACC. In situ evaluation of desensitizing toothpastes for protecting against erosive tooth wear and its characterization. Clin Oral Investig. 2021;25(12):6857–70.

Lussi A, Carvalho TS. The future of fluorides and other protective agents in erosion prevention. Caries Res. 2015;49(Suppl 1):18–29.

Lynch E, Brauer DS, Karpukhina N, Gillam DG, Hill RG. Multi-component bioactive glasses of varying fluoride content for treating dentin hypersensitivity. Dent Mater. 2012;28:168–78.

Lynch MC, Perfekt R, McGuire JA, Milleman J, Gallob J, Amini P, Milleman K. Potassium oxalate mouthrinse reduces dentinal hypersensitivity: a randomized controlled clinical study. J Am Dent Assoc. 2018;149(7):608–18.

Machado AC, Maximiano V, Yoshida ML, Freitas JG, Mendes FM, Aranha ACC, Scaramucci T. Efficacy of a calcium-phosphate/fluoride varnish and ionomeric sealant on cervical dentin hypersensitivity: a randomized, double-blind, placebo-controlled clinical study. J Oral Rehabil. 2022;49(1):62–70.

Madruga MM, Silva AF, Rosa WL, Piva E, Lund RG. Evaluation of dentin hypersensitivity treatment with glass ionomer cements: a randomized clinical trial. Braz Oral Res. 2017;31:e3.

Magalhães AC, Wiegand A, Rios D, Hannas A, Attin T, Buzalaf MA. Chlorhexidine and green tea extract reduce dentin erosion and abrasion in situ. J Dent. 2009;37(12):994–8.

Magno MB, Nascimento GC, Da Penha NK, Pessoa OF, Loretto SC, Maia LC. Difference in effectiveness between strontium acetate and arginine-based toothpastes to relieve dentin hypersensitivity. A systematic review. Am J Dent. 2015;28(1):40–4.

Mantzourani M, Sharma D. Dentine sensitivity: past, present and future. J Dent. 2013;41(Suppl 4):S3–S17.

Markowitz K. The original desensitizers: strontium and potassium salts. J Clin Dent. 2009;20(5):145–51.

Markowitz K, Bilotto G, Kim S. Decreasing intradental nerve activity in the cat with potassium and divalent cations. Arch Oral Biol. 1991;36(1):1–7.

Martins CC, Firmino RT, Riva JJ, Ge L, Carrasco-Labra A, Brignardello-Petersen R, Colunga-Lozano LE, Granville-Garcia AF, Costa FO, Yepes-Nuñez JJ, Zhang Y, Schünemann HJ. Desensitizing toothpastes for dentin hypersensitivity: a network meta-analysis. J Dent Res. 2020;99(5):514–22.

Martins CC, Riva JJ, Firmino RT, Schünemann HJ. Formulations of desensitizing toothpastes for dentin hypersensitivity: a scoping review. J Appl Oral Sci. 2022;30:e20210410.

Mason S, Hughes N, Sufi F, Bannon L, Maggio B, North M, Holt J. A comparative clinical study investigating the efficacy of a dentifrice containing 8% strontium acetate and 1040 ppm fluoride in a silica base and a control dentifrice containing 1450 ppm fluoride in a silica base to provide immediate relief of dentin hypersensitivity. J Clin Dent. 2010;21(2):42–8.

Massaro C, Miranda F, Janson G, Rodrigues de Almeida R, Pinzan A, Martins DR, Garib D. Maturational changes of the normal occlusion: a 40-year follow-up. Am J Orthod Dentofacial Orthop. 2018;154(2):188–200.

Mello SV, Arvanitidou E, Stranick MA, Santana R, Kutes Y, Huey B. Mode of action studies of a new desensitizing mouthwash containing 0.8% arginine, PVM/MA copolymer, pyrophosphates, and 0.05% sodium fluoride. J Dent. 2013;41(Suppl 1):S12–9.

Mensinkai PK, Ccahuana-Vasquez RA, Chedjieu I, Amaechi BT, Mackey AC, Walker TJ, Blanken DD, Karlinsey RL. In situ remineralization of white-spot enamel lesions by 500 and 1,100 ppm F dentifrices. Clin Oral Investig. 2012;16(4):1007–14.

Miglani S, Aggarwal V, Ahuja B. Dentin hypersensitivity: recent trends in management. J Conserv Dent. 2010;13(4):218–24.

Milleman JL, Milleman KR, Clark CE, Mongiello KA, Simonton TC, Proskin HM. NUPRO Sensodyne prophylaxis paste with NovaMin for the treatment of dentin hypersensitivity: a 4-week clinical study. Am J Dent. 2012;25(5):262–8.

Miller PD Jr. A classification of marginal tissue recession. Int J Periodontics Restorative Dent. 1985;5(2):8–13.

Mneimne M, Hill RG, Bushby AJ, Brauer DS. High phosphate content significantly increases apatite formation of fluoride-containing bioactive glasses. Acta Biomater. 2011;7(4):1827–34.

Mosquim V, Caracho RA, Zabeu GS, Condi LDS, Foratori-Junior GA, Borges AFS, Wang L. Resin-based materials to control human dentin permeability under erosive conditions in vitro: a hydraulic conductance, confocal microscopy and FTIR study. Dent Mater. 2022a;38(10):1669–78.

Mosquim V, Zabeu GS, Foratori-Junior GA, Borges AB, Rios D, Magalhães AC, Wang L. S-PRG-based toothpastes compared to NaF toothpaste and NaF varnish on dentin permeability in vitro. J Appl Oral Sci. 2022b;30:e20220082.

Mosquim V, Carneiro GU, Foratori-Junior GA, Honório HM, Gillam DG, Wang L. Knowledge and attitudes on preventing and treating dentin hypersensitivity and its predicting factors: a cross-sectional study with Brazilian citizens. Eur J Dent. 2023; 17(3):855–62.

Mosquim V, Zabeu GS, Jacomine JC, Santin DC, Honório HM, Wang L. Brazilian undergraduates' and dentists' knowledge on preventing, diagnosing and managing dentin hypersensitivity: A cross-sectional questionnaire study. Int J Dent Hyg. 2024 Jun 4. Epub ahead of print.

Müller HP, Heinecke A, Schaller N, Eger T. Masticatory mucosa in subjects with different periodontal phenotypes. J Clin Periodontol. 2000;27(9):621–6.

Nanjundasetty JK, Ashrafulla M. Efficacy of desensitizing agents on postoperative sensitivity following an in-office vital tooth bleaching: a randomized controlled clinical trial. J Conserv Dent. 2016;19(3):207–11.

Nongonierma AB, Fitzgerald RJ. Biofunctional properties of caseinophosphopeptides in the oral cavity. Caries Res. 2012;46(3):234–67.

O'Toole S, Bartlett D. The relationship between dentine hypersensitivity, dietary acid intake and erosive tooth wear. J Dent. 2017;67:84–7.

Olley RC, Pilecki P, Hughes N, Jeffery P, Austin RS, Moazzez R, Bartlett D. An in situ study investigating dentine tubule occlusion of dentifrices following acid challenge. J Dent. 2012;40(7):585–93.

Ongphichetmetha N, Lertpimonchai A, Champaiboon C. Bioactive glass and arginine dentifrices immediately relieved dentine hypersensitivity following non-surgical periodontal therapy: a randomized controlled trial. J Periodontol. 2022;93(2):246–55.

Orchardson R, Gillam DG. The efficacy of potassium salts as agents for treating dentin hypersensitivity. J Orofac Pain. 2000;14(1):9–19.

Orchardson R, Gillam DG. Managing dentin hypersensitivity. J Am Dent Assoc. 2006;137(7):990–8; quiz 1028–9.

Osmari D, Fraga S, Ferreira ACO, Eduardo CP, Marquezan M, Silveira BLD. In-office treatments for dentin hypersensitivity: a randomized split-mouth clinical trial. Oral Health Prev Dent. 2018;16(2):125–30.

Panagakos F, Schiff T, Guignon A. Dentin hypersensitivity: effective treatment with an in-office desensitizing paste containing 8% arginine and calcium carbonate. Am J Dent. 2009;22(Special Issue A):3A–7A.

Pashley DH. Potential treatment modalities for dentine hypersensitivity: in-office products. In: Addy M, Embery G, Edgar WM, Orchardson R, editors. Tooth wear and sensitivity. London: Martin Dunitz; 2000. p. 351–61.

Pashley DH, Carvalho RM, Pereira JC, Villanueva R, Tay FR. The use of oxalate to reduce dentin permeability under adhesive restorations. Am J Dent. 2001;14(2):89–94.

Patel VR, Shettar L, Thakur S, Gillam D, Kamala DN. A randomised clinical trial on the efficacy of 5% fluorocalcium phosphosilicate-containing novel bioactive glass toothpaste. J Oral Rehabil. 2019;46(12):1121–6.

Peacock JM, Orchardson R. Effects of potassium ions on action potential conduction in A- and C-fibers of rat spinal nerves. J Dent Res. 1995;74(2):634–41.

Pei D, Liu S, Huang C, Du X, Yang H, Wang Y, Deng D. Effect of pretreatment with calcium-containing desensitizer on the dentine bonding of mild self-etch adhesives. Eur J Oral Sci. 2013;121(3 Pt 1):204–10.

Pereira R, Chavas VK. Efficacy of a 3% potassium nitrate desensitizing mouthwash in the treatment of dentinal hypersensitivity. J Periodontol. 2001;72(12):1720–5.

Pereira JC, Segala AD, Gillam DG. Effect of desensitizing agents on the hydraulic conductance of human dentin subjected to different surface pre-treatments—an in vitro study. Dent Mater. 2005;21(2):129–38.

Petersson LG. The role of fluoride in the preventive management of dentin hypersensitivity and root caries. Clin Oral Investig. 2013;17(Suppl 1):S63–71.

Petrou I, Heu R, Stranick M, Lavender S, Zaidel L, Cummins D, Sullivan RJ, Hsueh C, Gimzewski JK. A breakthrough therapy for dentin hypersensitivity: how dental products containing 8% arginine and calcium carbonate work to deliver effective relief of sensitive teeth. J Clin Dent. 2009;20(1):23–31.

Petrović D, Galić D, Seifert D, Lešić N, Smolić M. Evaluation of bioactive glass treatment for dentin hypersensitivity: a systematic review. Biomedicines. 2023;11(7):1992.

Peumans M, Politano G, Van Meerbeek B. Treatment of noncarious cervical lesions: when, why, and how. Int J Esthet Dent. 2020;15(1):16–42.

Pini Prato G, Di Gianfilippo R. On the value of the 2017 classification of phenotype and gingival recessions. J Periodontol. 2021;92(5):613–8.

Pini NIP, Lima DANL, Luka B, Ganss C, Schlueter N. Viscosity of chitosan impacts the efficacy of F/Sn containing toothpastes against erosive/abrasive wear in enamel. J Dent. 2020;92:103247.

Pini-Prato G, Franceschi D, Cairo F, Nieri M, Rotundo R. Classification of dental surface defects in areas of gingival recession. J Periodontol. 2010;81(6):885–90.

Pion LA, Matos LLM, Gimenez T, Palma-Dibb RG, Faraoni JJ. Treatment outcome for dentin hypersensitivity with laser therapy: systematic review and meta-analysis. Dent Med Probl. 2023;60(1):153–66.

Polack MA, Mahn DH. Biotype change for the esthetic rehabilitation of the smile. J Esthet Restor Dent. 2013;25(3):177–86.

Pollard AJ, Khan I, Davies M, Claydon N, West NX. Comparative efficacy of self-administered dentifrices for the management of dentine hypersensitivity - A systematic review and network meta-analysis. J Dent. 2023;130:104433.

Pradeep AR, Sharma A. Comparison of clinical efficacy of a dentifrice containing calcium sodium phosphosilicate to a dentifrice containing potassium nitrate and to a placebo on dentinal hypersensitivity: a randomized clinical trial. J Periodontol. 2010;81(8):1167–73.

Pradeep AR, Agarwal E, Naik SB, Bajaj P, Kalra N. Comparison of efficacy of three commercially available dentifrices [corrected] on dentinal hypersensitivity: a randomized clinical trial. Aust Dent J. 2012;57(4):429–34.

Que K, Fu Y, Lin L, Hu D, Zhang YP, Panagakos FS, DeVizio W, Mateo LR. Dentin hypersensitivity reduction of a new toothpaste containing 8.0% arginine and 1450 ppm fluoride: an 8-week clinical study on Chinese adults. Am J Dent. 2010;23(Spec A):28A–35A.

Reynolds EC, Cai F, Cochrane NJ, Shen P, Walker GD, Morgan MV, Reynolds C. Fluoride and casein phosphopeptide-amorphous calcium phosphate. J Dent Res. 2008;87(4):344–8.

Rizzante FA, Maenosono RM, Duarte MA, Furuse AY, Palma-Dibb RG, Ishikiriama SK. In vitro evaluation of dentin hydraulic conductance after 980 nm diode laser irradiation. J Periodontol. 2016;87(3):320–6.

Rösing CK, Fiorini T, Liberman DN, Cavagni J. Dentine hypersensitivity: analysis of self-care products. Braz Oral Res. 2009;23(Suppl 1):56–63.

Sales-Peres SH, Reinato JV, Sales-Peres Ade C, Marsicano JA. Effect of iron gel on dentin permeability. Braz Dent J. 2011;22(3):198–202.

Sauro S, Mannocci F, Watson TF, Piemontese M, Sherriff M, Mongiorgi R. The influence of soft acidic drinks in exposing dentinal tubules after non-surgical periodontal treatment: a SEM investigation on the protective effects of oxalate-containing phytocomplex. Med Oral Patol Oral Cir Bucal. 2007;12(7):E542–8.

Scaffa PM, Vidal CM, Barros N, Gesteira TF, Carmona AK, Breschi L, Pashley DH, Tjäderhane L, Tersariol IL, Nascimento FD, Carrilho MR. Chlorhexidine inhibits the activity of dental cysteine cathepsins. J Dent Res. 2012;91(4):420–5.

Schiff T, Delgado E, Zhang YP, Cummins D, DeVizio W, Mateo LR. Clinical evaluation of the efficacy of an in-office desensitizing paste containing 8% arginine and calcium carbonate in providing instant and lasting relief of dentin hypersensitivity. Am J Dent. 2009;22(Spec A):8A–15A.

Schmidlin PR, Sahrmann P. Current management of dentin hypersensitivity. Clin Oral Investig. 2013;17(Suppl 1):S55–9.

Seong J, Macdonald E, Newcombe RG, Davies M, Jones SB, Johnson S, West NX. In situ randomised trial to investigate the occluding properties of two desensitising toothpastes on dentine after subsequent acid challenge. Clin Oral Investig. 2013;17(1):195–203.

Sgolastra F, Petrucci A, Severino M, Gatto R, Monaco A. Lasers for the treatment of dentin hypersensitivity: a meta-analysis. J Dent Res. 2013;92(6):492–9.

Sgreccia PC, Barbosa RES, Damé-Teixeira N, Garcia FCP. Low-power laser and potassium oxalate gel in the treatment of cervical dentin hypersensitivity-a randomized clinical trial. Clin Oral Investig. 2020;24(12):4463–73.

Sgreccia PC, Damé-Teixeira N, Barbosa RES, Araújo PF, Zanatta RF, Garcia FCP. Assessment of the Oral Health Impact Profile (OHIP-14) improvement of different treatments for dentin hypersensitivity in noncarious cervical lesions-a randomized clinical study. Clin Oral Investig. 2022;26(11):6583–91.

Sharif MO, Iram S, Brunton PA. Effectiveness of arginine-containing toothpastes in treating dentine hypersensitivity: a systematic review. J Dent. 2013;41(6):483–92.

Sharma D, McGuire JA, Amini P. Randomized trial of the clinical efficacy of a potassium oxalate-containing mouthrinse in rapid relief of dentin sensitivity. J Clin Dent. 2013a;24(2):62–7.

Sharma D, McGuire JA, Gallob JT, Amini P. Randomised clinical efficacy trial of potassium oxalate mouthrinse in relieving dentinal sensitivity. J Dent. 2013b;41(Suppl 4):S40–8.

Sharma D, Hong CX, Heipp PS. A novel potassium oxalate-containing tooth-desensitising mouthrinse: a comparative in vitro study. J Dent. 2013c;41(Suppl 4):S18–27.

Silveira C, Oliveira F, Dos Santos ML, de Freitas T, Imparato JC, Magalhães AC. Anacardic acid from Brazilian cashew nut trees reduces dentine erosion. Caries Res. 2014;48(6):549–56.

Sugumaran V, Krishnamoorthy E, Kamalakkannan A, Ramachandran RC, Subramanian B. Unscrambling the influence of sodium cation on the structure, bioactivity, and erythrocyte compatibility of 45S5 bioactive glass. ACS Appl Bio Mater. 2022;5(4):1576–90.

Talioti E, Hill R, Gillam DG. The efficacy of selected desensitizing OTC products: a systematic review. ISRN Dent. 2014;2014:865761.

Tao D, Ling MR, Feng XP, Gallob J, Souverain A, Yang W, Alavi A. Efficacy of an anhydrous stannous fluoride toothpaste for relief of dentine hypersensitivity: A randomized clinical study. J Clin Periodontol. 2020;47(8):962–9.

Tiskaya M, Shahid S, Gillam D, Hill R. The use of bioactive glass (BAG) in dental composites: a critical review. Dent Mater. 2021;37:296–310.

Tjäderhane L, Nascimento FD, Breschi L, Mazzoni A, Tersariol IL, Geraldeli S, Tezvergil-Mutluay A, Carrilho M, Carvalho RM, Tay FR, Pashley DH. Strategies to prevent hydrolytic degradation of the hybrid layer-a review. Dent Mater. 2013;29(10):999–1011.

Tjäderhane L, Buzalaf MA, Carrilho M, Chaussain C. Matrix metalloproteinases and other matrix proteinases in relation to cariology: the era of 'dentin degradomics'. Caries Res. 2015;49(3):193–208.

Tolentino AB, Zeola LF, Fernandes MRU, Pannuti CM, Soares PV, Aranha ACC. Photobiomodulation therapy and 3% potassium nitrate gel as treatment of cervical dentin hypersensitivity: a randomized clinical trial. Clin Oral Investig. 2022;26(12):6985–93.

Trushkowsky RD, Oquendo A. Treatment of dentin hypersensitivity. Dent Clin N Am. 2011;55(3):599–608.

Tschoppe P, Zandim DL, Martus P, Kielbassa AM. Enamel and dentine remineralization by nano-hydroxyapatite toothpastes. J Dent. 2011;39:430–7.

Umberto R, Claudia R, Gaspare P, Gianluca T, Alessandro del V. Treatment of dentine hypersensitivity by diode laser: a clinical study. Int J Dent. 2012;2012:858950.

Vandiver J, Dean D, Patel N, Bonfield W, Ortiz C. Nanoscale variation in surface charge of synthetic hydroxyapatite detected by chemically and spatially specific high-resolution force spectroscopy. Biomaterials. 2005;26(3):271–83.

Vanichvatana S, Auychai P. Efficacy of two calcium phosphate pastes on the remineralization of artificial caries: a randomized controlled double-blind in situ study. Int J Oral Sci. 2013;5(4):224–8.

Vatturu S, Ganugapanta VR, Teja NR, Singaraju GS, Mandava P, Priyanka JY. Comparative evaluation of the efficacy of the desensitizing and remineralizing agent in the reduction of dentin hypersensitivity after orthodontic debonding—a randomized clinical trial. Med Pharm Rep. 2021;94(2):229–38.

Vertuan M, Souza BM, Mosquim V, Silva CV, Freitas PM, Borges AFS, Rios D, Magalhães AC, Honório HM. Effect of TiF4 varnish after pre-treatment with proanthocyanidin or chlorhexidine on the progression of erosive dentin loss in the presence or absence of the demineralized organic matrix. J Mech Behav Biomed Mater. 2021;115:104287.

Viana ÍEL, Borges R, Marchi J, Feitosa S, Marques MM, Scaramucci T. A 58S bioactive glass for dentin hypersensitivity and erosive tooth wear: an in vitro study. J Dent. 2022;127:104343.

Walsh LJ. The effects of GC Tooth Mousse on cervical dentinal sensitivity: a controlled clinical trial. Int Dent S Afr. 2010;12(1):4–12.

Wang L, Magalhães AC, Francisconi-Dos-Rios LF, Calabria MP, Araújo D, Buzalaf M, Lauris J, Pereira JC. Treatment of dentin hypersensitivity using nano-hydroxyapatite pastes: a randomized three-month clinical trial. Oper Dent. 2016;41(4):E93–E101.

Wegehaupt FJ, Tauböck TT, Sener B, Attin T. Long-term protective effect of surface sealants against erosive wear by intrinsic and extrinsic acids. J Dent. 2012a;40(5):416–22.

Wegehaupt FJ, Tauböck TT, Stillhard A, Schmidlin PR, Attin T. Influence of extra- and intra-oral application of CPP-ACP and fluoride on re-hardening of eroded enamel. Acta Odontol Scand. 2012b; 70(3):177–83.

Wegehaupt FJ, Kummer G, Attin T. Prevention of erosions by a surface sealant and adhesives under abrasive conditions. Swiss Dent J. 2017;127(9):740–7.

West NX, Addy M, Jackson RJ, Ridge DB. Dentine hypersensitivity and the placebo response. A comparison of the effect of strontium acetate, potassium nitrate and fluoride toothpastes. J Clin Periodontol. 1997;24(4):209–15.

West NX, Lussi A, Seong J, Hellwig E. Dentin hypersensitivity: pain mechanisms and aetiology of exposed cervical dentin. Clin Oral Investig. 2013;17(Suppl 1):S9–S19.

Wojtowicz-Praga SM, Dickson RB, Hawkins MJ. Matrix metalloproteinase inhibitors. Investig New Drugs. 1997;15(1):61–75.

Yadav VS, Gumber B, Makker K, Gupta V, Tewari N, Khanduja P, Yadav R. Global prevalence of gingival recession: a systematic review and meta-analysis. Oral Dis. 2023;29(8):2993–3002.

Yamamoto D, Matsumoto K, Ohishi H, Ishida T, Inoue M, Kitamura K, Mizuno H. Refined x-ray structure of papain.E-64-c complex at 2.1-a resolution. J Biol Chem. 1991;266(22):14771–7.

Yang H, Lin XJ, Liu Q, Yu H. Effects of protease inhibitors on dentin erosion: an in situ study. Clin Oral Investig. 2023;27(3):1005–12.

Yates R, Owens J, Jackson R, Newcombe RG, Addy M. A split-mouth placebo-controlled study to determine the effect of amorphous calcium phosphate in the treatment of dentine hypersensitivity. J Clin Periodontol. 1998;25(8):687–92.

Yates RJ, Newcombe RG, Addy M. Dentine hypersensitivity: a randomised, double-blind placebo-controlled study of the efficacy of a fluoride-sensitive teeth mouthrinse. J Clin Periodontol. 2004;31(10):885–9.

Yoshida Y, Van Meerbeek B, Nakayama Y, Snauwaert J, Hellemans L, Lambrechts P, Vanherle G, Wakasa K. Evidence of chemical bonding at biomaterial-hard tissue interfaces. J Dent Res. 2000;79(2):709–14.

Zabeu GS, Mosquim V, Bastos-Bitencourt NA, Santin DC, Agulhari, MAS, Wang L. Dental cervical lesions: how the etiologies imply in different approaches for long-lasting performance. Arch Health Invest. 2022;11(1):125–33.

Zeola LF, Teixeira DNR, Galvão ADM, Souza PG, Soares PV. Brazilian dentists' perception of dentin hypersensitivity management. Braz Oral Res. 2020;33:e115.

Zhu M, Li J, Chen B, Mei L, Yao L, Tian J, Li H. The effect of calcium sodium phosphosilicate on dentin hypersensitivity: a systematic review and meta-analysis. PLoS One. 2015;10(11):e0140176.

Zweers J, Thomas RZ, Slot DE, Weisgold AS, Van der Weijden FG. Characteristics of periodontal biotype, its dimensions, associations, and prevalence: a systematic review. J Clin Periodontol. 2014;41(10):958–71.

8 Advances in the Management of the Patient with Dentine Hypersensitivity: Motivation and Prevention

David G. Gillam and Christoph A. Ramseier

8.1 Introduction

The aim of the first part of this chapter is to reflect on how the management of dentine hypersensitivity (DH) has been traditionally recommended in clinical practice and the steps taken to provide simple and practical guidelines for the busy clinician. The second part of this chapter will develop the recommendations on how to manage DH by concentrating on techniques (for example, motivational interviewing) used in both medicine and dentistry to effect behavioural changes when providing instructions to patients, enabling them to not only recognize the need for change but also to take ownership of their problem whether it is through an improvement in oral hygiene practice or taking steps to limit the effects of acidic food or drink on initiating DH.

8.2 Management of Dentine Hypersensitivity

The management of dentine hypersensitivity (DH) has been traditionally based on products that may either block the dentine tubules on the exposed root surface or desensitize the nerves in the pulp (Orchardson and Gillam 2006). The clinician when faced with a patient with DH would generally treat the condition based on the extent and severity of the problem. For example, if the patient complained of severe pain which was localized to one or two teeth, then the clinician would treat the problem in the dental office with a restorative product (Table 8.1). Alternatively, if the pain was generalized and of a mild to moderate in nature, then the clinician may consider recommending an over-the-counter (OTC) product (Table 8.1). Patients may also complain of pain following restorative procedures, for example, non-surgical and surgical periodontal procedures, and the clinician may depending on the extent and severity of the problem recommend a treatment regime that would resolve the problem (Orchardson and Gillam 2006; Gillam et al. 2013; Gillam 2017, 2020; Gillam and Chatzopoulou 2019). It is important however to acknowledge that the diagnosis of DH is somewhat problematic in nature, and therefore, it is essential that the clinician excludes all other clinical conditions that have a similar pain history to that of DH (Gillam et al. 2013; Olley and Bartlett 2015; Seong and West 2015). In a busy practice,

D. G. Gillam (✉)
Centre for Oral Bioengineering, Institute of Dentistry, Barts and the London School of Medicine and Dentistry, Queen Mary University of London, London, UK
e-mail: d.g.gillam@qmul.ac.uk

C. A. Ramseier
Department of Periodontology, School of Dental Medicine, University of Bern, Bern, Switzerland

D. G. Gillam (ed.), *Dentine Hypersensitivity*, https://doi.org/10.1007/978-3-031-74321-4_8

Table 8.1 Overall management strategy options for treating dentine hypersensitivity (Gillam et al. 2013 modified)

Gingival recession	Tooth wear	Periodontal treatment
Clinical evaluation	**Clinical evaluation**	**Clinical evaluation**
Clinical measurement of the gingival recession defect Take study casts and clinical photographs to monitor condition over time Check and monitor periodontal health Identification and correction of predisposing or precipitating factors Use of pain scores to assess and monitor DH (e.g., Visual Analogue Scores)	Identify cause of tooth wear (enamel loss) Record severity of lesions, if possible, using a recognized index (Smith and Knight 1984; Bartlett et al. 2008) Take study casts and clinical photographs to monitor condition over time Check and monitor periodontal health Use of pain scores to assess and monitor DH (e.g., Visual Analogue Scores)	Periodontal disease or periodontal treatment as the primary cause of exposure of dentine and associated DH Check and monitor periodontal health (6-point pocket charting) Use of pain scores to assess and monitor DH (e.g., Visual Analogue Scores)
Patient education (including preventive advice)	**Patient education (including preventive advice)**	**Patient education (including preventive advice)**
Show patient the affected site(s) Explain probable cause for recession Explain factors triggering sensitive teeth episodes Encourage patients to modify their oral hygiene regimen to reduce damage to gingivae (e.g., reducing brushing force, correction of toothbrush technique) Reduce excessive consumption of acid foods and drinks	Show patient the site(s) and explain probable cause of the tooth wear lesion(s) Recommend an oral hygiene regimen to minimize risk of further tooth wear Where appropriate recommend reducing frequency of consumption of acidic food and drink	Reinforce the need for good oral hygiene Show patient the site(s) affected by periodontal disease and explain probable cause of the exposed dentine Guide the patient to improve 'at home' oral hygiene regimen Instruction on measures of reducing periodontal risk factors, for example, diabetes, smoking, obesity
Corrective clinical outcomes	**Corrective clinical outcomes**	**Corrective clinical outcomes**
Reduce excessive consumption of acid foods and drinks Manufacture of silicone gingival veneers Orthodontic treatment Restorative correction of recession defect and subgingival margins of fillings and crowns Polymers: Sealants/varnishes/resins/dentine bonding agents Laser obturation of dentinal tubules. Use of desensitizing polishing pastes Pulpal extirpation (root canal treatment)	Provide high fluoride remineralizing treatment (pre-emptive phase) Provide professional desensitizing treatment to relieve DH Encourage patient to seek advice from medical practitioner, if tooth wear caused by working environment or reflux/excessive vomiting (psychiatric evaluation may also be appropriate) Restorative correction in the form of composite build up, crowns may also be appropriate	**Initial phase** Non-surgical periodontal procedure(s) DH treatment (including desensitizing polishing pastes/fluoride varnishes) **Re-evaluation** Follow-up assessment on periodontal status and dentine hypersensitivity **Corrective phase** Surgical periodontal procedure(s), e.g., guided tissue regeneration, coronally advanced flap + enamel matrix derivatives, connective tissue graft (flap), free gingival graft (acellular dermal matrix allograft) DH treatment (including desensitizing polishing pastes/fluoride varnishes) **Follow-up management** **Maintenance phase** Supportive periodontal therapy Ongoing monitoring of periodontal health Dentine hypersensitivity treatment (including desensitizing polishing pastes/fluoride varnishes) Oral hygiene advice

(continued)

Table 8.1 (continued)

Gingival recession	Tooth wear	Periodontal treatment
Recommendations for home use (including toothpaste/mouthrinses)	**Recommendations for home use (including toothpaste/ mouthrinses)**	**Recommendations for home use (including toothpaste/mouthrinses)**
Oral hygiene implementation as per recommendation Strontium chloride/strontium acetate Potassium nitrate/chloride/citrate/ oxalate Calcium compounds: Calcium carbonate and arginine and casein phosphopeptide+amorphous calcium phosphate Bioactive glass Nano/hydroxyapatite Fluoride in higher concentration (2800/5000 ppm F[prescription]) Amine/stannous fluoride	Oral hygiene implementation as per recommendation Toothpastes and mouthrinses (see Recommendations for Gingival Recession)	Oral hygiene implementation as per recommendation Regular brushing with an antibacterial toothpaste to aid plaque control Short period, the use of a 0.2% chlorhexidine solution for plaque control Use of a desensitizing mouthrinse twice daily for DH control (when appropriate)

this may be a challenge, but to successfully manage DH, it is essential for the clinician to take time and determine the correct diagnosis before providing treatment. There is often a tendency for the busy clinician to simply prescribe or recommend a treatment without determining the aetiological and predisposing factors that may have been instrumental in initiating the problem (Gillam and Ramseier 2015) and if not correctly managed or monitored will continue to impact on a patient's quality of life (oral health-related quality of life, OHRQoL) (Bekes et al. 2008; Bioko et al. 2010; Bekes and Hirsch 2013, 2015) (see Chap. 3). This approach would therefore involve not only educating the patient but also the clinician and it is important to recognize that the clinicians will need to adopt management strategies and goals that will effectively encourage behavioural changes in the lifestyle of their patients. To accomplish these goals, the clinician will need to motivate and engage the patient to effect the recommended changes in behaviour. The question, however, arises whether the clinician can effectively diagnose, manage, and monitor DH within the constraints of clinical practice (Gillam et al. 2013). There have been several treatment paradigms that have been previously reported in the published literature, and there is, however, a recognition that they may be impractical to implement in clinical environment practice (Addy and Urquhart 1992; Canadian Advisory Board on Dentin Hypersensitivity 2003; Orchardson and Gillam 2006; Gillam et al. 2013). New guidelines have also been published from a UK Expert Forum on DH (Gillam et al. 2013; Gillam 2017), which recognized that there was a need to promote simple guidelines that can be readily applied in general practice, although the forum acknowledged that a simple one strategy approach to the problem may not necessarily satisfy all patients. One of the key components from the guidelines document was that the authors linked recommended management strategies to three specific groups of patients rather than recommending a blanket management for all patients with DH. These patient groups included: (1) patients with gingival recession caused by mechanical trauma, (2) patients with tooth wear lesions, and (3) patients with periodontal disease and those receiving periodontal treatment (Table 8.1). It is also evident from most clinical studies for the treatment of DH that patient compliance with both oral hygiene and dietary regimens was paramount to achieve satisfactory treatment outcomes and predictable long-term success. The second part of the chapter will discuss how a clinician may attempt to engage their patients to follow an individualized oral care regimen which can be incorporated into the management strategy for treating DH. This will enable the patient to modify any risk factors associated with the development and progression of

DH and subsequently prevent or reduce these effects. For example, apart from the standard of care for oral hygiene practices, these regimens include dietary counselling as well as instructions to avoid brushing the teeth following the intake of acid containing drinks.

8.3 The Challenge of Changing Health Behaviour in the Management of Medical and Dental Conditions

It is generally recognized that one of the problems in clinical practice (medical or dental) is the lack of compliance or adherence to the instructions provided by the clinician during therapy. Compliance may be defined as the process of complying with a regimen of treatment, for example, taking medication (Merriam-Webster definition) although the term adherence may be the preferred term to use. Adherence may therefore be defined as the extent to which the patient continues the agreed-upon mode of treatment under limited supervision when faced with conflicting demands, as distinguished from compliance or maintenance (The American Heritage® Medical Dictionary 2010). This term may therefore be considered a more general term representing 'the extent to which a patient follows medical instructions' (Definition of Adherence 2001). The lack of compliance or adherence to instructions provided by a health care professional is not, however, unique to dentistry. According to Wertheimer and Santella (2003), non-compliance occurred in approximately 50–75% of patients taking prescribed medication, with the rate of non-compliance higher in patients with a chronic illness. For example, a problem that may arise is in relation to a patient with a diabetic condition with a sedentary lifstyle who simply complies with following the instructions relating to their prescribed medication without making any attempt to make changes in their behaviour and lifestle activity. Such inactivity will not necessarily improve their medical condition.

It may, however, be unrealistic to expect every patient to understand and comply with professionally driven instructions particularly when treating chronic diseases and health conditions, for example, diabetes, obesity, smoking, alcoholism, and periodontal disease. For example, the patient's attention and comprehension levels may be optimal during the first 15 min of a visit, but their ability to absorb and retain any further information may subsequently decline thereafter. It is therefore important to provide patients with simple clear instructions which they can understand and routinely implement as part of their day-to-day activities. This process may, however, take several visits and requires the clinician to build up a rapport with the patient, show empathy, and have a close working partnership with the patient to effect the changes in behaviour that would reduce or eliminate the underlying problems associated with DH (e.g., drinking erosive drinks) (Olley and Bartlett 2015, see also Chap. 4). Before illustrating how a clinician may work with a patient to effect a change in their daily intake of food and drink associated with DH, it may be beneficial to observe how clinicians in medicine and dentistry have attempted to effect changes in behaviour (Bischof et al. 2021). For example, according to Ramseier (2005), there was emerging evidence that the patient's individual behaviour may be influential or even critical for the success of periodontal therapy as evidenced by the limited success of periodontal therapy in patients lacking the appropriate behaviour to maintain their periodontal condition. It is also evident that the maintenance of periodontal health is supported by appropriate behaviours, for example, regularly self-performed plaque control, avoidance of tobacco, and glycaemic control with diabetes mellitus type 2. In contrary, patients with inadequate oral hygiene, tobacco usage, and uncontrolled glucose levels have been reported to have an unsatisfactory periodontal status. According to Ramseier (2005), both plaque control and smoking cessation are important measures in the management of chronic periodontitis. Therefore, it would appear to be appropriate to: (1) include assessments of patient behaviour and if necessary (2) apply effective behaviour change counselling methods in the maintenance of the patients' periodontal condition.

8.4 Reasons for the Lack of Compliance or Adherence Instructions Provided by the Medical and Dental Profession

As previously indicated, it was evident from the published literature that non-compliance of both medical and dental patients is a major problem when delivering health care guidance and instruction as part of the treatment process. This appeared to be a problem in patients with long-term or chronic conditions, for example, diabetes, hypertension, cardiovascular disease (Khan et al. 2012), and in the dental environment, chronic periodontal disease may also be associated with these systemic conditions (Loesche and Grossman 2001; Kim and Amar 2006). According to Khan et al. (2012), non-compliance can be due to several factors, for example, those that are (1) patient-centred, (2) therapy-related, or (3) health-care system-related.

The reasons for non-compliance are therefore complex in nature and may also vary not only between patients but also depend on the situation the patient may be experiencing at the time. For example, the reasons for non-compliance in the Khan et al. (2012) diabetes study included the unavailability of transport, forgetting the appointment, not attending the clinic since the visit was considered unnecessary as the patients were taking medicine from other sources, and failure to follow instructions on exercising regularly. According to Tan (2009), the fear of receiving dental treatment, economic factors, and indifferent behaviour on the dentist's part, as well as higher incidences of stressful life events or insecurity in personal relationships may be reasons for patient non-compliance. Mendoza et al. (1991) reviewed records of patients undergoing periodontal maintenance over a three-year period and reported that the most common reason given by patients for non-compliance was that their periodontal treatment was provided by a general dental practitioner. Some patients also considered the treatment too expensive, whereas a significant number of patients considered that they no longer need the recommended treatment.

Fardal (2006) also reported that patients gave a variety of reasons (for example, health reasons, lack of motivation, fear, financial reasons, own dentist providing the periodontal care, dissatisfied with the treatment, did not see the need for future treatment, and a faulty recall procedure) when he interviewed non-compliant patients who returned to his practice for periodontal maintenance.

8.5 Patient Education and Changing Behaviour in the Medical and Dental Environment

It is therefore evident that to successfully treat a patient's medical or dental condition, the clinician must establish a good rapport and close working partnership with the patient. One of the problems historically was the often-one-sided relationship between the clinician and the patient where the clinician simply gave instructions to the patient of what was expected for them to comply (the so-called clinician-centred approach) (Curro and Gillam 2015). For example, demonstrating a brushing technique or a flossing technique on a demonstration model will often fail to determine whether the patient could master a particular brushing technique or whether they have the dexterity to be able to floss their teeth. According to Freeman (1999), this failure to actively involve the patient in the treatment process essentially renders the patient as a passive listener of information which they were unable to assimilate into their day-to-day experience. This prescriptive approach failed to give the patient any opportunity to gain autonomy, motivation, competency, and a readiness for change (Williams and Bray 2011). One of the problems with this traditional clinician-centred approach was that the message was often considered judgemental in nature, and this subsequently meant that the patient became resistant to any prescribed recommendations for changing their lifestyle behaviour and may set up the patient for subsequent failure at the next appointment (Freeman 1999; Williams and Bray 2011). According to Freeman (1999), a readiness to change can provide a bridge between the clinician and the patient with respect to understanding a patients' perceived lack of motivation to change their lifestyle behaviour(s). The clinician should therefore be aware that when attempting to provide information designed to change a patient's oral hygiene practices or a major lifestyle behavioural change, the patient should be involved in the process and not be an impassive observer of information that does not encourage him to assess the advantages or disadvantages of accepting or not accepting the rationale for changing behaviour (ambivalence).

According to Partovi (2006), the patient must be motivated before the education process can take place, although motivation without compliance or adherence to a recommended procedure (e.g., changing oral hygiene practices: flossing) may lead to failure unless some form of preplanning of behavioural interventions has been discussed with the patient (Schuz, et al. 2006).

8.6 Introduction to Motivational Interviewing in the Management of Dentine Hypersensitivity: A Different Approach

According to Gillam and Yusuf (2019), motivational interviewing (MI) has been demonstrated to be effective for a wide range of health behaviours which has been utilized in both the medical and dental environment (e.g., dietary advice, smoking cessation, changes in oral health behaviour, alcohol advice, etc.) (Senft et al. 1995; Berg-Smith et al. 1999; Evensen et al. 2021). It is essentially an effective behaviour change method, which can be modified for use in dental practices as a brief intervention to increase motivation to improve patients' oral hygiene behaviours including advising patients to change harmful habits such as over-zealous tooth brushing and excessive dietary intake of acidic food and drink when managing dentine hypersensitivity (see below). These authors also suggested that MI could be utilized as a brief intervention delivered in a resource and time constrained environment over several appointments such as in general dental practice (Gillam and Yusuf 2019).

8.6.1 Definition of Motivation

Motivation has defined as (1) the act or an instance of motivating or providing with a reason to act in a certain way, (2) the state or condition of being motivated, and (3) something that motivates; inducement; incentive (Dictionary.com). One of the problems when discussing the concepts of compliance, motivating, and educating the patient is that we forget that the clinician also must embrace these qualities. It may be possible that the characteristics that may mark out the patient, for example, lack motivation, denial, failure to see the need (or relevancy) to change, and resistance to change may also affect the clinician. The consequence of this type of apathy will ultimately lead to disillusionment for both parties and the opportunity to initiate the changes that would benefit the patient will be lost.

8.6.2 Motivational Interviewing (MI)

As indicated above, the traditional health education approaches provided by clinicians were often considered to be ineffective in changing patient behaviour. For example, in periodontal care, conventional oral hygiene instructions frequently lack any long-term effect and therefore require continual reinforcement (Wilson Jr. et al. 1984a, b; Demetriou et al. 1995; Schuz et al. 2006). This would infer that there may be a false assumption inherent in the health education approach itself which would tend to suggest, that behaviour change was simply a function of the patient having a requisite knowledge or understanding, and that all the clinicians had to do was provide the relevant information.

Motivational interviewing (MI) in contrast is based on a different assumption of human behaviour change which concluded that knowledge was insufficient to bring about any behaviour change and that motivation to change was elicited 'from within the patient' rather than externally imposed upon the patient by a clinician. MI has also been defined as 'a client (patient)-centred, directive method for enhancing intrinsic motivation to change by exploring and resolving ambivalence'. According to Rollnick et al. (2008), MI was initially developed as a brief intervention for problem drinking in which patient motivation was an obstacle to a change in behaviour (e.g., refrain from drinking). It soon became evident that this model would be beneficial in dealing with other health problems, and subsequently, MI was reported to have positive results in the management of various chronic diseases.

Motivational interviewing has also been defined as a collaborative, goal-oriented method of communication with particular attention to the language of change. It is intended to strengthen personal motivation for, and commitment to, a specific goal by eliciting and exploring an individual's own reasons for change within an atmosphere of acceptance and compassion (Andrews 2012 citing Miller and Rollnick 2010). An easier definition that may benefit someone outside the medical or dental profession would be: 'Motivational interviewing is a collaborative conversation to strengthen a person's own motivation for and commitment to change' (Andrews 2012). In other words, the MI approach for effecting change and may provide an alternative strategy for promoting lifestyle changes that are essential for improving patient outcomes (Freudenthal 2013). MI has also been described as a skilful clinical style for eliciting from patients their own good motivations for making behaviour changes in the interests of their own health (Miller and Rollnick 2002; Rollnick et al. 2008). According to these investigators, the so-called spirit of MI has been described as collaborative, evocative, and honouring of patient autonomy. The use of MI in clinical practice was based on four general principles: (1) to listen with empathy in order to understand and explore the patient's own motivations, (2) to develop discrepancy between the patient's current behaviour and how they would ideally like to behave, (3) roll with resistance, e.g., by resisting the righting reflex, and (4) to empower the patient's self-efficacy, encouraging hope and optimism. A helpful acronym RULE (Resist, Understand, Listen, and Empower) has been suggested by Rollnick et al. (2008) to remember these principles. According to Miller and Rollnick (2009), it is important for clinicians to recognize that MI is not: (i) the trans-theoretical model of change (pre-contemplation, contemplation, preparation, action) (Prochaska and DiClemente 1983); (ii) a way of tricking people into doing what you want them to do; (iii) a specific technique; (iv) a decisional balance; (v) an assessment feedback; (vi) a cognitive-behaviour therapy; (vii) a client-centred therapy; (viii) easy to learn; (ix) practice as usual; and (x) a panacea.

8.6.3 Evidence for the Effectiveness of MI in Changing Behaviour in Medical and Dental Health Conditions

MI originated in the field of addictive behaviour therapy but has increasingly been applied to a wide variety of other behaviour change issues, including behaviours, for example, tobacco use, diet, and exercise (Burke et al. 2004; Hettema et al. 2005). The evidence from these studies appears to be robust and generally indicate that MI-based interventions are at least equivalent to other active treatments and superior to no-treatment or placebo controls for problems involving addictive behaviour (drugs, alcohol, smoking, and gambling), health behaviours such as diet and exercise, risk behaviours, and treatment engagement, retention, and adherence (Burke et al. 2003, 2004; Hettema et al. 2005; Rubak et al. 2005; Lundahl et al. 2010). For example, Rubak et al. (2005) reported that in brief encounters of 15 min, 64% of studies showed an effect. Furthermore, when the intervention was delivered by physicians, an effect was observed in approximately 80% of studies suggesting that it was reasonable for clinicians who are not counselling experts to effectively deliver MI in brief encounters. Data analysed in meta-analysis studies has also demonstrated positive impacts when using MI in tobacco use cessation programmes (Butler et al. 1999; Lai et al. 2010; Lundahl et al. 2010; Wakefield et al. 2004; Borrelli et al. 2005) as well as in changing dietary behaviour (dietary intake, fat intake, carbohydrate consumption, cholesterol intake, body mass index (BMI) weight, salt intake, consumption of fruit and vegetables, alcohol reduction, and exercise (Woollard et al. 1995; Mhurchu et al. 1998; Resnicow et al. 2001; Bowen et al. 2002; Richards et al. 2006). A recent systematic review by Carra et al. (2020) and subsequent published clinical guidelines from the EFP Workshop Treatment of stage I–III periodontitis (the EFP S3 level clinical practice guideline) (Sanz et al. 2020), however, indicated that there are benefits in employing psychological interventions based on cognitive constructs and motivational interviewing principles provided by oral health professionals. According to these authors, the available published evidence failed to demonstrate that these techniques improved the patient's oral hygiene performance as measured by the reduction of plaque and bleeding scores over time (Carra et al. 2020; Sanz et al. 2020).

Researchers have also investigated the impact of MI in the dental setting compared to traditional health education for motivating 240 mothers of young children with high risk for developing dental caries to use dietary and non-dietary behaviours for caries prevention (Weinstein et al. 2004, 2006). The results from this study would appear to be consistent with results from meta-analyses studies that reported MI to be efficacious for dietary change (Burke et al. 2003; Hettema et al. 2005; Lundahl et al. 2010). Other short- and long-term studies have also demonstrated a positive impact on (1) oral hygiene as measured by plaque indices, (2) gingival inflammation as assessed by gingival indices, and (3) association of greater patient satisfaction with improvement in oral hygiene (Almomani et al. 2009; Jönsson et al. 2009a, b, 2010; Godard et al. 2011). Several reviews have also indicated the potential of MI in improving dental care (Nalini and Punithavathy 2010; Gao et al. 2013), although the impact on improving periodontal health remains unclear (Brand et al. 2013; Gao et al. 2013). To date there does not appear to be any published studies on the role of MI in the management of dentine hypersensitivity an issue raised by Gillam and Ramseier (2015). According to these authors, such an approach would be beneficial in changing behaviours that may lead to the initiation of the condition (see also Olley and Bartlett 2015) as well as having a positive impact during the management and monitoring phases of treatment (Table 8.1).

8.7 The Implementation of Motivational Interviewing Over Single and Multiple Appointments in Order to Effect Changes in Behaviour in Patients with DH

The implementation of MI in the management of DH would be a promising approach to help change behaviours that have been implicated in the initiation and progression of the condition. It is also important to acknowledge that when treating the condition, the clinician should not lose sight of the behavioural causes of DH or the need to counsel patients on the effectiveness of treatment. This type of intervention may therefore be suitable for implementation into the management guidelines for specific patient groups with DH as proposed by Gillam et al. (2013; Gillam 2017). The question as to whether a single or multiple appointment strategy approach should be used may depend on a number of factors, for example, the extent and severity of problem, the availability of the patient, the frequency of monitoring during the maintenance phase, the readiness or willingness of the patient to engage in the consultation process and consider the advantages and disadvantages of accepting or rejecting the recommended changes in behaviour, and the motivation and subsequent adherence (compliance) to the clinician's recommendations to change behaviour. One of the problems in implementing any changes in patient behaviour in the management of DH is the busy schedule of the clinician within the clinical environment, and therefore, a pragmatic approach may need to be adopted to not only manage the patient's discomfort but also to change behaviour to reduce or prevent future effects of DH. It is also important for the clinician to set an agreed agenda (Rollnick et al. 1999a, b) with the patient as there may be more than one health behaviour issue that may impact on their DH. For example, incorrect tooth brushing techniques may damage both hard and soft tissue, excessive acidic food and drink in the diet, or smoking (Olley and Bartlett 2015, see also Chap. 4). The clinician therefore should be prepared to manage both his/her expectation as well as the patient when considering changes in behaviour. According to Bandura (1995), achieving small changes may make a patient feel more able and confident to make other changes and as such it is important to start where the patient feels most comfortable and encourage them to suggest what area they would like to talk about, rather than simply selecting what the clinician considers is right course of action. This may be achieved by using an agenda setting chart containing several circles with picture representations of the various issues in DH and some blank circles for other factors to be inserted by the patient. The patient then selects the issue that they would like to talk about first.

According to Miller and Rollnick (2002) to be an effective MI practitioner, the clinician needs to embody the underlying philosophy of MI over multiple appointments rather than simply applying a collection of counselling techniques. For example, Suvan et al. (2010) presented a specific patient activation fabric model implementing the spirit of MI into a single appointment to capture the inter-dependent elements of the dental visit using the concept of interwoven threads. This model attempts to blend communication, information exchange, and the use of behavioural change tools with the clinical assessment and treatment (Fig. 8.1).

8.8 Communication with the Patient with Dentine Hypersensitivity

There are several different styles that are used in conversation with other people in everyday life. However, in a clinical situation when dealing with a patient with DH, it would be more appropriate from time to time to specifically adapt to their individual behavioural needs and to allow them to communicate their chief complaints in their own way. A 3-style model for healthcare clinicians to communicate with their patients in daily practice has been recommended by Rollnick et al. (2007), which uses the following styles, e.g., directing, guiding, or following style. According to Rollnick et al. (2007), some patients may require 'direction'—particularly those who have stated that they want further advice or support when considering changing health care behaviour. Other patients (clients), however, may have more pressing concerns and therefore need to be "followed" more closely despite the fact that they appear to know what they need to do and yet have failed to manage their behavioral needs. These patients (clients) may be more receptive to a 'guiding' style. Furthermore, four main communication skills may be used by the clinician, and these can be summarized by the acronym OARS which stands for: (1) *open* (ended) questions, (2) *affirmations*, (3) *reflective* listening, and (4) *summarizing*. It is important, however, for the clinician to be aware or sensitive to any changes in the patient's reaction to a particular style of communication and it may be necessary if there is a breakdown within the communication process that the clinician uses a different style to maintain the rapport between both patient and clinician.

8.9 Giving Advice to Patients in the Clinical Environment

One of the problems that may be encountered in the clinical environment is that the clinician may attempt to provide the information regarding a

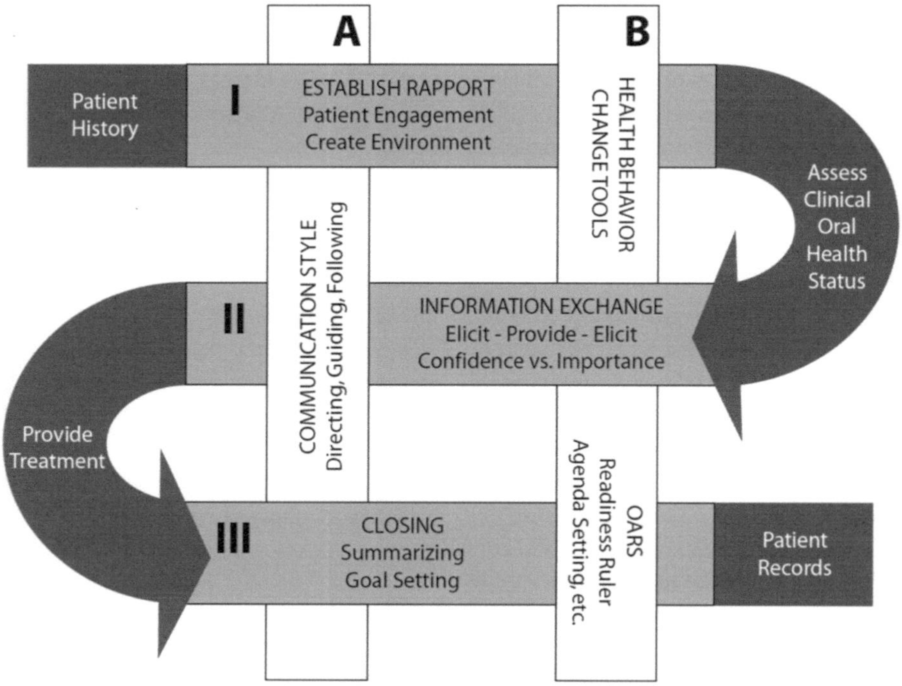

Fig. 8.1 The patient history and patient's records positioned at the start and end depict the critical elements of documentation that serve to weave one dental visit into the next. The horizontal bands depict the three core strands of conversations constituting the visit. These bands labelled as 'Establish Rapport', 'Information Exchange', and 'Closing' transition directly into the curves, representing the clinical assessment or treatment that takes place between the conversations as part of the flow of the appointment. The bands are woven together through the vertical ribbons that signify the specific elements of the communication and interaction characterizing the approach. These vertical ribbons represent communication style and health behaviour change tools and are consistent, yet flexible, recurring throughout the appointment ready to provide stability. (Acknowledgement: Patient Activation Fabric for the Dental Visit (Implementation Model) from Suvan et al. (2010))

clinical condition (e.g., dietary advice to reduce the effects of acidic drinks in association with the timing of tooth brushing) far too early in the consultation process. This may convey to the patient that the clinician has a particular agenda to pursue and therefore the patient may feel pressurized to accept the recommendation even though they may not have been ready to accept this information at such an early stage in the consultation. It is also important to recognize in this context the difference between advice-oriented health education and MI as it may be appropriate to simply provide information to address the patient's questions, misapprehensions, or lack of knowledge. It is therefore essential for the clinician (in the MI process) to provide information when the patient is willing and interested in receiving the information (the so-called advice with permission) (Moyers et al. 2003). A 3-step process that may be used as a framework for providing advice in an MI consistent style has been outlined by Rollnick et al. (1999a) as follows: (1) *elicit* the patient's readiness and interest in hearing the information, (2) *provide* the information in a neutral fashion as possible, and (3) *elicit* the patient's reaction to the information presented. In practice when addressing the patient's perspective of a particular clinical problem, the clinician may reveal gaps in the patient's knowledge, questions and concerns, and misapprehensions which in turn may lead to the patient being more willing to accept the relevant information.

As indicated above, it may take several visits for the patient to make any significant changes in health behaviour and the clinician must be careful not to force the pace of change; otherwise, both parties may become frustrated by the lack of change particularly with highly ambivalent patients.

It is critical for the clinician to acknowledge the problems in assessing a patient's readiness to change their behaviour as this will involve learning about both the patient's motivation and self-efficacy to change (Rollnick et al. 1999b). Several scales that assess both motivation and self-efficacy enabling the clinician to discover the patient's specific motivators and values in order to link them to the desired behaviour change have also been described in the published literature (Rollnick et al. 1999b).

8.10 Clinical Scenario Incorporating MI Principles in a Patient with DH Who Drinks Excessive Orange Juice

The following clinical scenario demonstrates the way MI may be used in conjunctive with a management strategy designed to reduce and prevent the impact of DH on patient's day-to-day lifestyle by changing behaviour that may influence the aetiological causes and predisposing factors implicated in DH (Olley and Bartlett 2015, see also Chap. 4). As previously indicated, the clinician may decide on a specific communication style depending on the individual patient and implement the various behaviour changes by judging the response of the patient during the consultation visit. It may therefore be possible for the clinician to implement MI during the initial stages of the management strategy as previously outlined (Table 8.2).

8.11 Conclusions

One of the problems that the busy clinician may face when managing DH is to simply prescribe or recommend a treatment without determining the aetiological and predisposing factors that may have been instrumental in initiating the problem which if not managed or corrected may continue to impact on a patient's quality of life. Traditionally, clinicians expect their patients to change their health behaviour because it is good for their overall health and any information exchanged between the clinician and patient was based on a clinician directed philosophy which not only failed to empower the patient but was also ineffective in motivating the patient to change behaviour. It is therefore important for the clinician to adopt management strategies and goals that will effectively encourage behavioural changes in the lifestyle of their patients. The introduction of patient-centred approaches, for example, brief motivational/motivational interviewing that actively encourages the involvement of the patient in taking ownership of their oral condition is therefore essential in current dental practice. It is acknowledged that for many clinicians in a busy practice, this approach may be difficult to implement due to several different constraints in the practice environment. This approach may also be very challenging for some patients and the clinician will need to show patience and empathy with the patient during the duration of the treatment. The introduction of brief motivational/motivational interviewing may, however, be of great benefit in motivating patients with DH, particularly in the early stages of management of the condition.

Table 8.2 Example of an individual management strategy using MI principles for a patient with DH who drinks excessive orange juice

Clinician	Patient	Strategy
Initial visit		
May I share with you some information about dentine hypersensitivity?	Yes	**Ask permission/elicit**
Aetiology of DH Treatment options Options to limit erosive drinks in the diet		**Providing information**
What do you think about all of this?	I was not aware of the effect of erosive drinks on my teeth	**Elicit**
From the dental examination today, it appears that you consume acid food on a regular basis	Yes, I drink orange juice a lot	
May I speak to you about your diet? Do you understand that drinking juices may damage your teeth and cause you pain? May I ask you whether you could cease drinking orange juices?	Yes I do not care, I enjoy drinking orange juice it is good for me Honestly, no. I don't want to quit even if you wanted me to	**Ask permission** **Agenda setting chart**
I hear that you don't want to quit. How do you feel about talking a little bit about your habit?	No, I don't want to speak about it right now.	**Rolling with resistance**
I hear that you don't want to speak about it right now. May I ask you again at a next visit	That's ok	
Follow-up visit		
May I ask you to speak about your habit of drinking juices?	Well, I know that it is harmful for my teeth. But I am kind of used to it, you know. So I probably won't change	**Ask permission**
So you kind of want to change but you can't change right now…?	Well, yes, kind of	**Reflection**
What may be your personal advantages if would change?	Well, I may have less sensitive teeth	**Ambivalence** **Pros (and cons)** *Advantages to change?* *Disadvantages to change?* *Advantages not to change?* *Disadvantages not to change?*
On a scale of 0 to 10 when 10 will be the highest motivation, how motivated would you be to change?	Maybe a 4	**Use of a readiness scale** *Asking about motivation* *Asking about self-efficacy*
On a scale of 0 to 10 when 10 will be the highest confidence, how confident would you be to you succeed?	I think that I am at a 3	
Well, according to the previous achievements you already made I feel that you will succeed to change your diet after all	Thanks, it feels good to hear that	**Increasing self-efficacy**
Well, how could you help yourself reducing dental erosions?	Well, I might want to wait a bit before brushing my teeth again… OR I might take a straw when drinking my orange juice	**Reflecting and summarizing**

References

Addy M, Urquhart E. Dentine hypersensitvity: its prevalence, aetiology and clinical management. Dent Update. 1992;19(10):407-8, 410-2.

Almomani F, Brown T, Williams K, Catley D. Effects of an oral health promotion program in people with mental illness. J Dent Res. 2009;88:648.

Andrews S. Motivational interviewing: a guided dialogue. www.hetimaine.org/Literature/MI_A_Guided_Dialogue.doc; 2012

Bandura AE. Self-efficacy in changing societies. New York: Cambridge University Press; 1995.
Bartlett D, Ganss C, Lussi A. Basic Erosive Wear Examination (BEWE): a new scoring system for scientific and clinical needs. Clin Oral Investig. 2008;12(Suppl 1):65–8.
Bekes K, Hirsch C. What is known about the influence of dentine hypersensitivity on oral health-related quality of life. Clin Oral Invest. 2013;17(Suppl 1):S45–51.
Bekes K, Hirsch C. Chapter 9. The impact of dentine hypersensitivity on oral-health-related quality of life. In: Gillam DG, editor. Dentine hypersensitivity: advances in diagnosis, management, and treatment. Cham: Springer; 2015. p. 133–42. https://doi.org/10.1007/978-3-319-14577-8.
Bekes K, John MT, Schaller H-G, Hirsch C. Oral health-related quality of life in patients seeking care for dentin hypersensitivity. J Oral Rehabil. 2008;36(1):45–51.
Berg-Smith SM, Stevens VJ, Brown KM, Van Horn L, Gernhofer N, Peters E, Greenberg R, Snetselaar L, Ahrens L, Smith K. A brief motivational intervention to improve dietary adherence in adolescents. The Dietary Intervention Study in Children (DISC) Research Group. Health Educ Res. 1999;14(3):399–410. https://doi.org/10.1093/her/14.3.399. PMID: 10539230.
Bioko OV, Baker SR, Gibson BJ, Locker D, Sufi F, Barlow APS, Robinson PG. Construction and validation of the quality of life measure for dentine hypersensitivity (DHEQ). J Clin Periodontol. 2010;37:973–80.
Bischof G, Bischof A, Rumpf HJ. Motivational interviewing: an evidence-based approach for use in medical practice. Dtsch Arztebl Int. 2021;118(7):109–15. https://doi.org/10.3238/arztebl.m2021.0014. PMID: 33835006; PMCID: PMC8200683.
Borrelli B, Novak S, Hecht J, Emmons K, Papandonatos G, Abrams D. Home health care nurses as a new channel for smoking cessation treatment: outcomes from project CARES (Community-nurse Assisted Research and Education on Smoking). Prev Med. 2005;41:815–21.
Bowen D, Ehret C, Pedersen M, Snetselaar L, Johnson M, Tinker L, Hollinger D, Ilona L, Bland K, Sivertsen D, Ocke D, Staats L, Beedoe JW. Results of an adjunct dietary intervention program in the Women's Health Initiative. J Am Diet Assoc. 2002;102:1631–7.
Brand VS, Bray KK, MacNeill S, Catley D, Williams K. Impact of single-session motivational interviewing on clinical outcomes following periodontal maintenance therapy. Int J Dent Hyg. 2013;11(2):134–41.
Burke BL, Arkowitz H, Menchola M. The efficacy of motivational interviewing: a meta-analysis of controlled clinical trials. J Consult Clin Psychol. 2003;71:843–61.
Burke BL, Dunn CW, Atkins DC, Phelps JS. The emerging evidence base for motivational interviewing: a meta-analytic and qualitative inquiry. J Cogn Psychother. 2004;18:309–22.
Butler CC, Rollnick S, Cohen D, Bachmann M, Russell I, Stott N. Motivational consulting versus brief advice for smokers in general practice: a randomized trial. Br J Gen Pract. 1999;49:611–6.
Canadian Advisory Board on Dentin Hypersensitivity. Consensus-based recommendations for the diagnosis and management of dentin hypersensitivity. J Can Dent Assoc. 2003;69(4):221–6.
Carra MC, Detzen L, Kitzmann J, Woelber JP, Ramseier CA, Bouchard P. Promoting behavioural changes to improve oral hygiene in patients with periodontal diseases: a systematic review. J Clin Periodontol. 2020;47(Suppl 22):72–89. https://doi.org/10.1111/jcpe.13234. PMID: 31912530
Curro FAC, Gillam DG. Chapter 7: Challenging the traditional approach to the conduct of dentine hypersensitivity studies: person-centric studies connecting the patient with their practitioner to optimize the clinical outcome. In: Gillam DG, editor. Dentine hypersensitivity: advances in diagnosis, management, and treatment. Cham: Springer; 2015. p. 85–99. https://doi.org/10.1007/978-3-319-14577-8.
Definition of Adherence. Adherence to Long-term Therapies: Policy for Action, Meeting Report, World Health Organization, June 4–5, 2001. Referenced in: Understanding and Improving Adherence for Specialty Products; 2001. www.imshealth.com/deployedfiles/ims/Global/Content/. Accessed Aug 2013.
Definition of Adherence. The American Heritage® Medical Dictionary; 2010. http://medical.yourdictionary.com/adherence. Accessed Aug 2013.
Definition of Compliance. http://www.merriam-webster.com/medical/compliance. Accessed Aug 2013.
Definition of Motivation. Dictionary.com. http://dictionary.reference.com. Accessed 2013.
Demetriou N, Tsami-Pandi A, Parashis A. Compliance with supportive periodontal treatment in private periodontal practice. A 14-year retrospective study. J Periodontol. 1995;66:145–9.
Evensen KB, Bull VH, Ness L. A health promotion intervention to improve oral health of prisoners: results from a pilot study. Int J Prison Health. 2021;17(4):546–59. https://doi.org/10.1108/IJPH-11-2020-0085.
Fardal Ø. Interviews and assessments of returning non-compliant periodontal maintenance patients. J Clin Periodontol. 2006;33:216–20.
Freeman R. The psychology of dental patient care: strategies for motivating the non-compliant patient. B Dent J. 1999;187:307–12.
Freudenthal JJ. Motivational interviewing. Dimens Dent Hyg. 2013;11(3):19–22.
Gao X, Man Lo EC, Ching Ching Kot S, Wai Chan KC. Motivational interviewing in improving oral health: a systematic review of randomized controlled trials. J Periodontol. 2013; [Epub ahead of print].
Gillam DG. Current diagnosis of dentin hypersensitivity in the dental office: an overview. Clin Oral Invest. 2013;17(Suppl 1):S21–9.
Gillam DG. A new perspective on dentine hypersensitivity-guidelines for general dental practice. Dent Update. 2017;44:33–42. Update on the 2013 dental paper and

a presentation at a National Conference, Manchester (BDA).

Gillam DG. Management of postoperative sensitivity. Dent Health. 2020;59:36–40.

Gillam DG, Chatzopoulou D. Post-operative pain following non-surgical and surgical periodontal procedures. Periodontol Dent Implantol, Jane Manakil, IntechOpen. 2019; https://doi.org/10.5772/intechopen.78728. Available from: https://www.intechopen.com/chapters/62139.

Gillam DG, Ramseier CA. Chapter 10: Advances in the management of the patient with dentine hypersensitivity: motivation and prevention. In: Gillam DG, editor. Dentine hypersensitivity: advances in diagnosis, management, and treatment. Cham: Springer; 2015. p. 143–56. https://doi.org/10.1007/978-3-319-14577-8.

Gillam DG, Yusuf H. Brief motivational interviewing in dental practice. Dent J. 2019;7(2):E51.

Gillam DG, Chesters RK, Attrill DC, Brunton P, Slater M, Strand P, Whelton H, Bartlett D. Dentine hypersensitivity-guidelines for the management of a common oral health problem. Dent Update. 2013;40:514–24.

Godard A, Dufour T, Jeanne S. Application of self-regulation theory and motivational interview for improving oral hygiene: a randomized controlled trial. J Clin Periodontol. 2011;38:1099–105.

Hettema J, Steele J, Miller WR. Motivational interviewing. Annu Rev Clin Psychol. 2005;1:91–111.

Jönsson B, Ohrn K, Oscarson N, Lindberg P. The effectiveness of an individually tailored oral health educational programme on oral hygiene behaviour in patients with periodontal disease: a blinded randomized-controlled clinical trial (one-year follow-up). J Clin Periodontol. 2009a;36:1025–34.

Jönsson B, Ohrn K, Oscarson N, Lindberg P. An individually tailored treatment programme for improved oral hygiene: introduction of a new course of action in health education for patients with periodontitis. Int J Dent Hyg. 2009b;7:166–75.

Jönsson B, Ohrn K, Lindberg P, Oscarson N. Evaluation of an individually tailored oral health educational programme on periodontal health. J Clin Periodontol. 2010;37:912.

Khan AR, Al-Abdul Lateef ZN, Al Aithan MA, et al. Factors contributing to non-compliance among diabetics attending primary health centers in the Al Hasa district of Saudi Arabia. J Family Community Med. 2012;19(1):26–32.

Kim J, Amar S. Periodontal disease and systemic conditions: a bidirectional relationship. Odontology. 2006;94(1):10–21.

Lai DT, Cahill K, Qin Y, Tang JL. Motivational interviewing for smoking cessation. Cochrane Database Syst Rev. 2010;CD006936

Loesche WJ, Grossman NS. Periodontal disease as a specific, albeit chronic, infection: diagnosis and treatment. Clin Microbiol Rev. 2001;14(4):727–52.

Lundahl BW, Kunz C, Brownell C, Tollefson D, Burke BL. A meta-analysis of motivational interviewing: twenty-five years of empirical studies. Res Soc Work Pract. 2010;20:137–60.

Mendoza AR, Newcomb GM, Nixon KC. Compliance with supportive periodontal therapy. J Periodontol. 1991;62:731–6.

Mhurchu CN, Margetts BM, Speller V. Randomized clinical trial comparing the effectiveness of two dietary interventions for patients with hyperlipidaemia. Clin Sci. 1998;95:479–87.

Miller WR, Rollnick S. Motivational interviewing: preparing people for change. 2nd ed. New York: Guillford Press; 2002.

Miller WR, Rollnick S. Ten things that motivational interviewing is not. Behav Cogn Psychother. 2009;37:129–40.

Moyers TB, Martin T, Catley D, Harris K, Ahluwalia JS. Assessing the integrity of motivational interviewing interventions: reliability of the motivational interviewing skills code. Behav Cogn Psychother. 2003;31:177–84.

Nalini HE, Punithavathy R. Motivational interviewing in improving oral hygiene—a review of literature with possible application in periodontics. JIADS. 2010;1(1):12–5.

Olley R, Bartlett D. Chapter 4: Aetiology and clinical features of dentine hypersensitivity. In: Gillam DG, editor. Dentine hypersensitivity: advances in diagnosis, management, and treatment. Cham: Springer; 2015. p. 49–62. https://doi.org/10.1007/978-3-319-14577-8.

Orchardson R, Gillam D. Managing dentin hypersensitivity. J Am Dent Assoc. 2006;137(7):990–8.

Partovi M. Compliance and your patient; 2006. http://www.rdhmag.com/articles/print/volume-30/issue-11/features/compliance-and-your-patients.html.

Prochaska JO, DiClemente CC. Stages and processes of self-change of smoking: toward an integrative model of change. J Consult Clin Psychol. 1983;51:390–5.

Ramseier CA. Potential impact of subject-based risk factor control on periodontitis. J Clin Periodontol. 2005;32(Suppl 6):283–90.

Resnicow K, Jackson A, Wang T, De AK, McCarty F, Dudley WN, Baranowski T. A motivational interviewing intervention to increase fruit and vegetable intake through Black churches: results of the Eat for Life trial. Am J Public Health. 2001;91:1686–93.

Richards A, Kattelmann KK, Ren C. Motivating 18- to 24-year-olds to increase their fruit and vegetable consumption. J Am Diet Assoc. 2006;106:1405–11.

Rollnick S, Mason P, Butler C. Health behaviour change: a guide for practitioners. Edinburgh: Harcourt Brace; 1999a.

Rollnick S, Mason P, Butler CC. Health behavior change: a guide for practitioners. Edinburgh: Churchill Livingstone; 1999b.

Rollnick S, Miller W, Butler C. Motivational interviewing in healthcare. New York: Guilford Press; 2007.

Rollnick S, Miller WR, Butler CC. Motivational interviewing in health care: helping patients change behavior. New York: The Guilford Press, A Division of Guilford Publications Inc.; 2008.

Rubak S, Sandbaek A, Lauritzen T, Christensen B. Motivational interviewing: a systematic review and meta-analysis. Br J Gen Pract. 2005;55:305–12.

Sanz M, Herrera D, Kebschull M, Chapple I, Jepsen S, Beglundh T, Sculean A, Tonetti MS, EFP Workshop Participants and Methodological Consultants. Treatment of stage I-III periodontitis-The EFP S3 level clinical practice guideline. J Clin Periodontol. 2020;47(Suppl 22):4–60. https://doi.org/10.1111/jcpe.13290. Erratum in: J Clin Periodontol. 2021;48(1):163. PMID: 32383274; PMCID: PMC7891343.

Schuz B, Sniehotta FF, Wiedemann A, Seemann R. Adherence to a daily flossing regimen in university students: effects of planning when, where, how and what to do in the face of barriers. J Clin Periodontol. 2006;33:612–9.

Senft RA, Polen MR, Freeborn DK, Hollis JF. Drinking patterns and health: a randomized trial of screening and brief intervention in a primary care setting. Final report to the National Institute on Alcohol Abuse and Alcoholism. Portland: Center for Health Research, Kaiser Permanente; 1995.

Seong J, West N. Chapter 4: Advances in the diagnosis of dentine hypersensitivity. In: Gillam DG, editor. Dentine hypersensitivity: advances in diagnosis, management, and treatment. Cham: Springer; 2015. p. 63–70. https://doi.org/10.1007/978-3-319-14577-8.

Smith B, Knight J. An index for measuring the wear of teeth. Br Dent J. 1984;156:435–8.

Suvan J, Fundak A, Gobat N. Implementation of health behavior change principles in dental practice. In: Ramseier C, Suvan J, editors. Health behavior change in the dental practice, vol. 1. 1st ed. Oxford: Wiley-Blackwell; 2010. p. 113–44.

Tan AES. Periodontal maintenance. Aust Dent J. 2009;54(1 Suppl):S110–7.

Wakefield M, Olver I, Whitford H, Rosenfeld E. Motivational interviewing as a smoking cessation intervention for patients with cancer: randomized controlled trial. Nurs Res. 2004;53:396–405.

Weinstein P, Harrison R, Benton T. Motivating parents to prevent caries in their young children: one-year findings. J Am Dent Assoc. 2004;135:731–8.

Weinstein P, Harrison R, Benton T. Motivating mothers to prevent caries: confirming the beneficial effect of counseling. J Am Dent Assoc. 2006;137:789–93.

Wertheimer AI, Santella TM. Medication compliance research: still so far to go. J Appl Res Clin Exper Therap. 2003;3(3) http://jrnlappliedresearch.com/articles/Vol3Iss3/index.htm. Accessed Aug 2013.

Williams KB & Bray K (2011) Motivational interviewing: a patient-centered approach to elicit positive behavior change. Crest®/Oral-B® at dentalcare.ca Continuing Education Course. Accessed Aug 2013.

Wilson TG Jr, Glover ME, Schoen J, et al. Compliance with maintenance therapy in a private periodontal practice. J Periodontol. 1984a;55:468–73.

Wilson TG Jr, Glover ME, Schoen J, Baus C, Jacobs T. Compliance with maintenance therapy in a private periodontal practice. J Periodontol. 1984b;55:468–73.

Woollard J, Beilin L, Lord T, Puddey I, MacAdam D, Rouse I. A controlled trial of nurse counselling on lifestyle change for hypertensives treated in general practice: preliminary results. Clin Exp Pharmacol Physiol. 1995;22:466–8.

9 Future Strategies for the Development of Desensitizing Products

Robert Hill and David G. Gillam

9.1 Introduction and Brief Overview of This Chapter

Dentine hypersensitivity (DH) is a clinical problem that may impact on the quality of life of individuals who experience discomfort when eating and drinking hot and cold food and drink during their day-to-day activities. Currently, there is no ideal desensitizing product (Over the counter [toothpaste, gel or mouthwash] or dentist applied) that provides both fast acting and long-lasting protection against the pain associated with DH. Currently, toothpastes, gels and mouthwashes are designed to reduce or relieve pain arising from DH based on either their (1) tubular occluding components (e.g., silica, calcium carbonate, various apatites, oxalates or bioactive glass) or (2) nerve desensitization properties (e.g., potassium ions) based on the hydrodynamic theory (see Chap. 5). Several novel products have either been reformulated from existing products or developed as biomimetic materials as an alternative to the traditional desensitizing products for treating DH, inhibiting caries and promoting remineralization. This chapter will focus attention on the physical and chemical properties of both traditional and novel products recommended for the treatment of DH as well as introducing more recent advances into the development of biomimetic products for the treatment of DH.

R. Hill (✉)
Department of Dental Physical Sciences, Centre for Oral Bioengineering, Queen Mary University of London, London, UK
e-mail: r.hill@qmul.ac.uk

D. G. Gillam
Centre for Oral Bioengineering, Institute of Dentistry, Barts and the London School of Medicine and Dentistry, Queen Mary University of London, London, UK
e-mail: d.g.gillam@qmul.ac.uk

9.2 The Rationale for Treatment

Although the Brännström Hydrodynamic hypothesis (Brännström 1963; Brännström and Åström 1972) does not necessarily explain all aspects of the mechanism of pain associated with DH (see Chap. 5), nevertheless it does underpin the development of new product formulations and therefore forms the rationale for measuring dentine fluid flow or hydraulic conductance and tubule occlusion in the in vitro environment prior to clinical evaluation (see Chap. 7).

As previously mentioned in Chap. 5, the hypothesis is based on the concept that the parallel dentine tubules act as a capillary bore which enables fluid flow to move bi-directonally in relation to stimuli. Implicit in the mechanism of hydrodynamic fluid flow through the open dentine tubules are several important features contained in the Hagen Poiseuilles Equation, namely variations in pressure, the radius of the tubule, the viscosity of the fluid and the length of the tubule.

D. G. Gillam (ed.), *Dentine Hypersensitivity*, https://doi.org/10.1007/978-3-031-74321-4_9

Dentine, however, is composed on numerous dentine tubules approximately 5000–20,000/mm^2 in number and their radius and length will vary depending on the region of the dentine (mid-coronal/root dentine). Dentine tubules may therefore vary from approximately 1–5 μm in diameter. In the mid-coronal region of dentine which is often used for fluid flow studies there are about 15,000 tubules/mm^2. The tubules near the dentine enamel junction (DEJ) are generally smaller in size approximately 2 μm, whereas the tubules nearest to the pulp may be as large as 5 μm. The tubules in root dentine close to the cervical margins of the crown-root area of the tooth where clinically DH has been reported to be more prevalent (see Chap. 2) are generally smaller in diameter (approximately 1 μm). Ideally dentine from this area of the tooth should be utilized for in vitro studies to determine the potential of desensitizing products and their ability to block the open dentine tubules. However, there are a number of reasons that have traditionally precluded Investigators using sections from this area of dentine, namely the anatomy, size, number of the dentine tubules and the perceived difficulty in cutting sections from cervical dentine compared to mid-coronal sections.

As previously discussed in Chap. 5, the importance and significance of determining the effects of a desensitizing product or an acid challenge based on the Hagen Poiseuiles equation may be demonstrated by the observation that an increase by a factor of two in the radius of the tubule will result in a 2^4 or 16 fold increase in the fluid flow. Conversely, a reduction in fluid flow through partially occluding the dentine tubules will result in a dramatic reduction in fluid flow and dentine permeability and it may therefore not always be necessary to have complete tubule occlusion following the application of a desensitizing product. Although the dentine disk has been utilized in in vitro studies for both tubular occluding properties and dentine permeability studies nevertheless due to the regional variation in numbers of tubules and variations in fluid flow depending on the proximity of the tubules to the pulp this may account for the large experimental scatter observed in the various published in vitro studies. A further observation may also be appropriate in that saliva is often absent in these in vitro studies and therefore certain desensitizing products that rely on the interaction of the saliva, for example, bioactive glasses toothpaste formulations should ideally include an immersion period in artificial saliva prior to testing to mimic the clinical environment. In addition, it would also be of benefit to include an acid challenge post-tooth brushing to simulate either a caries challenge or the consumption of an acidic beverage and then assess the durability of the tubule occlusion of the desensitizing product. A further observation when interpreting the results from these studies is that the apparent surface coverage of the dentine following an application of a desensitizing product may not actually reduce the fluid flow, whereas an apparently scarce surface coverage may have profound effects on fluid flow values. This observation may initially be confusing but can be explained by the example of Potassium Oxalate application where the tubule occlusion is not necessary on the dentine surface but rather subsurface (see Chap. 5). Similarly, toothpastes that occlude the dentine tubules not just at the surface but also occlude the tubules deep beneath the surface may be postulated to provide a more durable longer lasting treatment. From a practical viewpoint, toothpaste that simply cover the dentine surface without any penetration into the dentine tubules are more likely to be removed more readily either by acid dissolution or abrasive wear.

9.3 Current Approaches

The current treatment approaches in the management of DH have been addressed in Chaps. 7 and 8 and therefore the focus of the following section will be on the physical and chemical characteristics of the selected components and the significance of their inclusion into desensitizing products in the management of DH.

9.4 Pro Arginine-Based Products

Arginine is a natural amino acid, and it is found in saliva. Arginine has been postulated to form a calcium arginine complex with calcium carbonate on the tooth surface and within the dentine tubules (Kleinberg 2002; Cummins 2010). Typical commercial toothpastes contain 8% w/w arginine (Docimo et al. 2009). The chemistry of this process is poorly understood and has not been characterized in any detail. Despite this Arginine toothpastes containing calcium carbonate particles are very effective at tubule occlusion (see Fig. 9.1). In many cases, the "arginine calcium complex" appears to form preferentially on the surface of the enamel. Arginine bicarbonate which is the most frequent form used in toothpastes is an amino acid found naturally in saliva and has adhesive properties that are attractive for occluding the dentine tubules. Arginine bicarbonate is prepared from arginine (a basic amino acid) by titrating the arginine with gaseous carbon dioxide until a pH of about 7 is reached at this pH the arginine is completely converted to arginine bicarbonate the pH is then adjusted to between 8 and 9, which facilitates complex formation and binding of the arginine to the tooth surface. The presence of a slightly soluble calcium salt, which is generally calcium carbonate facilitates the tubule occlusion however a variety of calcium phosphate salts can also be used (Kleinberg 2002; Kleinberg et al. 2003).

9.5 Strontium Salts

Strontium salts have been used in desensitizing toothpastes for over 50 years (Markowitz 2009) (see also Chaps. 6 and 7). Originally strontium chloride was used but more recently strontium acetate at a loading of 8% w/w has been used. The acetate form has been used to reduce the risk of strontium precipitating as strontium fluoride when a fluoride source is included in the toothpaste formulation. The main mode of action of Strontium formulations (Acetate/Chloride) as discussed in Chaps. 6 and 7 has been suggested to be by tubular occlusion (Fig. 9.2) although the actual effect attributed to strontium in clinical studies has yet to defined (Rösing et al. 2009). When applied to tooth surfaces, it is believed that an adsorption of strontium ions occurs on the odontoblastic processes or in the dentine tubules thus blocking the transmission or neural impulses

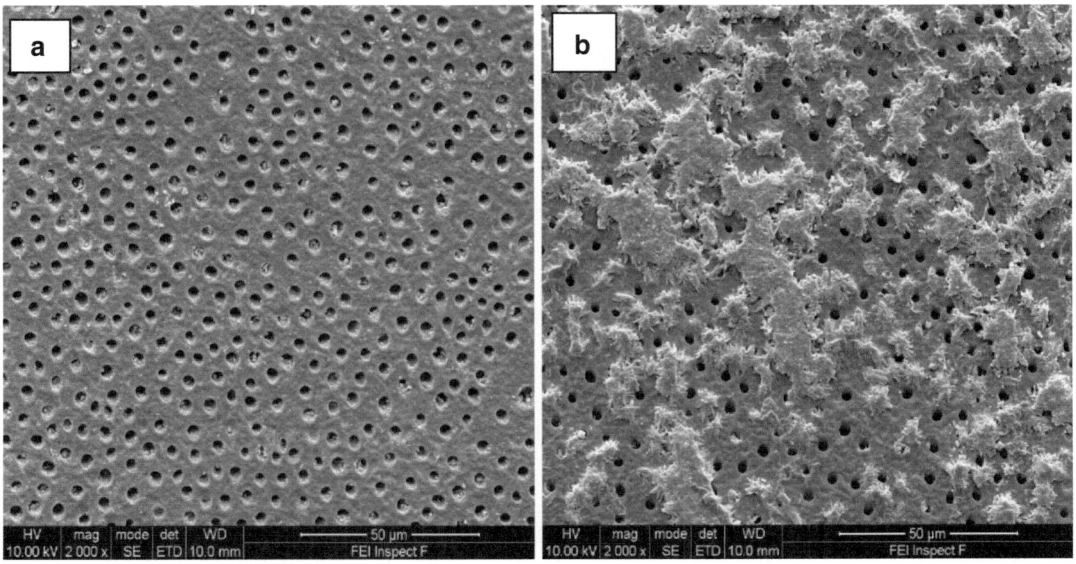

Fig. 9.1 SEM of Mid-coronal dentine section (**a**) before brushing and (**b**) after brushing with Colgate ProRelief Toothpaste

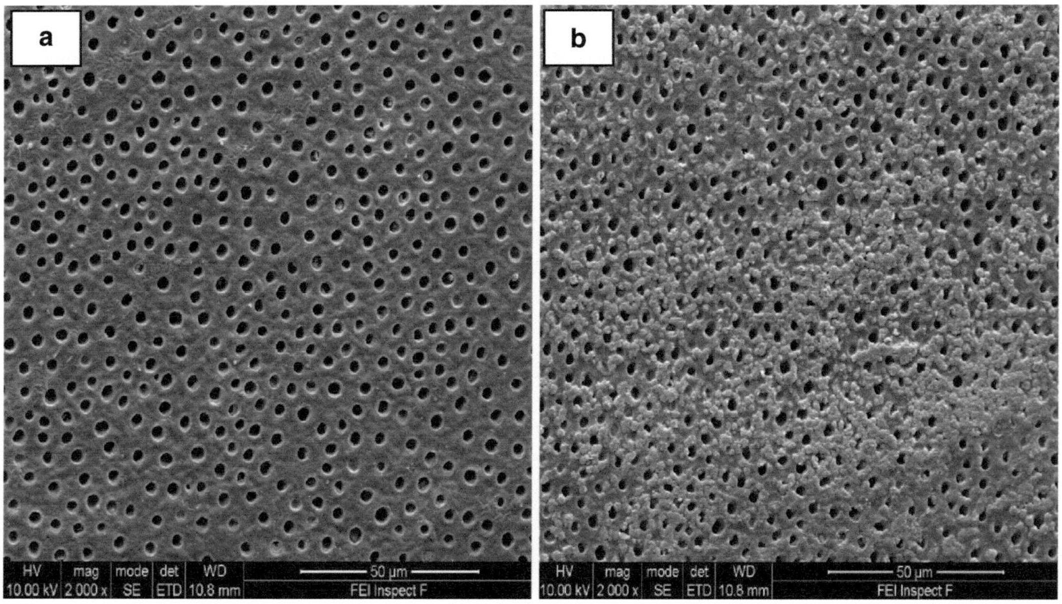

Fig. 9.2 SEM of mid-coronal dentine section (**a**) before brushing and (**b**) after brushing with Sensodyne Rapid Relief Toothpaste

from the dentine surface to the dental pulp. The strontium ion is a normal constituent of tooth structure at trace element concentrations and has a low systemic toxicity. In fact, in recent years, strontium salts have been approved for the treatment of osteoporosis where 1–2 g/day are administered. It is thought that this mechanism of strontium binding provides a mechanism to control and manage DH. It is also thought that detergents or surface wetting agents in the toothpaste enhance the effectiveness of soluble strontium ions by facilitating the penetration of strontium ions into the tooth structure.

Another possibility is that soluble strontium ions may aid apatite formation. The strontium ion is only slightly larger than the calcium ion and strontium can completely replace calcium in the apatite crystal structure. It is thought that the solubility product of a mixed calcium strontium apatite may be lower than that of calcium hydroxyapatite or strontium hydroxyapatite (Pan et al. 2009; Ni et al. 2012).

Consequently, soluble forms of strontium in toothpaste may cause apatite to precipitate from saliva. This may be aided by the presence of fluoride. The original strontium chloride toothpastes did not contain fluoride since the fluoride was thought to initiate the precipitation of strontium fluoride (SrF_2), however, this problem can be reduced by using strontium acetate as the source of strontium. However, much of the initial tubule occlusion and reduction in dentine fluid flow may be due not to the strontium ion per se but rather to the presence of small silica particles added as an abrasive that can enter the dentine tubules.

9.6 Hydroxyapatite

Hydroxyapatite $Ca_{10}(PO_4)_6(OH)_2$ is the basis of the mineral phase of enamel and dentine. Enamel contains approximately 98% by weight apatite, whilst dentine contains approximately 60% by weight. Hydroxyapatite (Ha) has been used as a remineralizing additive in toothpastes for many years, particularly in Asia, but only recently been recently used for DH toothpastes (Park et al. 2005; Kang et al. 2009; Kim et al. 2009; Yuan et al. 2012; Amaechi et al. 2021). Most Ha toothpastes, however, do not contain fluoride, since the

Ha is promoted as an alternative remineralizing additive to fluoride. The apatite crystal structure is shown in Fig. 9.3.

The open nature of the crystal lattice makes it relatively easy to substitute other ions in the crystal lattice. Manufacturers in recent years have taken advantage of this feature to produce substituted hydroxyapatites. These include strontium substituted hydroxyapatite $Ca_{(10-X)}Sr_x(PO_4)_6(OH)_2$ zinc substituted hydroxyapatite $Ca_{10-x}Zn_x(PO_4)_6(OH)_2$ and hydroxycarbonated apatite (HCA), where carbonate ions are substitute for orthophosphate ions.

Some of these toothpastes presented in Table 9.1 are currently promoted as nanohydroxyapatites nanoHA, whilst some are promoted as being natural or biomimemetic. In most of these products, the crystallite size is typically 20–100 nm. However, the hydroxyapatite particle size is always much larger and consists of many hundreds of aggregated nanocrystals. This is shown schematically in Fig. 9.4a, whilst Fig. 9.4b shows a transmission electron micrograph of the aggregated crystals. The nanosized crystals exhibit the broader diffraction lines (XRD patterns) and this is shown for Enamel and a Ultradex® hydroxyapatite toothpaste. These toothpastes generally contain polymers with carboxylic acid functional groups that are capable of chelating calcium ions in the apatite particles and the apatite in enamel and serve to stick the particles to the tooth surface and prevent them being washed away by salivary flow. The fine nanoHA crystals dissolve preferentially at the expense of the enamel apatite when the pH is reduced and thus have a sacrificial and protective function. To be effective for occluding the dentine tubules for treating dentine hypersensitivity, particles <5 µm are required (in the formulation) that can enter the dentine tubules (Fig. 9.5).

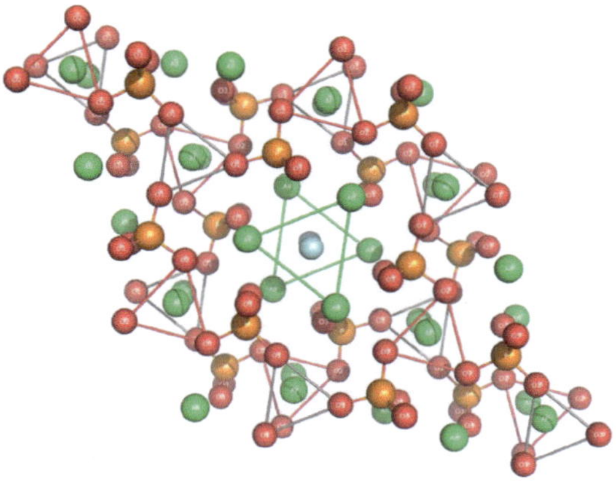

Fig. 9.3 The crystal structure of apatite. The green spheres represent calcium, the orange phosphorus and the red oxygen, whilst the light blue are hydroxyl. (Acknowledgement: Figure from Powerpoint presentation by Wolfram Hoeland, Ivoclar Lichtenstein)

Figure 9.6 shows the particle size distribution of a nanoHA toothpaste suitable for treating DH. The shaded area indicates the particles smaller than the dentine tubule size.

The crystallite size for nanoHA can be obtained from Scherrer line broadening analysis of the X-ray diffraction pattern. Crystallites larger than about 200 nm result in broadening of the diffraction lines. Figure 9.5 shows the X-ray diffraction patterns for (a) enamel (b) a microcrystalline HA and (c) a nanoHA. The broadening of the diffraction lines is clearly seen on comparing the microcrystalline and nanocrystalline HAs. It is worth noting the similarity of the nanoHA diffraction pattern with that of enamel.

Table 9.1 Commercially Available Hydroxyapatite Toothpastes

Toothpaste I	Company	Principal active ingredients
UltraDEX Recalcifying and Whitening®	Periproducts	Hydroxyapatite Sodium Monofluorophosphate
BioRepair Plus®	BioRepair/ACDOCO	Zinc substituted Hydoxyyapatite
Pepsodent Ultra Complete Sensitive®	Unilever	Hydroxyapatite
MentaDent P®	Unilever	Hydroxyapatite
Megasonex®	Goldspire	Hydroxyapatite
Apagard®	Sangi co	Hydroxyapatite

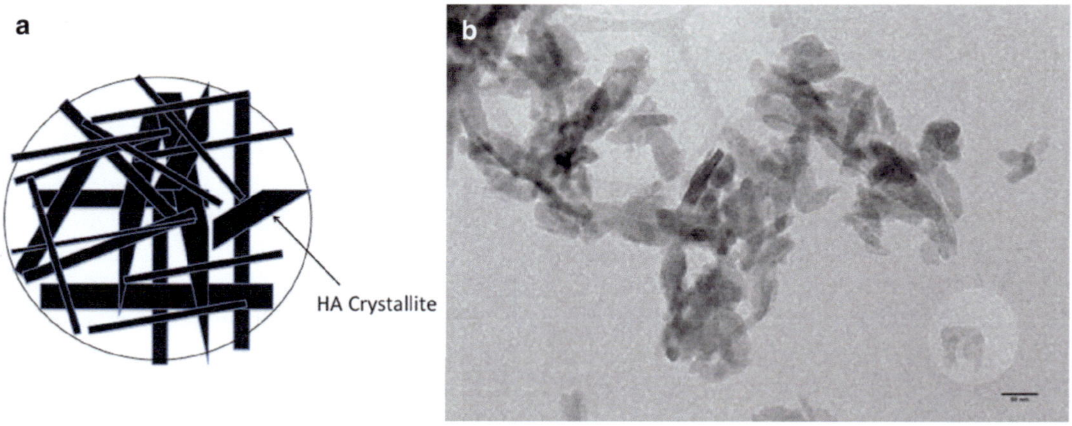

Fig. 9.4 (**a**) Schematic of aggregated nanocrystals of hydroxyapatite forming a large particle. (**b**) Transmission electron micrograph of nano-HA crystals. The crystallites about 50 nm in size based on scale bar—80× smaller than the particle size. Note that the nano-HA crystals form large aggregates of many hundreds of crystals that are much larger than the individual crystals. Scherrer line broadening analysis gave 24.6 nm for the crystallite size of this sample

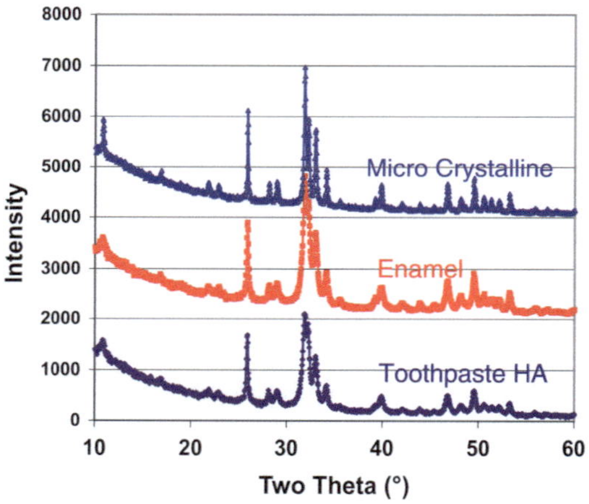

Fig. 9.5 XRD patterns for a microcrystalline hydroxyapatite, Enamel and Ultradex. Note the broader diffraction lines for Enamel and the Ultradex hydroxyapatite indicating nanocrystals. Note the almost identical diffraction patterns for Ultradex and Enamel

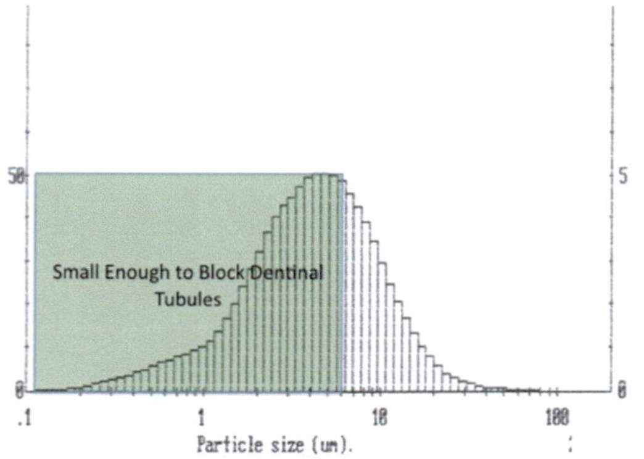

Fig. 9.6 Ultradex hydroxyapatite particle size distribution

$$D = 0.9\lambda / (\beta_{002} \cos\theta)$$

where D is the crystallite size in nm; λ is the wavelength of the incident X-rays, (0.154 nm); β_{002} is the width at half height of the 002 reflection and cos θ is the cosine of the X-ray incident angle.

Most nanoHA toothpastes do not contain a source of fluoride. However, incorporation of fluoride is beneficial. Upon acid dissolution of the nanoHA particles in the presence of fluoride reprecipitate as a fluoridated apatite. This reprecipitation process probably aids both remineralization and tubule occlusion.

Figure 9.7 shows the ^{19}F MAS-NMR spectra of a tooth treated demineralized at the surface then treated with a nanoHA toothpaste with 1000 ppm fluoride under acidic conditions (0.1M Acetic Acid pH = 4.5). There is no significant fluoride in the tooth before treating and after demineralization. However, after treating with the Ha toothpaste with fluoride the ^{19}F spectrum shows a peak at −103 ppm corresponding to the formation of fluorapatite (FAP).

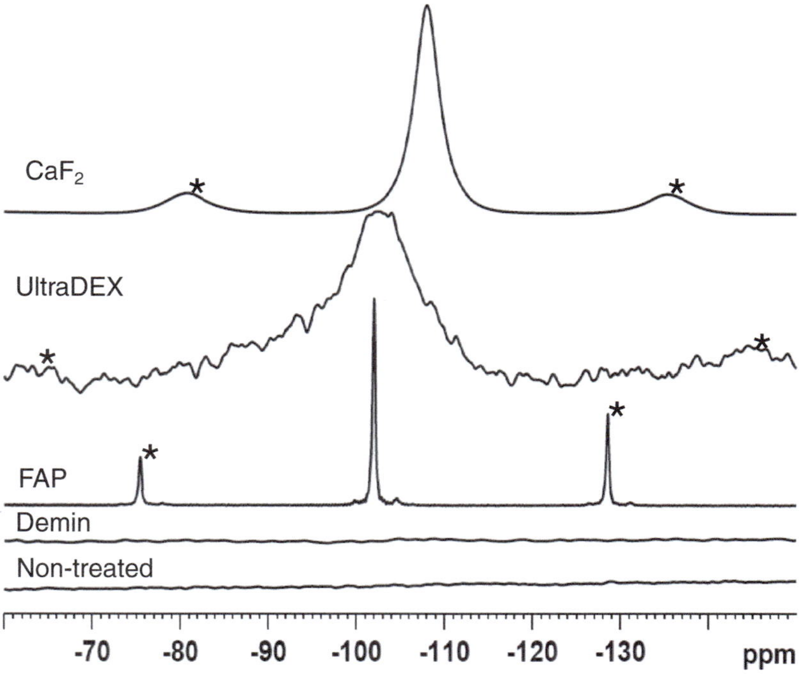

Fig. 9.7 ^{19}F MAS-NMR Spectra for the enamel samples (non-treated, demineralised and nHA oral rinse treated)

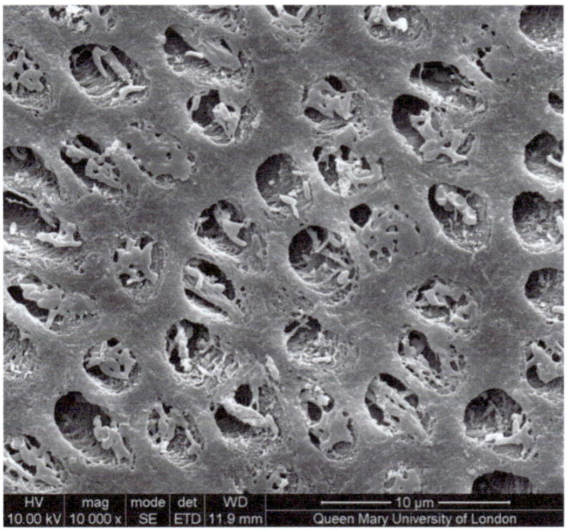

Fig. 9.8 Occlusion of dentine tubules following exposure to a nanoHA oral rinse

In addition to Ha toothpastes, there is also one oral rinse that contains both nanoHA and fluoride. Figure 9.8 shows the tubule occlusion that occurred following a series of Demineralization-Remineralization and oral rinse cycles with a nanoHA mouthrinse. The tubules which were initially open in this etched mid-coronal section are partially occluded by needle like crystals of fluoridated apatite.

Table 9.2 45S5 Glass Composition in Mole Percent

SiO_2	P_2O_5	CaO	Na_2O	NC
46.10	2.50	26.90	24.4	2.10

9.7 Calcium Phospho-Silicate (NovaMin®)

NovaMin®, which is based on the 45S5 bioactive glass composition (Table 9.2), has been used successfully in toothpastes as a re-mineralising additive and for treating DH (Zhu et al. 2015; Petrović et al. 2023), although its efficacy in remineralization has recently been questioned (Khijmatgar et al. 2020) (see Chaps. 8 and 9). The 45S5 glass particles dissolve in the mouth releasing Ca^{2+} and PO_4^{3-} ions and are thought to form hydroxycarbonated apatite (HCA) on the tooth surface.

It is worth pointing out that the 45S5 composition (see Table 9.2) was designed as a bone substitute and was never designed or intended for use originally as an additive for DH toothpastes.

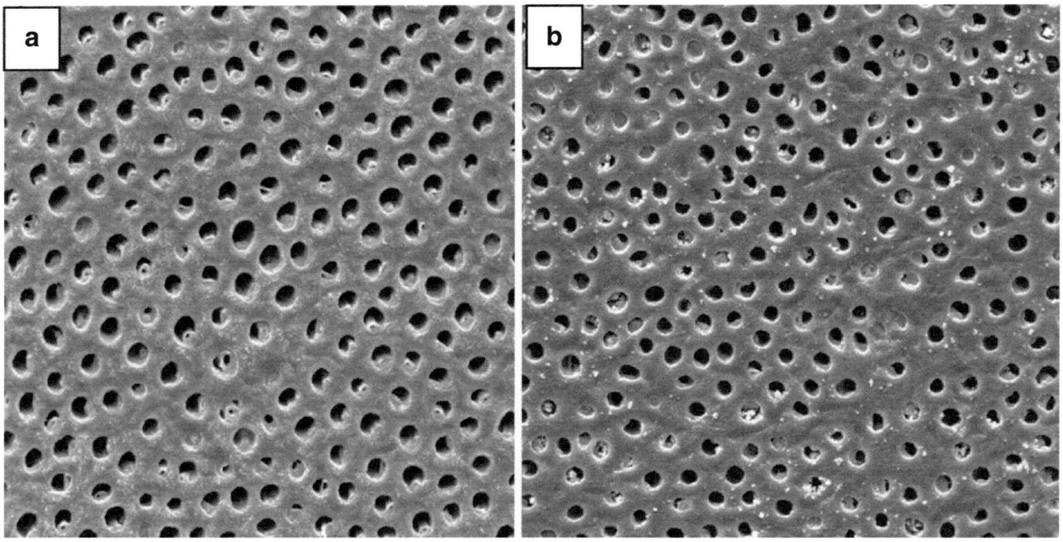

Fig. 9.9 SEM of the open dentine tubules from a mid-coronal section (**a**) before and (**b**) after brushing with a bioactive glass toothpaste

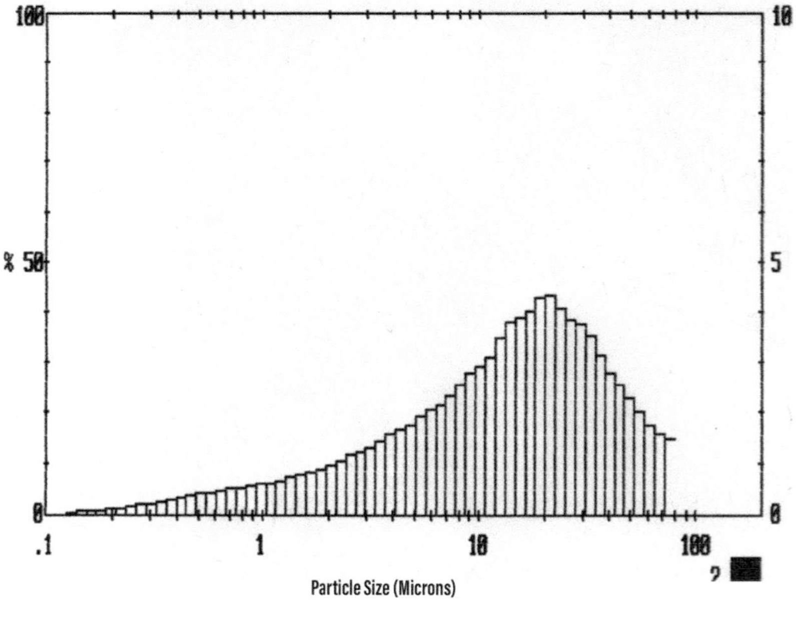

Fig. 9.10 Particle size distribution of NovaMin

In NovaMin® toothpastes some of the bioactive glass particles are small enough (<5 μm) to enter the dentine tubules and occlude them (Fig. 9.9). In the presence of saliva, which is a supersaturated calcium phosphate solution the bioactive glass particles dissolve releasing Ca^{2+} and PO_4^{3-} ions, which is believed to result in the formation of HCA (Jones 2013). The NovaMin® particle size distribution is broad and shown in Fig. 9.10. Particles smaller than about 5 μm can occlude dentinal tubules, whilst the larger particles in the distribution take much longer to dissolve and provide longer term release of Ca^{2+} and PO_4^{3-} ions. Studies suggest that better tubule

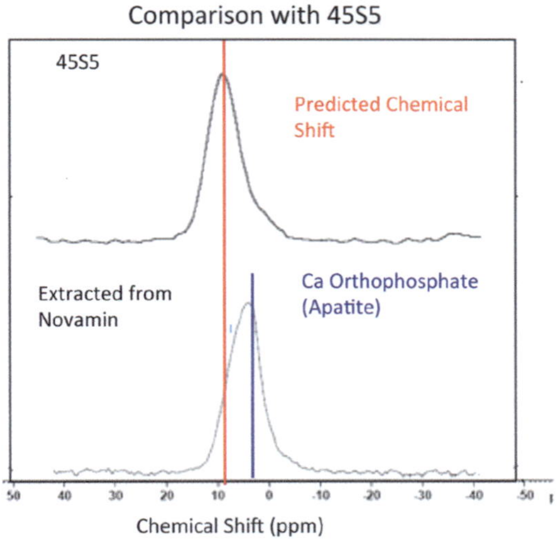

Fig. 9.11 ^{31}P ssNMR spectra of 45S% glass and glass extracted from NovaMin® Toothpaste

occlusion with NovaMin can be achieved by using a much smaller particle size to enable more particles to enter the dentinal tubules.

The NovaMin® toothpastes are like the HA pastes and contain a carboxyl functional polymer to provide the required viscosity to the toothpaste. However, the polymer also plays important role in chelating calcium ions in apatite and calcium ions in the NovaMin® glass and acts to promote the adhesion of the glass particles to the tooth and prevents them being washed away by salivary flow. In most cases, the polymer used is poly (acrylic acid) which is the same polymer used in glass ionomer cements and which enables them to bond to the apatite phase of enamel and dentine.

The NovaMin® toothpastes are glycerol, rather than water based and this is to prevent the glass reacting with water during storage in the toothpaste tube before use. In the early NovaMin® toothpastes, the 45S5 glass reacted with small amounts of water in the glycerol during storage. Approximately, 50% of the phosphate content of the glass can convert to HCA in the toothpaste during storage. ^{31}P solid-state nuclear magnetic resonance spectra for the glass extracted from the toothpaste and the 45S5 glass synthesized in the laboratory are shown in Fig. 9.11.

The latest test versions of NovaMin® toothpastes contain a fine particulate silica gel to preferentially absorb any water in the toothpaste thereby preventing it from reacting with the bioactive glass.

There is increasing evidence that bioactive glasses preferentially form an apatite-like material both on the tooth surface and within the dentine tubules. The apatite-like material grows preferentially on the highly mineralized peritubular dentine on the inside of the dentine tubule. It is postulated that the HCA in the peritubular dentine preferentially nucleates apatite crystals. Bioactive glasses have also been shown to remineralise demineralised dentine (Mneimne et al. 2014; Mneimne 2014) (Figs. 9.12, 9.13 and 9.14).

There is also increasing evidence that bioactive glasses dissolve more rapidly and forms apatite more rapidly at acidic pHs associated with caries rather than at pH = 7 or higher. This feature is particularly attractive as bioactive glasses will act to mitigate the pH fall during a caries or acid erosion challenge and will simultaneously release Ca^{2+} and PO_4^{3-} ions. In this sense, bioactive glasses are smart materials that respond to their environment.

9.8 Self-assembly Peptides

The self-assembly of biological macromolecules is widespread in nature. Examples include the spontaneous folding of proteins and the formation of a double helix from two strands of DNA. Molecular self-assembly enable production on the nanometre scale and is a form of nanotechnology and therefore may have potential for several applications in dentistry. Biological mineralization and especially odontogenesis involves biological self-assembly of proteins prior to mineralization.

Enamel formation, for example, occurs via the 3D self-assembly of amelogenin which then acts as a nucleating template for apatite crystal formation. There is therefore enormous scope for self-

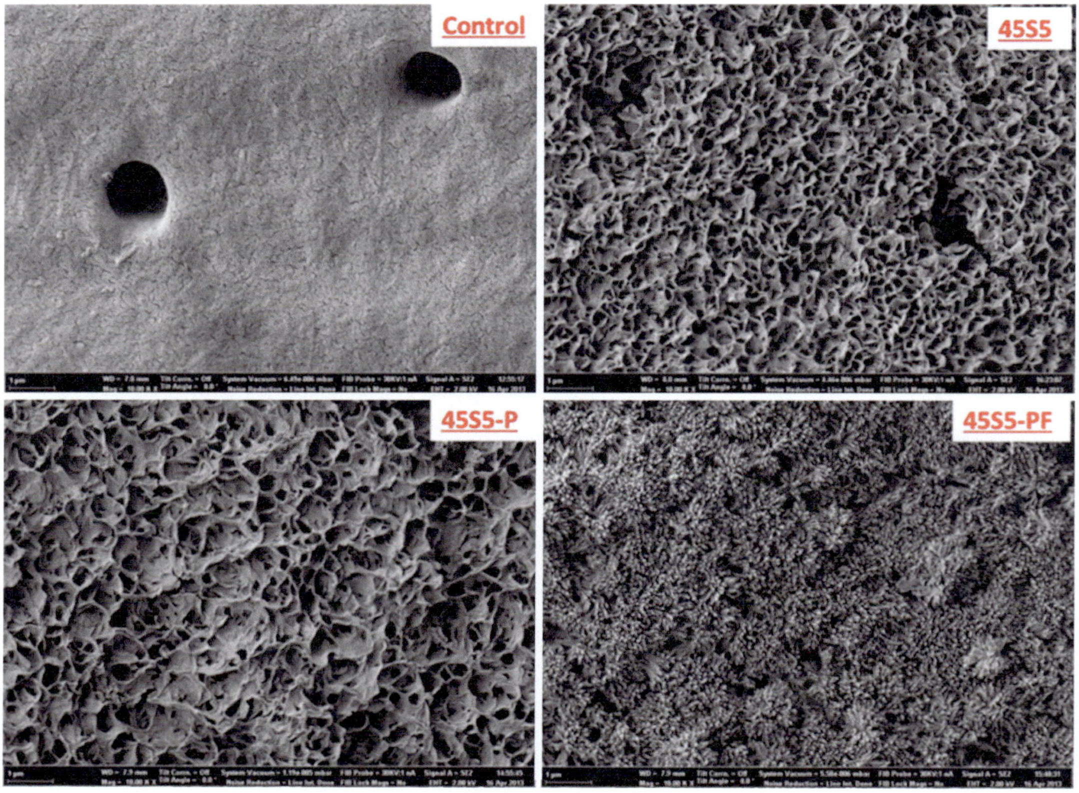

Fig. 9.12 Dentine surfaces treated with different bioactive glass toothpaste formulations

Fig. 9.13 Remineralization of etched dentine surfaces following application of a bioactive glass and immersion in artificial saliva

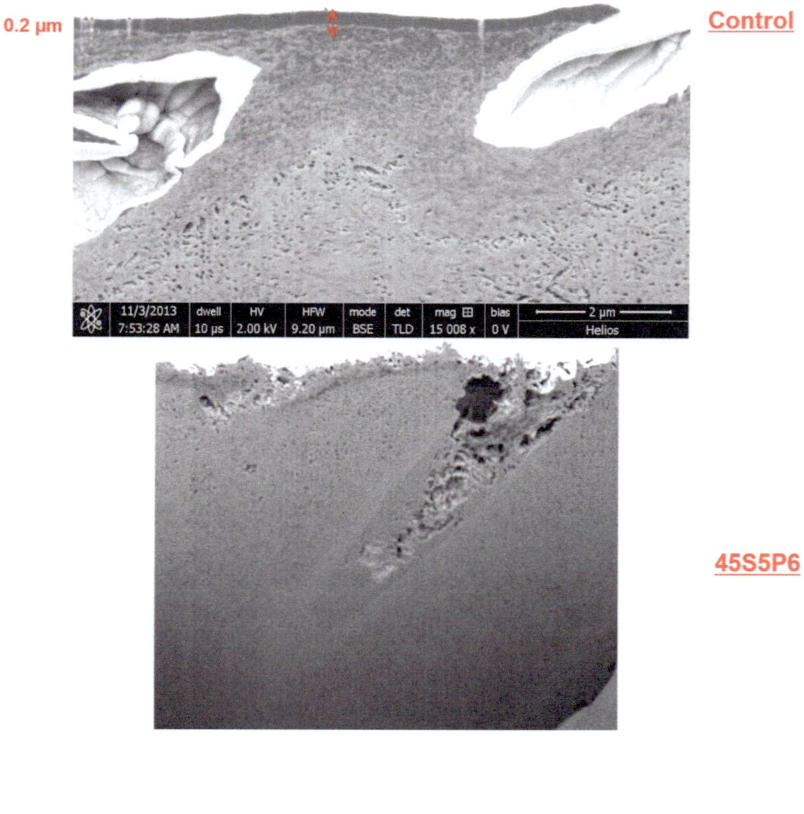

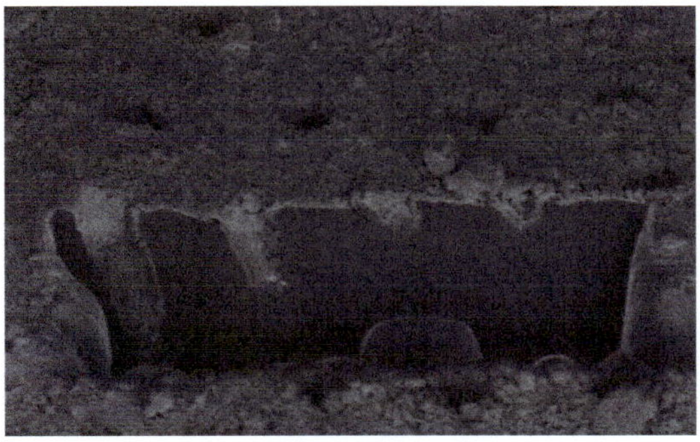

Fig. 9.14 Focused Ion Beam Scanning Electron Micrograph (FIB-SEM) showing tubule occlusion following the application of a bioactive glass toothpaste

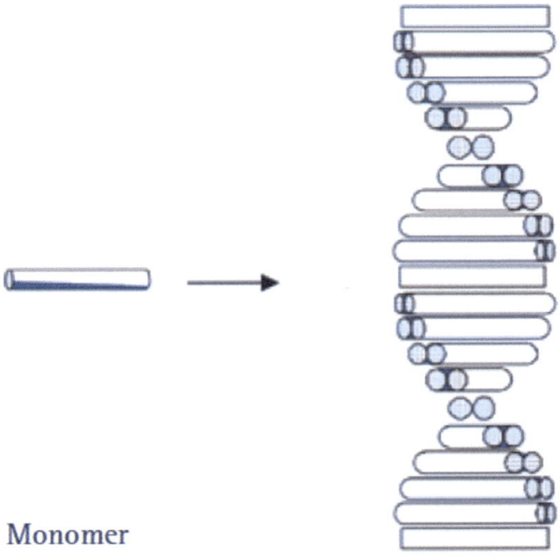

Fig. 9.15 Schematic of the Self-assembling Process

assembling proteins that promote mineralization.

A self-assembling peptide system was recently introduced as a non-invasive treatment for early-stage dental caries (Kirkham et al. 2007; Brunton et al. 2013). The self-assembling peptides diffuse into the subsurface micro-pores and forms a 3D scaffold mimicking the proteins' function during tooth development to support apatite crystallization, and reverse early tooth decay (Fig. 9.15).

The peptide P11-4 (Ace-Gln-Gln-Arg-Phe--Glu-Trp-Glu-Phe-Glu-Gln-Gln-NH2) can self-assemble into a matrix triggering a biomimetic mineralization and repair mechanism. The glutamic acid residues on the surface act as nucleation sites for apatite formation and result in remineralization of the lesion. The process of self-assembly is, however, quite sensitive to pH and ionic strength. Within the carious lesion, the pH and ionic strength favour the self-assembly process.

Recently the first self-assembled peptide product for DH has been launched called Curodont DeSenz®. This product is thought to use the same peptide as used in the remineralization and repair of carious lesion, but because the conditions for self-assembly of the peptide at the tooth surface and within dental tubules may not be ideal the current product uses pre-self-assembled particles.

However, it may be possible that following treatment with the self-assembled peptide that most tubules are occluded as there was a 64% reduction in hydraulic conductance following the application of Curodont DeSenz® on to the dentine section (Fig. 9.16) (Chen et al. 2014; Hill et al. 2020).

Figure 9.17 shows a SEM cross-section as opposed to a top-down view of a self-assembled peptide particle occluding a dentine tubule following immersion in artificial saliva. The particle contains numerous plate like crystals with a Ca:P ratio close to the apatite stoichiometry which indicates the self-assembled peptide particle is providing a surface for the preferential nucleation of apatite.

9.9 Future Innovations

There are relative few options for improving on the existing desensitizing products, for example, Arginine, Strontium and Ha toothpastes as these are well-established technologies. However, there is considerable potential for improving on the existing calcium phospho-silicate or bioactive glass toothpastes. This is largely a result of the bioactive glass that is currently used having been developed and optimized as a bone substitute.

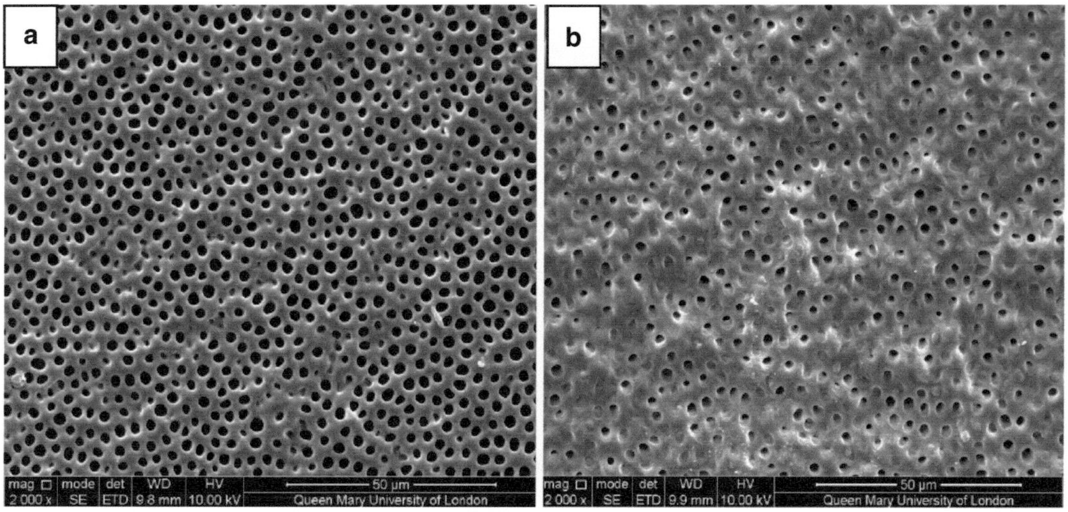

Fig. 9.16 SEM of etched mid-coronal dentine (**a**) before and (**b**) after treatment with Curodont DeSenz®

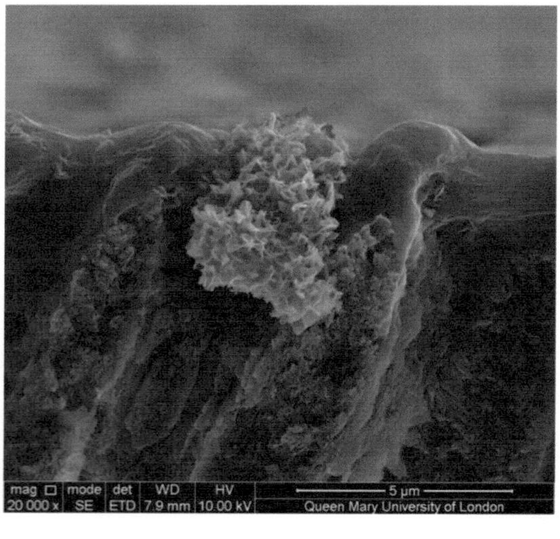

Fig. 9.17 SEM showing a Remineralised Curodont DeSenz®particle occluding a dentine tubule following immersion in artificial saliva

9.10 Consideration of the Ideal Design Criteria for a Desensitizing Product Including Toothpastes

Both Grossman (1935) and Gillam (1997) previously attempted to provide recommendations for an ideal desensitizing product from a clinical perspective, however, it is clear from the literature that there does not appear to be an ideal desensitizing product that is suitable for every clinical actuality (Gillam et al. 2013). However, it may be possible to consider this from a physical/chemical viewpoint and the following example is based on the design criteria for a calcium phosphosilicate or bioactive glass toothpaste for treating DH (Table 9.3).

9.11 The Development of Improved Calcium Phospho-Silicates Toothpaste Formulations

Although the 45S5 or NovaMin® performs remarkably well as an additive for toothpastes and has been reported to be clinically effective it was, however, never designed for this purpose. There is therefore enormous scope for designing improved glass compositions for the treatment of DH. For example, the current NovaMin® toothpaste has several major drawbacks:

(i) The apatite formed is generally thought to be an HCA. HCA is, however, more soluble than HA consequently the HCA formed will not be particularly resistant to acids in the mouth. A fluorapatite (FAP) formation would therefore be more durable.
(ii) The 45S5 glass has a hardness of about 4.7 GPa compared to enamel at about

Table 9.3 Recommendations for an ideal desensitizing product based on a calcium phospho-silicate or bioactive glass toothpaste

Rapid apatite formation (<6 h) in the mouth.
Rapid apatite formation (<6 h) in the mouth.
Formation of FAp rather than HCA.
Particle size distribution that includes small <3-μm particles for entering the dentine tubules that give rise to tubule occlusion and larger particles for more sustained release.
Strontium for its caries inhibition and remineralizing potential as well as for its possibility of binding to the odontoblast surface.
Fluoride releasing.
Potassium releasing to reduce nerve sensation.
pH rise <8.0.
No harder than enamel at 3.5 GPa.
Inexpensive to produce (note that strontium compounds are expensive).

3.5 GPa. In terms of abrasive wear during tooth brushing, it would be desirable to have a glass that is like the hardness values of natural enamel to minimize the loss of enamel.

The 45S5 glass is, however, too hard for a DH toothpaste where a softer dentine surface may be (1) exposed and (2) where the enamel is thinner (as in the cervical region) and therefore it is desirable to have a very low abrasivity toothpaste. The move in development in recent years has been towards toothpastes with lower abrasivity although NovaMin® based toothpastes are almost certainly abrasive to some degree and therefore it would be desirable to produce a glass that was softer and ideally no harder than enamel (3.7 GPa).

(iii) The NovaMin® glass generates a high pH upon dissolution. This was a major concern, but it is now considered that saliva effectively buffers the pH rise. However, whereas a high pH is desirable for hydroxyapatite formation and was considered necessary by some researchers for glass degradation, via the alkaline hydrolysis of Si-O-Si bonds of the glass network, pHs >8.0 are still considered excessive. Furthermore, even where there is an insignificant global pH rise localized pH rises could theoretically still occur.

(iv) It would be desirable that a re-mineralising glass for treating DH to have an additional bacteriocidal feature. Although this was claimed for NovaMin® toothpaste, one view is that this was largely a result of the pH rise. Therefore, there is probably no inherent bacteriocidal action of NovaMin® other than through a pH rise. If the pH rises sufficiently in order to kill or inactivate the bacteria it may also have an adverse effect on the oral soft tissues. Assuming NovaMin® is effectively buffered by oral fluids then there would be no significant bacteriocidal action.

(v) It is desirable that a toothpaste has some anti-caries activity, for example, by delivering fluoride ions or strontium ions as NovaMin® by itself appears to lack this feature.

(vi) It would be desirable if the glass acted to reduce nerve transmission to deal with the scenario where there was ineffective blocking of the dentine tubules.

(vii) Apatite formation and blocking of the dentine tubules may, however, take several weeks (in the in vivo environment) with NovaMin®. Patients are looking for an immediate relief of DH and pain. A toothpaste that acts more quickly to block the dentine tubules is likely therefore to provide more noticeable benefits to the individual and this may equate to a greater uptake in toothpaste products for DH.

All these deficiencies of NovaMin® can be overcome by designing new bioactive glass compositions specifically tailored for dental applications.

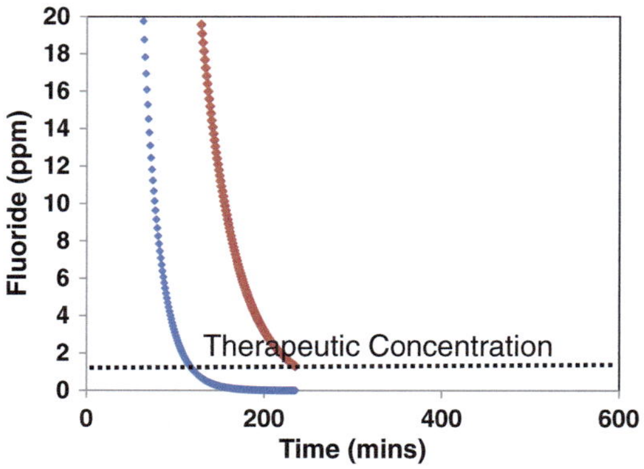

Fig. 9.18 Calculated salivary fluoride concentrations in saliva following brushing with a 1450 ppm fluoride toothpaste (blue) and a 5000 ppm prescription toothpaste (red)

For example, these compositions may include the following:

(i) fluoride containing bioactive glasses that form fluorapatite as well as releasing fluoride over the time between tooth brushings. Fluoride is thought to knock out octacalcium phosphate (OCP) formation and favours direct formation of apatite even at concentrations as low as 0.05 ppm. The solubility product of FAP is lower than that of HAP so its formation occurs more readily and at a lower pH. The ability to release fluoride in addition to Ca^{2+} and PO_4^{3-} ions is particularly attractive. Conventional fluoride containing toothpastes use soluble sources of fluoride, which are eluted away rapidly by the salivary flow in the mouth. Figure 9.18 shows calculated fluoride concentrations of fluoride in saliva following brushing with toothpastes containing different concentrations of water-soluble fluoride. The calculations have been performed assuming a salivary flow of 2.5 $ml.min^{-1}$ and a salivary volume of 2.5 ml and that at time zero immediately after brushing the fluoride concentration is one tenth of the original concentration in the toothpaste. These calculated figures agree well with the limited published studies. The fluoride concentration falls exponentially with time (for a 1450 ppm fluoride toothpaste) below the level required to inhibit caries (approximately 1 ppm) in under 2 h. In contrast a fluoride containing bioactive glass dissolves slowly releasing a controlled level of fluoride above the minimum effective dose and can maintain this concentration for longer than the time between tooth brushing (12 h).

(ii) Compositions that release bacteriocidal elements, for example, zinc and release zinc preferentially when subjected to an acidic or cariogenic challenge.

(iii) High phosphate content bioactive glasses that result in a reduced pH rise and more rapid apatite formation.

(iv) Nerve desensitizing compositions where sodium is fully or partially replaced by potassium in the glass composition.

(v) Glass compositions that contain chloride that dissolve faster and are softer and less abrasive towards tooth enamel.

9.12 Improvements in the Science and Technology of the Development of Toothpastes, and How Drawbacks in Current Toothpaste Formulations May Be Overcome

If we use the example of a NovaMin® toothpaste, then we can consider above-mentioned criteria in turn remembering that many of these points are interrelated. For example, if we recognize that HCA is more resistant to acid dissolution than OCP (that is also proposed to form with calcium phospho-silicate) and FAp is even more acid resistant how can we favour the formation of FAp at the expense of HCA or OCP?

Strontium exhibits complete solid substitution in all apatites but cannot, however, substitute fully into OCP. Octastrontium phosphate does not exist. It is likely that some strontium can substitute for calcium and possibly up to 25% of the calcium. It may be that more strontium than this destabilizes OCP and favours HCA. A mixed calcium/strontium hydroxyapatite with about 9/1 ratio has a lower solubility product than CaHA or SrHA. Replacing strontium for calcium in the glass will therefore both favour HCA formation and destabilize OCP formation. Furthermore, strontium surprisingly expands the glass network and results in faster glass dissolution, which also speeds up HCA formation. The downside to strontium incorporation into the glass is that the faster glass dissolution also results in a more rapid and undesirable pH rise. Strontium also has the disadvantage that the more expanded more weakly bonded glass structure is more prone to crystallization.

Given that FAp is more acid resistant than hydroxyapatite and HCA it would be desirable to form FAp.

There are two routes to achieving this.

(i) soluble fluoride salts can be incorporated into the formulation along with the glass.
(ii) Fluorine can be incorporated into the glass structure.

Option (i) fluoride could be added as sodium fluoride or sodium monofluorophosphate. Of these two species, the latter is the more attractive option, since simply adding a source of fluoride ions alone is more likely to result in fluorite formation. Body fluids and saliva at rest have a Ca:P ratio of approximately 2.6 compared to the apatite stoichiometry of 1.67. Once the phosphate in saliva has been consumed excess fluoride will form calcium fluoride, whose formation is undesirable. High fluoride concentrations in the saliva may also lead to direct fluorite formation. Using sodium monofluorophosphate in the formulation will add to the phosphate concentration and will therefore help mitigate against these problems.

Option (ii) however is a much better strategy. For example, incorporating a soluble fluoride into the formulation results in an initially very high fluoride concentration in saliva which is needed because we require a reasonable high fluoride concentration many hours after tooth brushing and as a result of salivary exchange (probably about every 1–5 min during the day), but salivary flow and salivary volumes very variable depending on the individual, However, there will be a virtually exponential decay in the fluoride concentration. The high concentration initially is undesirable and may lead to fluorite formation. What is required is a constant but relatively low fluoride concentration in the mouth, which can be achieved by using a fluoride containing glass in particulate form that sticks to the teeth and gingivae slowly releasing fluoride along with calcium and phosphate in ratios that favour FAp formation and preferably with a slight excess of fluoride since calcium and phosphate will also be supplied from the saliva. Recognizing that body fluids/saliva has a Ca:P ratio of about 2.6 compared to 1.67 for apatite it is probably more important that the glass delivers phosphate than Ca. The existing NovaMin® has a Ca:P ratio of close to 5 and thus releases more Ca than phosphorus.

Increasing the phosphate content of bioactive glasses (providing this is completed in the correct manner for example, keeping the NC close to 2 which is not necessarily obvious), results in (1) faster apatite formation and (2) an increase in apatite formation.

9.13 Reducing the Abrasivity of the Toothpaste

The finer the particle size and the less angular the particle the less abrasive the glass will be. The analogy here is of glass/sandpaper. The harder the glass is the more abrasive it will be.

Reducing the particle size reduces the abrasive wear, but this would knock out the long-term release of ions from the glass that would be probably undesirable. Although it would be possible to blend two or more glasses, for example, a small particle size less soluble glass with a particle size <45 μm with a more soluble glass with a particle size also <45 μm to give the same release kinetics as a single glass with a particle size <90 μm (the size range of NovaMin®). Having a particle size <50 μm would also remove the "gritty texture" of the existing NovaMin® tooth-

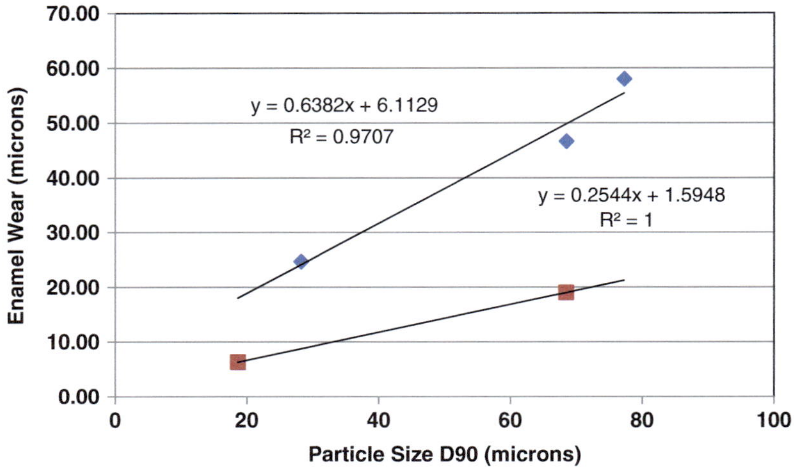

Fig. 9.19 Enamel wear of 45S5 Bioactive glass toothpastes as a function of D90 particle size. The red squares are round ball milled samples, and the blue points are percussion milled samples that give rise to more angular particles (Mahmood et al. 2014)

paste and would therefore result in a better tactile sensation to the toothpaste, e.g., a smoother feel rather than a gritty feel as with existing NovaMin® toothpastes (Fig. 9.19).

The grinding route will also influence particle shape and vibratory milling gives sharp angular particles, whilst ball milling gives rounded particles. Rounded particles should give less abrasive wear. Particle shape can be altered by post-grinding treatments, for example, dropping the particles through a high temperature furnace at a temperature above glass transition temperature (Tg) or through a plasma torch will result in the glass particles minimizing their surface energy by forming perfect spheres. However, these treatments, however, would add to the cost of production. It is also important to note that such treatments post grinding will reduce the surface area and will relax strains in the glass particle surface that have a significant influence on glass reactivity. Strained bonds put the glass into a more reactive state.

A simpler option and a less expensive option would be to reduce the hardness of the glass so that it is closer to the hardness of enamel. The hardness of glasses is related to the strength of bonding in the glass structure. There are very few published hardness values in the published literature for low network connectivity bioactive type glasses. However, there is a strong linear correlation between the glass transition temperature and hardness (Farooq et al. 2013). The more disrupted the glass the lower the, Tg and the lower the hardness. Tg reduces with:

(i) Increasing alkali metal content.
(ii) Moving down a group in the periodic table. Potassium containing glasses are softer than the equivalent sodium containing glasses. Replacing strontium for calcium results in slightly lower Tgs and hardness values.
(iii) Mixing alkali metals.
(iv) Reducing SiO_2 content.
(v) Increasing P_2O_5 content.
(vi) Increasing fluorine content.

Of these (i) and (vi) give large reductions in Tg. Alkali metal content, however, cannot be increased very much without risking the glass crystallizing. Replacing sodium for potassium does not change the glass dissolution kinetics significantly and having a little sodium, for example, a mixed glass gives a further slight reduction. Incorporation of potassium is also valuable for giving potassium ion release for the eliminating the pain associated with DH and therefore may be worth pursuing.

Incorporation of fluoride drops the Tg dramatically, as well as resulting in faster and quicker apatite formation, formation of apatite at a lower pH and formation of FAP and fluoride release.

The correlation between Tg and hardness for bioactive glasses must be regarded as a guide because it is (i) an extrapolation into an area outside the normal compositional range, for example, lower SiO_2 content and (ii) bioactive glasses may have two glass transition temperatures, the first is thought to correspond to the silicate glass phase and the second to the orthophosphate phase. In the case of very rapidly quenched glasses, the phase separation process may be suppressed, and the scale of phase separation may be exceedingly small and the first glass transition may be a combined glass transition temperature. As the glass is heated past the first Tg it may well phase separate further resulting in a second Tg. In the case of the 45S5 composition, the second Tg is not apparent because it is masked by crystallization. Since the first Tg probably corresponds to the silicate matrix glass phase, it would be expected to dominate the hardness.

9.14 Reducing the pH Rise in the Oral Environment

The pH rise can be reduced by reducing the alkali metal content, but this will result in a harder more abrasive glass. Increasing the phosphate content reduces the pH rise significantly as does increasing the fluorite content. Phosphate content has the most significant effect. The phosphate in bioactive glasses is probably present as a separate nanosized phase and as an amorphous orthophosphate. The phosphate phase is dispersed in the silicate phase. Phosphate glasses when they dissolve give an acidic pH and silicate glasses a basic pH. By adjusting the volume fraction of the phosphate phase relative to the silicate phase the pH rise can be manipulated. Again, care has to be taken to put in additional phosphate without altering the degradable silicate matrix glass composition.

9.15 Providing a Real Bacteriocidal Action in a Toothpaste Formulation

Strontium has a mild bacteriocidal action against many of the bacteria involved in caries (Guida et al. 2003) Fluoride has also a bacteriocidal action at acidic pHs (Malts and Emilson 1982).

9.16 Caries Inhibitory Properties

Fluoride has well-documented caries inhibitory properties. Strontium also has been associated with a caries inhibitory role and together their action is supposedly synergistic. Caution has, however, to be exercised with fluoride—more is not always better. Excess is more likely to result in CaF_2 formation or even SrF_2 or mixed Ca/SrF_2 where strontium is present. It is also important to note that whereas FAp is more stable than hydroxyapatite to acid dissolution there can be no hydrogen bonding along the c-axis channel in pure FAp and it has been argued that a mixed 50/50 fluoro/hydroxyapatite will be more stable because of hydrogen bonding between fluorine and the hydrogen of the hydroxyl group (Elliott 1994). There may therefore be an optimum fluoride content in the apatite corresponding to a fluoride content less than the stoichiometric amount.

Not only can bioactive glasses prevent caries, but they may also prevent acid erosion. Bioactive glasses can also promote remineralization in carious lesions or acid erosion lesions and the evidence indicates that high phosphate and fluoride containing glasses can do this more effectively than the conventional low phosphate glass (Mneimne 2014).

A very useful feature of bioactive glasses is their ability to dissolve more rapidly under acidic conditions. Since the first step in glass degradation of bioactive glasses is the ion exchange of Na^+ and Ca^{2+} ions for H^+ ions a lower pH accelerates glass dissolution and the release of Ca^{2+} and PO_4^{3-} ions for remineralization. In a practical sense bioactive glasses are "smart materials and respond to their chemical environment. The pH sensitivity of bioactive glasses can be enhanced further by incorporating zinc oxide into the glass. Zinc is incorporated into the glass structure as an intermediate oxide forming ZnO_4 tetrahedra and forming Zn-O-Si bonds. These bonds can be acid hydrolysed in a similar fashion to the Al-O-Si bonds in glass (ionomer) polyalkenoate cements, where Al_2O_3 also acts as an intermediate oxide.

9.17 Blocking Nerve Transmission

Replacing Na_2O by K_2O will result in K^+ ion release and may serve to aid in blocking nerve transmission without changing the key properties of the glass and as already mentioned previously will reduce glass hardness slightly (Tiskaya et al. 2021). Glass particles that are small enough to enter the dentine tubules are likely to deliver potassium ions more effectively than larger particles.

9.18 Increased Speed and Amount of Apatite Formation

Increasing the phosphate content and fluorine content dramatically increase the speed of apatite formation as well as the amount of apatite formation in the case phosphate. If the glass is more efficient in producing apatite, the glass fraction in the formulation may be reduced giving a considerable cost saving. The dissolution of bioactive glasses is generally very rapid, and the slow step is the nucleation of apatite. Glasses that have crystallized to small quantities of apatite form further apatite faster and pre-existing apatite crystals formed during glass formation, or because of reaction with water from the atmosphere at the glass surface can act as seed crystals or nuclei. Similarly glass powders/toothpastes may be seeded with small typically less than 3 μm FAP or HA crystals to nucleate apatite within the dentinal tubules more effectively. HA is readily available and considerably cheaper than bioactive glasses (6 Euros/kg compared to 50–100 Euros/kg). HA as discussed earlier is already used in DH toothpastes for tubule occlusion.

9.19 Water-Based Toothpaste Formulations

Unfortunately, it is not feasible to produce a water-based version of a calcium phosphorsilicate toothpaste. The problems of water absorption during manufacture and the reaction of the glass in the tube and subsequent apatite formation can probably be avoided by incorporating silica gel to preferentially absorb water and prevent it reacting with the glass. Water absorption by the glycerol once opened by the consumer is a significant concern. For example, if the toothpaste cap is left open, how long does it take for the glycerol to absorb water and apatite formation to commence? A further concern would be with regard to whether this influences the effectiveness of the toothpaste. More sophisticated packaging, for example, a self-closing tube or simply selling in smaller tubes might also be useful. There is a growing interest in toothpaste tablets largely driven by sustainability and environmental concerns with recycling of aluminium laminated toothpaste tubes. The development of toothpaste tablets containing bioactive glass powders would be an attractive option for the following reasons:

(i) Manufacture of glycerol-based toothpastes is technically challenging.
(ii) Glycerol is much more expensive than water.

Nanohydroxyapatite containing toothpaste tablets are already commercially available.

9.20 Anti-gingivitis Properties

It has been previously reported that NovaMin® has an anti-plaque and anti-gingivitis action (Allen et al. 2001; Tai et al. 2006) but there is no obvious mechanism of action. Zinc oxide can be incorporated into bioactive glasses formulations and zinc salts notably zinc citrate and zinc chloride have also been widely used in toothpastes for their bacteriocidal and anti-gingivitis action (Lynch 2011). Zinc oxide has been widely used in skin creams, wound dressings as well as dental cements where it has a well-documented bacteriocidal and wound healing role (Lansdown et al. 2007). It must be noted that whilst zinc has a well-documented antibacterial action it also inhibits apatite nucleation and crystal growth.

9.21 Octacalcium Phosphate (OCP)

Octacalcium phosphate, $Ca_8(PO_4)_6H_2.5H_20$ (OCP) is thought to be a precursor to HCA formation when the pH is <9. It is a precursor phase in biological apatite formation. OCP is thermodynamically less stable than hydroxyapatite (Ha) or HCA, but its formation is kinetically favoured probably because of having a lower activation energy for nucleation. OCP is structurally and crystallographically like hydroxyapatite and can co-crystallize with Ha. OCP is calcium deficient compared to Ha contains two acidic phosphate groups and a water layer. The X-ray diffraction patterns for OCP and HA are almost identical, but OCP contains an additional diffraction line at 4.6 two theta corresponding to a water layer. OCP converts with time in an aqueous environment to a calcium deficient apatite and where carbonate is present to a calcium deficient carbonated apatite. Fluoride ions are known to aid the conversion of OCP to apatite. OCP is therefore attractive as a potential remineralizing additive in toothpastes. However, to the knowledge of the authors, OCP has never been incorporated into toothpaste.

OCP tends to form as thin plate like crystals with similar aspect ratios to flake glass which make it attractive for treating DH. The conversion process is a solid-state transformation so the plate like morphology is retained after conversion to the apatite. OCP is much more soluble than HCA and it is likely therefore any toothpastes containing OCP will incorporate a source of fluoride for catalysing the transformation of OCP to apatite and for the formation of a more acid durable fluoridated apatite.

Whereas as mentioned above, there are no known OCP-based toothpastes OCP may, however, be formed as a transitory precursor phase with some existing toothpastes (including bioactive glass-based toothpastes) and in natural tooth remineralization processes with saliva.

9.22 Systems Involving Formation of Apatite-Like Phases from Calcium Phosphate Salts

One attractive solution to treating DH is to form the tooth mineral within the dentine tubule and on the tooth surface. Calcium phosphate cements have been developed at the Paffenberger Dental Institute, which have largely been used as a bone cement and grafting material in orthopaedics have recently been used for treating DH (Komath and Varma 2003; Ambard and Mueninghoff 2006).

A much higher water content and a finer particle size for the powder is used than would be the case for a classic calcium phosphate cement for the cement paste to have a low viscosity and be able to enter the dentine tubules.

The product Teethmate Densensitiser® consists of a mixture of tetracalcium phosphate ($Ca_4P_2O_9$) and dicalcium phosphate anhydrous ($CaHPO_4$) to which water is added. The two salts dissolve and are claimed to reprecipitate as Ha the mineral phase of tooth (see Fig. 9.20).

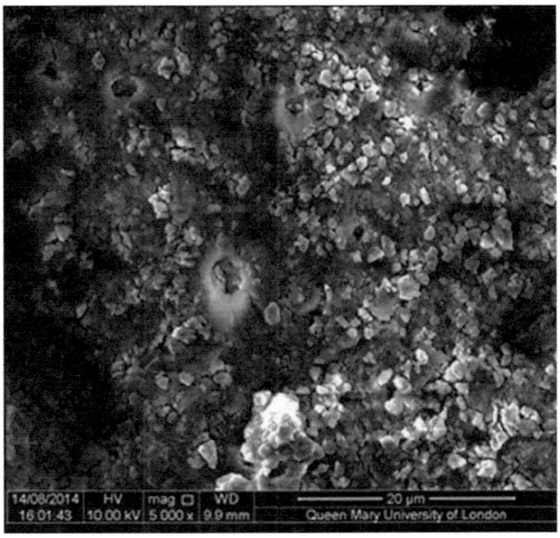

Fig. 9.20 SEM of a dentine disk section following the application of Teethmate Desensitizer®

However, the phase formed initially is actually OCP, $Ca_8H_2(PO_4)_6.5H_2O$, which has a very similar X-ray diffraction pattern to Ha but has an additional diffraction line due to the water layer in its structure at 4.68° two theta. The phase formed within the tubules has a plate like appearance which is typical of OCP.

Teethmate Desensitizer® provides good tubule occlusion and it has been reported (Thanatvarakorn et al. 2013a, b; Eyüboğlu and Naiboğlu 2020; Maillard et al. 2023) that it provides a tensile bond strength to dentine close to 10 MPa however calcium phosphate cements particularly with high water contents have compressive strengths lower than this figure and the tensile strength would be expected to be a fraction of their compressive strength. OCP is much more acid soluble than Ha and the long-term durability of this product when faced with an acid challenge remains to be evaluated. Despite these criticisms there is potential in this type of product for treating DH and it does avoid issues of toxicity associated with resin-based systems (Choudhary et al. 2012; Mehta et al. 2014).

Recently researchers at QMUL have developed calcium phosphate cements based on fluoride containing bioactive glasses as an alternative to using calcium phosphate salts and the phase formed is a fluoridated apatite which would be expected to be much more durable than the OCP in the Teethmate Desensitizer® product.

9.23 Polymers and Peptides That Promote the Formation of a Pellicle Like Layer

There is a lot of interest in polymers that promote the formation of a pellicle like layer that could be beneficial regarding preventing both acid erosion and dentine hypersensitivity (Reis et al. 2023). The use of synthetic statherin peptides has been shown to promote the formation of a pellicle like layer that protects the tooth particularly against acid erosion and it has been suggested that statherin like peptides could be incorporated into oral health care products. However, statherin like peptides are not economically feasible for this purpose. Polygamma glutamic acid is the basis of fermented soyabeans known as Natto. The carboxylate groups chelate Ca^{2+} cations in the apatite crystals of enamel in a similar way to statherin and inhibit the dissolution of enamel (Parati et al. 2022), Furthermore, polygamma glutamate is sold both as a food additive and as a component of cosmetic skin creams and is commercially available at reasonable cost. It is already used in Japan for xerostomic patients, as a mouth moisuriser. Polygamma glutamate, since it is based only on glutamic acid does not elicit an immune response and furthermore unlike statherin is not hydrolysed and degraded readily by salivary proteases in the mouth, making it last longer in the mouth.

9.24 Systems Designed to Stimulate Odontoblast and Tertiary Dentine Formation

One aspect that has been rarely considered in DH is the natural response of the tooth to damage and open tubules. Tertiary dentine is produced by odontoblasts in the pulp chamber in response to open dentinal tubules. This tertiary dentine lacks the organized orientated dentine tubule structure of primary dentine. The formation of tertiary dentine acts to seal the sensitive pulp from external stimuli and bacterial infection. Because tertiary dentine has no organized dentine tubule structure, it effectively acts to occlude the dentinal tubules from within. Odontoblasts are like osteoblasts in bone and produce collagen and form apatite. Osteoblasts are up regulated by various factors including strontium, zinc and fluoride ions as well as by bioactive glasses. Silicon release in the form of soluble silicates has been shown to activate many of the genes involved in bone formation. It is possible that odontoblasts too may be stimulated to produce tertiary dentine by components from DH toothpastes that are capable of diffusing down the dentinal tubules. It is important to note that the process of tertiary dentine formation is likely to be slower than surface tubule occlusion. However, treatments that result tertiary dentine formation are likely to have long-term efficacy compared to treatments that give only surface occlusion of dentinal tubules. It is surprising given the well-known influence of strontium ions on up regulation of osteoblasts and the prevalence of strontium in many dental restorative materials including toothpastes that the influence of strontium on odontoblasts has not been investigated.

9.25 Hybrid Materials

9.25.1 Flake Glass Varnish

A flake glass varnish would not be sold as an over-the-counter product, for example, a toothpaste but would be used as an In office treatment as an alternative to existing varnish treatments. Flake glasses are thin plates of glass that can be from 0.1 to 10 μm thick and vary in width from 10 to 500 μm. A scanning electron micrograph of flake glass particles is shown in Fig. 9.21.

Flake glass epoxy composites are currently used as corrosion and wear resistant coatings on the inside of crude oil pipelines. The flake particles align parallel to the surface of the pipe. This is shown schematically in Fig. 9.22. The flake particles act as a barrier to water ingress. The flake glass particles also dramatically improve the abrasive wear behaviour and since they are much harder than the resin protect the composite coating from abrasive wear by small sand particles in the crude oil.

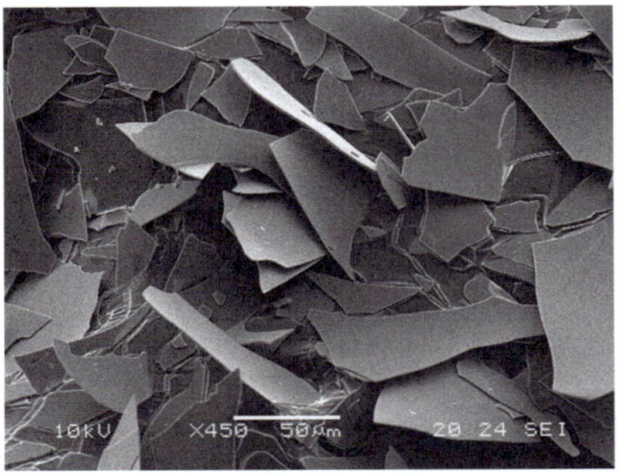

Fig. 9.21 Scanning electron micrograph of flake glass particles

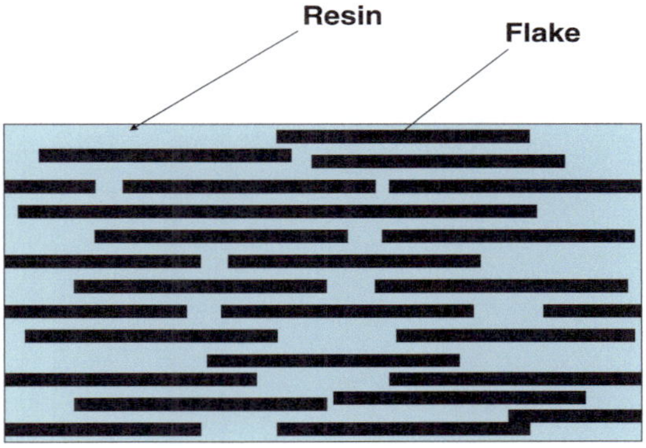

Fig. 9.22 Schematic of an aligned flake glass composite

Figures 9.23a, b show the microstructure of an aligned flake glass varnish developed for dental use. Such a varnish is likely to be much more durable in the mouth than conventional unfilled varnishes. Another advantage of these varnishes is the flake particles act as barriers to oxygen diffusion into the coating and this dramatically reduces the formation of the oxygen inhibited layer, resulting in a very high degree of polymerization. Such flake glass varnishes are particularly attractive for a long term in office treatment for DH.

9.26 The Development of a Novel Fluoride Containing Bioactive Glass-Based Toothpastes (Biomin F)

As indicated above Fluorine containing bioactive glasses have been developed in recent years. These new glass compositions are like the NovaMin composition. Table 9.4 compares the NovaMin composition with the BioMinF composition containing fluorine.

The BioMinF composition developed at QMUL differs from the NovaMin composition in that it contains fluorine in the glass and the glass is a sodium calcium fluoro phosphor-silicate. Incorporating fluorine in the glass results in a

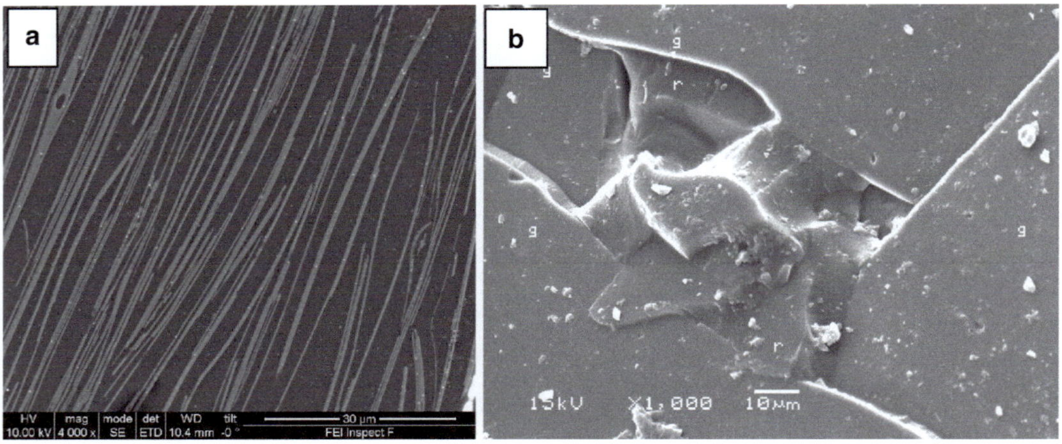

Fig. 9.23 (**a**) (left) SEM Cross-section of aligned flakes in a flake glass coating and (**b**) SEM of top-down view

Table 9.4 Comparison of BioMinF and NovaMin glass compositions

Glass	SiO2	P2O5	CaO	Na2O	CaF2	D50 particle size microns	Hardness (GPa)
BioMinF	39–41	5–6	28–30	23–24	1–2	≈8	4.4
NovaMin /45S5	46.1	2.5	26.9	24.4	0	≈16	4.7

slow sustained release of fluoride avoiding the problem of soluble NaF being washed away exponentially by salivary flow.

The BioMinF not only releases fluoride but also large amounts of calcium and orthophosphate. Since the first stage of the reaction of a bioactive glass with water is an ion exchange of Na + and Ca2+ cations for H+ ions which results in a significant pH rise which is of benefit in preventing acid erosion and caries. The glass is engineered to dissolve at pH 7 over 10–12 h the time between tooth brushings (BDJ In Practice 2023).

The fluorine in the glass results in fluoride release and the formation of fluorapatite in contrast to hydroxyapatite formed with the NovaMin composition. This is shown very clearly by 19F solid-state Nuclear Magnetic Resonance Spectroscopy (Fig. 9.24). The initial glass has a relatively broad-spectrum reflecting fluorine being present as F-M(n) where M is Ca/Na. A peak at −103 ppm appears in the spectrum of the glass immersed in artificial saliva pH 7 after about 30 min and grows intensity with time. This peak corresponds to the F-(Ca)3 site in calcium fluorapatite.

The BioMinF glass has a smaller particle size to enable more glass particles to enter the dentinal tubules to treat dentine hypersensitivity. The smaller particle size also helps to reduce the abrasivity of the toothpaste against both enamel and dentine. The higher P2O5 or phosphate content in the BioMinF results in both faster formation of the apatite and more apatite being formed.

Figure 9.25 shows the remineralization rate determined by scanning microradiography for four different re-mineralising toothpastes. Here Enamel blocks are placed in a cell and 0.1 M acetic acetic acid at pH 4 flowed through the cell to demineralise the block. The block is then brushed twice a day with the chosen paste and placed in flowing Artificial Saliva (0.9 ml min^{-1}) at pH 7.

The BioMinF toothpaste results in a high remineralization rate over twice that of artificial saliva. There are many studies in the literature investigating the remineralization of enamel using BioMinF by measuring surface hardness recovery following a demineralization treatment. In addition, BioMinF has been found to be potentially good for treating White Spot Lesions (Salah et al. 2022).

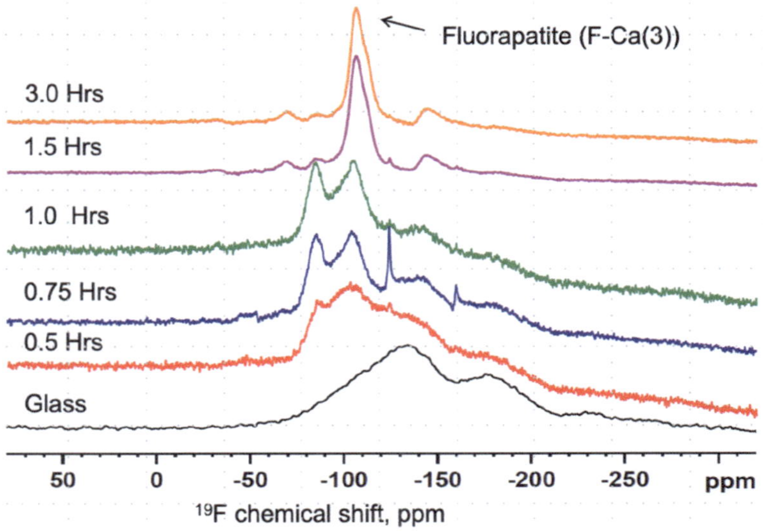

Fig. 9.24 19F solid-state NMR spectroscopy of the BioMinF glass immersed in AS7

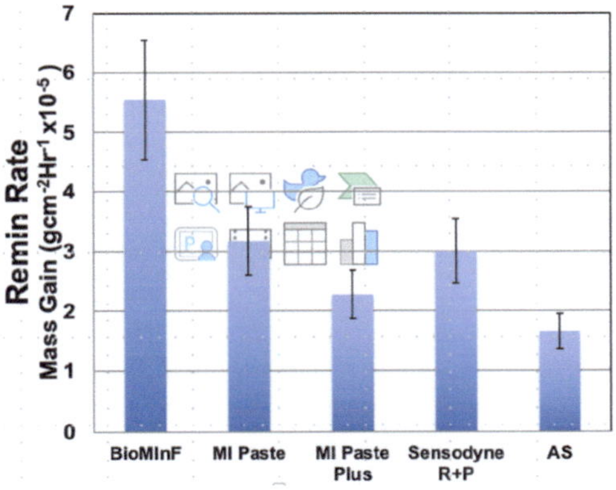

Fig. 9.25 Remineralization rates of demineralised enamel blocks treated with BioMinF toothpaste MI paste, MI PastePlus, Sensodyne Repair, and Protect with NovaMin and Artificial Saliva AS

The smaller glass particles in BioMinF can go into the dentinal tubules where they react and form fluorapatite. This fluorapatite nucleates and grows preferentially on the apatite rich wall of the peritubular dentine. This results in excellent tubule occlusion with a single application. More importantly since the apatite formed is fluorapatite it has much reduced solubility compared to the hydroxyapatite formed with NovaMin. Consequently, it is much more resistant to an acid challenge providing the pH does not go lower than pH 4.5. Figure 9.26 show the tubule occlusion achieved with BioMinF.

The tubule occlusion with the BioMinF toothpaste seen in Fig. 9.26 results in a very marked reduction in fluid flow through the dentinal tubules with the BioMinF toothpaste. This can be seen in Fig. 9.27 where the BoMinF is compared against other toothpastes.

There is a growing body of evidence, both from in vitro studies as well as clinical studies regarding the effectiveness of Biomin F for the treatment of Dentine Hypersensitivity (Petrović et al. 2023) and its antibacterial effect on bacteria such as strep mutans (Doura et al. 2024).

9.27 Conclusion

There are as discussed, a diverse range of treatments for DH, some of these treatments are relatively mature technologies that offer relatively few options for further optimisation. The newer treatments based on the formation of apatite-like phases may, however, offer a greater scope for improved treatments. Amorphous calcium phospho-silicate based technologies appear to offer the greatest potential for future development of products due in part to their ability to (1) incorporate a wide range of additional therapeutic ions into an amorphous glass and (2) control their release over time.

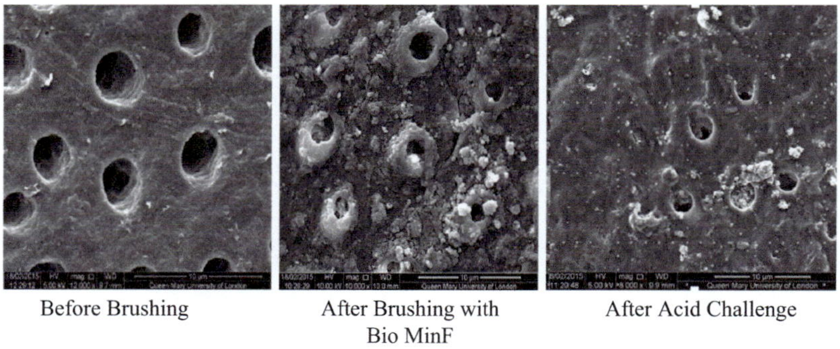

Fig. 9.26 Scanning Electron Micrographs of Dentinal Tubules Before Brushing After Brushing and Immersion in AS7 for 1 h and after brushing with an Acid Challenge

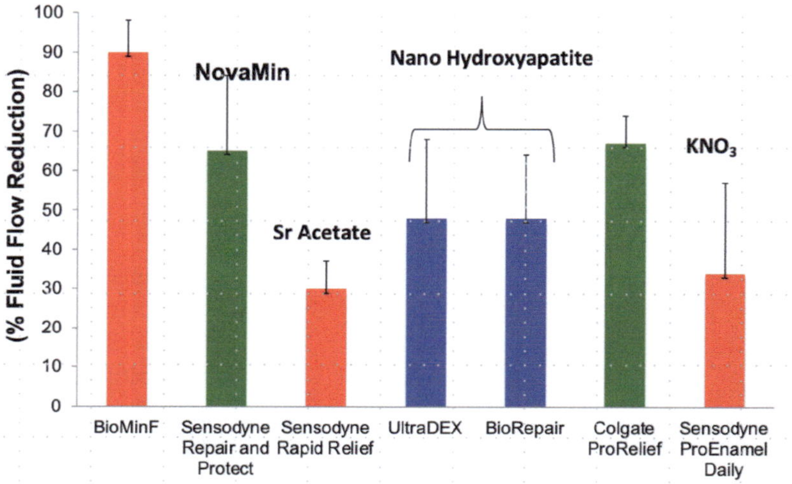

Fig. 9.27 Percentage Reduction of Fluid Flow in a Hydraulic Conductance Test after application of various toothpastes

Acknowledgements The authors would like to acknowledge the contributing of our colleagues in the preparation of the SEM images namely: Dr. Delia Brauer, Dr. Natalia Karpukhina, Dr. Mohammed Mneimne, Dr. Xiaohui Chen, Dr. Saroash Shahid, Dr. Asad Mahmood, Dr. Allesia D'Onofrio and Dr. Tomas Duminis.

Disclosure Statement The authors have one or more patents on the bioactive glass formulations and other oral care products and are currently directors of BioMin Technology Ltd, UK.

References

Allen I, Newman H, Wilson M. Antibacterial activity of particulate Bioglass® against supra- and subgingival bacteria. Biomaterials. 2001;22(12):1683–7.

Alomari HA, Tolibah YA, Kouchaji C. Efficacy of BioMin F and NovaMin toothpastes against streptococcus mutans: an in vitro study. BDJ Open. 2024;10:20. https://doi.org/10.1038/s41405-024-00202.

Amaechi BT, Lemke KC, Saha S, et al. Clinical efficacy of nanohydroxyapatite-containing toothpaste at relieving dentin hypersensitivity: an 8 weeks randomized control trial. BDJ Open. 2021;7:23. https://doi.org/10.1038/s41405-021-00080-7.

Ambard AJ, Mueninghoff L. Calcium phosphate cement: review of mechanical and biological properties. J Prosthodont. 2006;15(5):321–8.

Increase acid resistance of teeth by 1000%. BDJ In Pract. 2023;36:40. https://doi.org/10.1038/s41404-023-2164-x.

BDJ in practice increase acid resistance of teeth by 1000%. BDJ In Pract. 2023;26:40.

Brännström M. A hydrodynamic mechanism in the transmission of pain-produced stimuli through the dentine. In: Anderson DJ, editor. Sensory mechanisms in dentine. Oxford: Pergamon; 1963. p. 73–9.

Brännström M, Åström A. The hydrodynamics of the dentin; its possible relationship to dentinal pain. Int Dent J. 1972;22(2):219–27.

Brunton PA, Davies RPW, Burke JL, Smith A, Aggeli A, Brookes SJ, Kirkham J. Treatment of early caries lesions using biomimetic self-assembling peptides—a clinical safety trial. Br Dent J. 2013;215:1–6.

Chen X, Gillam DG, Mustafa HA, Lysek D, Hill RG. Dentine tubule occlusion of a novel self-assembling peptide containing gel. Cape Town: Abstract Presentation IADR; 2014. (Abstract no 1347).

Choudhary P, Tandon S, Ganesh M, Mehra A. Evaluation of the remineralization potential of amorphous calcium phosphate and fluoride containing pit and fissure sealants using scanning electron microscopy. Indian J Dent Res. 2012;23(2):157–63.

Cummins D. Recent advances in dentin hypersensitivity: Clinically proven treatments for instant and lasting sensitivity relief. Am J Dent. 2010;23 Sp Is A:3A–13A.

Docimo R, Montesani L, Maturo P, Costacurta M, Bartolino M, DeVizio W, Zhang YP, Cummins D, Dibart S, Mateo LR. Comparing the efficacy in reducing dentin hypersensitivity of a new toothpaste containing 8.0%arginine, calcium carbonate, and 1450 ppm fluoride to a commercial sensitive toothpaste containing 2% potassium ion: An eight-week clinical study in Rome, Italy. J Clin Dent. 2009;20(Spec Iss):17–22.

Doura Alomari H, Alsayed Tolibah Y, Kouchaji C. Efficacy of BioMin F and NovaMin toothpastes against streptococcus mutans: an in vitro study. BDJ Open. 2024;10(1):20. https://doi.org/10.1038/s41405-024-00202-x. PMID: 38467637; PMCID: PMC10928140.

Eyüboğlu GB, Naiboğlu P. Clinical efficacy of different dentin desensitizers. Oper Dent. 2020;45(6):E317–33. https://doi.org/10.2341/19-258-C. PMID: 32516395.

Elliott JC Structure and Chemistry of the Apatites and Other Calcium Orthophosphates 1st Edition, Volume 18 - April 28, 1994 Hardback ISBN: 9780444815828.

Farooq I, Tylkowski M, Muller S, Tomasz Janicki T, Brauer DS, Hill RG. Influence of sodium content on the properties of bioactive glasses for use in air abrasion. Biomed Mater. 2013;8:1–9.

Gillam DG. Clinical trial designs for testing of products for dentine hypersensitivity—a review. Periodontal Abstr. 1997;45:37–46.

Gillam D, Chesters R, Attrill D, Brunton P, Slater M, Strand P, Whelton H, Bartlett D. Dentine hypersensitivity—guidelines for the management of a common oral health problem. Dent Update. 2013;40(7):514–6, 518–20, 523–4.

Grossman L. A systematic method for the treatment of hypersensitive dentine. J Am Dent Assoc. 1935;22:592–602.

Guida A, Hill RG, Towler M, et al. Preliminary work on the antibacterial effect of strontium in glass-ionomer cements. J Mater Sci Letts. 2003;22:1401–3.

Hill RG, Chen H, Mustafa HA, Lysek DA, Gillam D. An in vitro comparison of a novel self-assembling peptide matrix gel and selected desensitizing toothpastes in reducing fluid flow by dentine tubular occlusion. JDMR. 2020;3(1):1–11.

Jones JR. Review of bioactive glass: from Hench to hybrids. Acta Biomater. 2013;9:4457–86.

Kang S-J, Kwon Y-H, Park J-B, Herr Y, Chung J-H. The effects of hydroxyapatite toothpaste on tooth hypersensitivity. J Korean Acad Periodontol. 2009;39:9–16. (Korean).

Khijmatgar S, Reddy U, John S, Badavannavar AN, DSouza T. Is there evidence for Novamin application in remineralization: a systematic review. J Oral Biol Craniofac Res. 2020;10(2):87–92. https://doi.org/10.1016/j.jobcr.2020.01.001. Epub 2020 Jan 22. PMID: 32190542; PMCID: PMC7068624.

Kim SH, Park JB, Lee CW, Koo KT, Kim TI, Seol YJ, et al. The clinical effects of a hydroxyapatite containing toothpaste for dentine hypersensitivity. J Korean Acad Periodontol. 2009;39(1):87–94. Korean

Kirkham J, Firth A, Vernals D, Boden N, Robinson C, Shore RC, Brookes SJ, Aggeli A. Self-assembling peptide scaffolds promote enamel remineralisation. J Dent Res. 2007;86:426–30.

Kleinberg I. SensiStat, a new saliva-based composition for simple and effective treatment of dentinal sensitivity pain. Dentistry Today. 2002;21:42–7.

Kleinberg I, Acevebo AM, Chatteriee R. Dental anti hypersensitivity composition and method. US 2003/013385.

Komath M, Varma HK. Development of a fully injectable calcium phosphate cement for orthopedic and dental applications. Bull Mater Sci. 2003;26(4):415–22.

Lansdown AB, Mirastschijski U, Stubbs N, Scanlon E, Agren MS. Zinc in wound healing: theoretical, experimental, and clinical aspects. Wound Repair Regen. 2007;15(1):2–16.

Lynch RJ. Zinc in the mouth, its interactions with dental enamel and possible effects on caries; a review of the literature. Int Dent J. 2011;61(Suppl 3):46–54.

Mahmood A, Mneimne M, Zou L-F, Hill RG, Gillam DG. Abrasive wear of enamel by bioactive glass-based toothpastes. Am J Dent. 2014;27:263–7.

Maillard M, Bandiaky ON, Maunoury S, Alliot C, Alliot-Licht B, Serisier S, Renard E. The effectiveness of calcium phosphates in the treatment of dentinal hypersensitivity: a systematic review. Bioengineering (Basel). 2023;10(4):447. https://doi.org/10.3390/bioengineering10040447. PMID: 37106634; PMCID: PMC10135917.

Malts M, Emilson CG. Susceptibility of oral bacteria to various fluoride salts. J Dent Res. 1982;61(6):786–90.

Markowitz K. The original desensitizers: strontium and potassium salts. J Clin Dent. 2009;20(5):145–51.

Mehta D, Gowda VS, Santosh A, Finger WJ, Sasaki K. Randomized controlled clinical trial on the efficacy of dentin desensitizing agents. Acta Odontol Scand. 2014 Nov;72(8):936–41.

Mneimne M. Ph.D Thesis, Queen Mary University of London. 2014.

Mneimne M, Hill RG, Langford R, Gillam DG, Earl J. FIB-SEM depth profiling of dentine treated with novel bioactive glasses. Cape Town: Abstract Presentation IADR; 2014. (Abstract no 679).

Ni GX, Shu B, Huang G, Lu WW, Pan HB. The effect of strontium incorporation into hydroxyapatites on their physical and biological properties. J Biomed Mater Res B Appl Biomater. 2012 Feb;100(2):562–8.

Pan HB, Li ZY, Lam WM, Wong JC, Darvell BW, Luk KD, Lu WW. Solubility of strontium-substituted apatite by solid titration. Acta Biomater. 2009;5(5):1678–85.

Parati M, Clarke L, Anderson P, Hill R, Khalil I, Tchuenbou-Magaia F, Stanley MS, McGee D, Mendrek B, Kowalczuk M, et al. Microbial Poly-γ-Glutamic Acid (γ-PGA) as an effective tooth enamel protectant. Polymers. 2022;14:2937. https://doi.org/10.3390/polym14142937.

Park JJ, Park JB, Kwon YH, Herr Y, Chung JH. The effect of microcrystalline hydroxyapatite containing toothpaste in the control of tooth hypersensitivity. J Korean Acad Periodontol. 2005;35:577–90.

Petrović D, Galić D, Seifert D, Lešić N, Smolić M. Evaluation of bioactive glass treatment for dentin hypersensitivity: a systematic review. Biomedicines. 2023;11(7):1992. https://doi.org/10.3390/biomedicines11071992. PMID: 37509631; PMCID: PMC10377612

Reis FN, Francese MM, da Silva NDG, Pelá VT, Câmara JVF, Trevizol JS, Honório HM, Crusca E, Marchetto R, Buzalaf MAR. Solutions containing a Statherin-derived peptide reduce enamel erosion in vitro. Caries Res. 2023;57(1):52–8. https://doi.org/10.1159/000529016. Epub 2023 Jan 11. PMID: 36630932

Rösing CK, Fiorini T, Liberman DN, Cavagni J. Dentine hypersensitivity: analysis of self-care products. Braz Oral Res. 2009;23Suppl 1:56–63.

Salah R, Afifi RR, Kehela HA, Aly NM, Rashwan M, Hill RG. Efficacy of novel bioactive glass I the treatment of enamel white spot lesions. A randomised controlled trial. J Evid Based Dent Pract. 2022;22(4):101725. https://doi.org/10.1016/j.jebdp.2022.101725. Epub 2022 Mar 19. PMID: 36494113

Tai BJ, Bian Z, Jiang H, Greenspan DC, Zhong J, Clark AE, Du MQ. Anti-gingivitis effect of a dentifrice containing bioactive glass (NovaMin) particulate. J Clin Periodontol. 2006;33:86–91.

Thanatvarakorn O, Nakashima S, Sadr A, Prasansuttiporn T, Thitthaweerat S, Tagami J. Effect of a calcium-phosphate based desensitizer on dentin surface characteristics. Dent Mater J. 2013a;32(4):615–21.

Thanatvarakorn O, Nakashima S, Sadr A, Prasansuttiporn T, Ikeda M, Tagami J. In vitro evaluation of dentinal hydraulic conductance and tubule sealing by a novel calcium–phosphate desensitizer. J Biomed Mater Res Part B. 2013b;101B:303–9.

Tiskaya M, Gillam D, Shahid S, Hill R. A potassium based fluorine containing bioactive glass for use as a desensitizing toothpaste. Molecules. 2021;26(14):4327. https://doi.org/10.3390/molecules26144327. PMID: 34299602; PMCID: PMC8304061

Yuan P, Shen X, Liu J, Hou Y, Zhu M, et al. Effects of dentifrice containing hydroxyapatite on dentinal tubule occlusion and hexavalent chromium cations sorption: a preliminary study. PLoS One. 2012;7(12):e45283. https://doi.org/10.1371/journal.pone.0045283.

Zhu M, Li J, Chen B, Mei L, Yao L, Tian J, et al. The effect of calcium sodium phosphosilicate on dentin hypersensitivity: a systematic review and meta-analysis. PLoS One. 2015;10(11):e0140176. https://doi.org/10.1371/journal.pone.0140176.

10 Remineralization of the Early Carious Lesion with Emphasis on Available Materials Used to Aid Remineralization Namely: Self-assembling Peptides, Hydroxyapatite Toothpastes, Riva Star, ACP, Calcium Phosphate, LDH, Glass Ionomers, Bioactive Glass, Fluoride Releasing Composites

Robert Hill and David G. Gillam

10.1 Introduction

According to Olley and Bartlett (Chap. 4), Erosion (acid dissolution) is the most common and important etiological factor for tooth wear globally as well as important etiological factor in the development of Dentine Hypersensitivity (see West et al. 2013). These processes occur due to the superficial demineralization of hard tissue and the subsequent chemical dissolution of the apatite crystals in enamel following an acidic challenge (Bartlett 2005). It is evident from the published literature that so-called acid erosion is caused by relatively small acidic challenges (sometimes in conjunction with other etiological factures such as attrition and abrasion, aided by dietary intake, etc.) leading to the loss of enamel and dentine and subsequently exposing the dentine tubules and initiate DH (see Chap. 4). According to Zero and Lussi (2005), the protective role of a mature salivary pellicle is key in the prevention against an erosive challenge, its removal, therefore may be the first step in the demineralization of the underlying enamel and dentine. It comes as no surprise, therefore that products developed for the treatment of dentine hypersensitivity are also effective in the treatment. These products have been extensively reviewed by Victor Mosquim and colleagues (see Chap. 7) as well as in Chaps. 5 and 6 and as such this chapter will focus on the available published literature that supports the efficacy of these products in treating demineralization (see Table 10.1).

The products outlined in Table 10.1 are designed to treat several clinical conditions and despite various claims made for the effectiveness in treating the loss of mineral tissue from the tooth surface the consensus from the published reviews such as systematic reviews with/without meta-analysis appears somewhat inclusive for some of the products. Part of the problem as expressed in several reviews is the lack of standardization of both in vitro and in vivo studies and perhaps this should be addressed in the future.

R. Hill (✉)
Department of Dental Physical Sciences, Centre for Oral Bioengineering, Queen Mary University of London, London, UK
e-mail: r.hill@qmul.ac.uk

D. G. Gillam
Centre for Oral Bioengineering, Institute of Dentistry, Barts and the London School of Medicine and Dentistry, Queen Mary University of London, London, UK
e-mail: d.g.gillam@qmul.ac.uk

D. G. Gillam (ed.), *Dentine Hypersensitivity*, https://doi.org/10.1007/978-3-031-74321-4_10

Table 10.1 reviews selected commercial and experimental products that claim to remineralize enamel in the early caries lesions (including white spot lesions)

Authors	Type of study	Authors comments
Self-assembling peptides Wierichs et al. (2021)	Systematic review and meta-analysis on the efficacy of a self-assembling peptide compared to any other (placebo) treatment or untreated/ standard control.	"Self-assembling peptides may be a viable option to remineralize enamel caries. However, results should be interpretated with caution due the low number of clinical trials, the short follow-up periods and the limiting grade of evidence."
Gohar et al. (2023)	Randomized controlled trial on post-orthodontic white spot lesions. Biomimetic self-assembling peptides compared to fluoride-based delivery systems:	"The visual assessment using ICDAS reveals that the biomimetic remineralization using self-assembling peptides and the fluoride-based varnish material showed a similar effect in masking post-orthodontic white spot lesions. However, the laser fluorescence using DIAGNOpen showed that the self-assembling peptides reveal higher performance in subsurface remineralization than the fluoride-based varnish material. Therefore, self-assembling peptides are considered a promising material for lesion regression in post-orthodontics white spot lesions".
Atteya et al. (2024)	Randomized controlled clinical trial on the effect of nanosilver fluoride, self-assembling peptide and sodium fluoride varnish on salivary cariogenic bacteria:	"In general, the antimicrobial effect of P11-4 and NSF on salivary S. mutans and Lactobacilli was not significantly different from NaF varnish. P11-4 induced greater reduction more quickly than the two other agents and NSF antibacterial effect was lost after one month. *Clinical relevance*: NSF varnish and P11-4 have antimicrobial activity that does not significantly differ from NaF by 3 months. P11-4 has the greatest antibacterial effect after one month with sustained effect till 3 months. The antibacterial effect of NSF lasts for one month. NaF remains effective till 3 months."
Keeper et al. (2023)	Systematic review and meta-analysis on the effect of self-assembling peptide P_{11}-4 on arrest, cavitation, and progression of initial caries lesions	"Six clinical trials met the inclusion criteria. Results of this review represent 2 primary and 2 secondary outcomes. When compared with parallel groups, use of CR likely results in a large increase in caries arrest (relative risk [RR], 1.82 [95% CI, 1.32 to 2.50]; 45% attributable risk [95% CI, 24% to 60%]; number needed to treat [NNT], 2.8) and likely decreases lesion size by a mean (SD) of 32% (28%). The evidence also suggests that use of CR results in a large reduction in cavitation (RR, 0.32 [95% CI, 0.10 to 1.06]; NNT, 6.9) and is uncertain about lowering merged International Caries Detection and Assessment System score (RR, 3.68 [95% CI, 0.42 to 32.3]; NNT, 19). No studies used Curodont Repair Fluoride Plus. No studies reported adverse esthetic changes. *Practical implications:* CR likely has clinically important effects on caries arrest and decreased lesion size. Two trials had nonmasked assessors, and all trials had elevated risks of bias. The authors recommend conducting longer trials. CR is a promising treatment for initial caries lesions"

(continued)

Table 10.1 (continued)

Authors	Type of study	Authors comments
*Hydroxyapatite toothpastes*Bossù et al. (2019)	In vitro and in vivo comparison: enamel remineralization and repair results of biomimetic hydroxyapatite toothpaste on deciduous teeth: an effective option to fluoride toothpaste	"The study was performed in vitro and in vivo, comparing the hydroxyapatite toothpaste with two others toothpaste containing different fluorine concentrations. The coating effect of the micro-structured Hydroxyapatite nanoparticles reintegrates the enamel with a biomimetic film reproducing the structure and the morphology of the biologic Hydroxyapatite of the enamel. As demonstrated, the coating is due to the deposit of a new layer of apatite, which presents fewer particles than the natural enamel, not based on the chemical-physical changes occurring in fluorinated toothpastes. Moreover, it shows resistance to brushing as a consequence of chemical bonds between the synthetic and natural crystals of the enamel. *Conclusions:* The use of Biomimetic Hydroxyapatite toothpastes has proven to be a valuable prevention measure against dental caries in primary dentition since it prevents the risk of fluorosis."
Sari et al. (2022)	Development of a hydroxyapatite nanoparticle-based gel for enamel remineralization -A physico-chemical properties and cell viability assay analysis	"Nano-hydroxyapatite (nHA) was synthesized from abalone mussel shells (Haliotis asinina) using a precipitation method, and gel HA-Abalone was developed using the carbomer materials with concentrations of 0, 10, 20, 30, and 40 wt%. The specimens used were 25 freshly extracted caries-free premolar teeth, and the treatment was done twice a day for 14 days. Gel HA-Abalone 20 wt%, with a crystallite size of 14.70 ± 1.21 nm, was the best concentration to achieve the best remineralization (~863 VHN) of the superficial layer. Based on the results of cell viability assay on gel HA-Abalone 20 wt%, the growth of NIH/3T3 cells was inhibited beginning at a gel concentration of 1000 μg/mL, and the half maximal inhibitory concentration (IC_{50}) value was 1497 μg/mL. Based on to the one-way analysis of variance (ANOVA), the result reflected statistically significant differences in the average of the cell viability and enamel surface microhardness values ($p < 0.05$)."
Wierichs et al. (2022)	Systematic review and meta-analysis on nano-hydroxyapatite on caries prevention	"The low number of clinical studies, the relatively short follow-up periods, the high risks of bias, and the limiting grade of evidence do not allow for conclusive evidence on the efficacy of nHA. *Clinical relevance:* No conclusive evidence on the efficacy of nHA could be obtained based on the low number of clinical studies, the relatively short follow-up periods, the high risks of bias, the limiting grade of evidence, and study conditions that do not reflect the everyday conditions."

(continued)

Table 10.1 (continued)

Authors	Type of study	Authors comments
Silver diamine fluoride McReynolds and Duane 2018	Systematic review on the effectiveness of silver diamine fluoride for both root caries prevention and arrest in older adults	"Results Three randomised controlled trials were identified that addressed the effectiveness of SDF on root caries in older adults, but none addressed coronal caries. Root caries prevented fraction and arrest rate for SDF were significantly higher than placebo. The prevented fraction for caries prevention for SDF compared to placebo was 71% in a 3-year study and 25% in a 2-year study. The prevented fraction for caries arrest for SDF was 725% greater in a 24-month study and 100% greater than placebo in a 30-month study. No severe adverse effects were observed. *Conclusions* Existing reports of SDF trials support effectiveness in root caries prevention and arrest, remineralization of deep occlusal lesions and treatment of hypersensitive dentine."
Crystal and Niederman (2019)	Evidence-based dentistry update on silver diamine fluoride: review	"This article reviews current evidence on the effectiveness of silver diamine fluoride (SDF) as a caries arresting and preventive agent. It provides clinical recommendations around SDF's appropriate use as part of a comprehensive caries management program. Systematic reviews confirm that SDF is effective for caries arrest on cavitated lesions in primary teeth and root caries in the elderly. It may also prevent new lesions. Application is easy, noninvasive, affordable, and safe. Although it stains the lesions dark as it arrests them, it provides clinicians with an additional tool for caries management when esthetics are not a primary concern."
Oliveira et al. (2019)	Systematic review and meta-analysis on the effect of silver diamine fluoride in preventing caries in the primary dentition:	"Searches yielded 2366 unique records; 6 reports of 4 trials that randomized 1118 and analyzed 915 participants were included. Two trials compared SDF to no treatment, 1 compared SDF to placebo and sodium fluoride varnish (FV), and 1 compared SDF to high-viscosity glass ionomer cement (GIC). All studies had at least 1 domain with unclear or high risk of bias. After 24 months of follow-up, in comparison to placebo, no treatment, and FV, SDF applications significantly reduced the development of new dentin caries lesions (placebo or no treatment: WMD = −1.15, PF = 77.5%; FV: WMD = −0.43, PF = 54.0%). GIC was more effective than SDF after 12 months of follow-up but the difference between them was not statistically significant (WMD, dmft: 0.34, PF: −6.09%). *Conclusion:* When applied to caries lesions in primary teeth, SDF compared to no treatment, placebo or FV appears to effectively prevent dental caries in the entire dentition. However, trials specifically designed to assess this outcome are needed."

(continued)

Table 10.1 (continued)

Authors	Type of study	Authors comments
Muntean et al. (2024)	Systematic review on silver diamine fluoride in pediatric dentistry: effectiveness in preventing and arresting dental caries	"*Results:* The inclusion criteria identified 16 randomized controlled trials involving patients aged 18 months to 13 years and followed over a period of 12–30 months. *Conclusions*: SDF is a practical, accessible and effective noninvasive way to prevent and arrest caries in temporary and permanent teeth. Its application requires regular monitoring. The resulting black spot is diminished by immediate application of potassium iodide but this may affect its effectiveness."
Calcium phosphate Combinations ACP-CPP Llena et al. (2015)	CPP-ACP and CPP-ACFP versus fluoride varnish in remineralization of early caries lesions. A prospective study (randomized clinical trial)	"DIAGNOdent values were significantly reduced in Group B at 4 weeks, and in Groups A and C at 8 weeks. Mean values in Group B were lower than in Groups A and C at 4 weeks, and lower than Group C at 8 weeks. CPP-ACFP appeared to have a specific effect on smooth-surface caries, but no significant effect on caries in pits and fissures. *Conclusion:* At 4 weeks, CPP-ACFP is superior to fluoride varnish at remineralizing smooth-surface WSLs. CPP-ACP is not superior to fluoride varnish by any of the measures studied."
Li et al. (2014)	Systematic review. On the long-term remineralizing effect of casein phosphopeptide-amorphous calcium phosphate (CPP-ACP) on early caries lesions in vivo:	"CPP-ACP has a long-term remineralizing effect on early caries lesions in comparison with placebo, although this does not appear to be significantly different from that of fluorides. The advantage of using CPP-ACP as a supplement to fluoride-containing products is still unclear. High-quality, well-designed clinical studies in this area are still required before definitive recommendations can be made. *Clinical significance:* CPP-ACP is a promising remineralizing agent with a significant remineralizing effect that has been demonstrated in both in vivo and in vitro studies. The evidence to support its synergistic effect with fluoride is insufficient based on the current existing long-term human randomized controlled trials."

(continued)

Table 10.1 (continued)

Authors	Type of study	Authors comments
Golzio et al. (2024)	A meta-analysis on the combined casein phosphopeptide-amorphous calcium phosphate and fluoride is not superior to fluoride alone in early carious lesions:	"21 studies were included for qualitative synthesis, and 15 studies were eligible for quantitative analysis. No significant difference was found between CPP-ACP and fluoride versus fluoride alone in LF at 1, 3, and 6 months of use: SMD −0.30 (−0.64; 0.04); SMD −0.47 (−1.02; 0.07); SMD −0.49 (−1.13; 0.15), respectively. For QLF, the analysis did not demonstrate significant differences between these two kinds of treatment at 1 and 6 months of use: MD 0.21 (−0.30;0.71); MD 0.60 (−1.70;2.90), but at 3 months, higher QLF values were found in the fluoride-only group compared to the CPP-ACP and fluoride combination was shown regarding the WSLs: MD 0.58 (0.25;0.91). On the contrary, data showed a small but statistically significant decrease in the lesion area in favor of the CPP-ACP plus fluoride versus fluoride alone at 6 months MD -0.38 (−0.72; −0.04). None of these observed changes indicated substantial clinical relevance. The combination of CPP-ACP and fluoride did not overcome the effect of fluoride given alone. Our data suggest that fluoride itself is effective in improving WSLs. However, the certainty of evidence was very low. These results indicate that further studies and future development of more effective products than CPP-ACP are needed in addition to fluoride to achieve robust amelioration of WSLs."
Rahmath Meeral et al. (2024)	Systematic review and meta-analysis on the efficiency of casein phosphopeptide-amorphous calcium phosphate versus topical fluorides on remineralizing early enamel carious lesions	"Conflicting evidence exists on the clinical efficacy of CPP-ACP compared to the various fluoride forms tested, and no adverse effect associated with CPP-ACP use was discovered in comparison to fluorides that had certain detrimental health impacts. Although, the review results in favor of both fluorides and CPP-ACP with similar clinical efficiency, when ill effects are considered the CPP-ACP can be a choice of remineralizing early enamel lesions. However, before concrete suggestions can be given, high-quality, well-designed clinical research studies in this area are still necessary. *Clinical significance:* A considerable remineralizing impact has been shown in both in vitro and in vivo experiments, making CPP-ACP/CPP-ACPF a more promising remineralizing agent than fluorides. Therefore, this can be applied clinically to early enamel carious lesion."

(continued)

Table 10.1 (continued)

Authors	Type of study	Authors comments
Calcium phosphate Ekambaram et al. (2017)	Review of enamel remineralization potential of calcium- and phosphate-based remineralization systems	"Several studies including laboratory-based studies, in situ and randomized controlled clinical trials showed casein phosphopeptide-amorphous calcium phosphate (CPP-ACP)-containing remineralization agents to have superior remineralization potential compared to other forms of calcium- and phosphate-based remineralization agents, such as functionalized tri-calcium phosphate (fTCP) and amorphous calcium phosphate (ACP). *Conclusions*: More long-term clinical studies are necessary to compare the enamel remineralization potential of calcium- and phosphate-based agents that contain fTCP and ACP with those containing CPP-ACP. Additional well-designed randomized controlled clinical trials are also necessary to justify long-term clinical supplemental use of products containing CPP-ACP."
LDH Wei et al. (2019)	In vitro study on novel dental resin composites containing LiAl-F layered double hydroxide (LDH) filler: Fluoride release/recharge, mechanical properties, color change, and cytotoxicity	"The LDH-contained resin composites show significantly increased fluoride release and recharge capability. Among them, R3 and R5 have more stable and long-term fluoride release than R3W, R5W, R3D, R5D, and CC. The LDH filler did not induce cytotoxicity, although few amounts of Al^{3+}/Li^{+} ions were detected on the first day. The LDH filler did not alter the flexural strength of RX, and the microhardness (R3, R5, R3D, and R5D) was significantly higher than the CC group ($P < 0.01$). The LDH filler slightly increased the color of the composite in red (a* values) and yellow (b* values)." **Significance:** The LiAl-F LDH can be a fluoride reservoir filler for dental resin composites that increases the anti-caries ability."
Hoxha et al. (2020)	In vitro study on novel fluoride rechargeable dental composites containing MgAl and CaAl layered double hydroxide (LDH).	"CaAl LDH and MgAl LDH-composites significantly increased the amount of fluoride released in both media ($P < 0.05$). In AS, the mean release after every recharge was greater for MgAl LDH-composites compared to CaAl LDH-composites ($P < 0.05$). After every recharge, the fluoride release was greater than the previous release cycle ($P < 0.05$) for all LDH-composites. Physico-mechanical properties of the LDH-composites demonstrated similar values to those reported in literature. The solubility and cation release showed a linear increase with LDH loading. *Significance:* LDH-composites repeatedly absorbed/released fluoride and maintained desired physico-mechanical properties. A sustained low-level fluoride release with LDH-composites could lead to a potential breakthrough in preventing early stage carious lesions."

(continued)

Table 10.1 (continued)

Authors	Type of study	Authors comments
Hoxha et al. (2019)	Systematic review. On layered double hydroxide fluoride release in dental applications:	"LDH has been used as antacids, water purification in removing excess fluoride in drinking water and drug delivery. It has great potential for controlled fluoride release in dentistry, e.g., varnishes, fissure sealants and muco-adhesive strips, etc. LDHs incorporated in dental materials have been previously evaluated for fluoride release and proven to be clinically safe. LDHs have the potential to sustain a controlled release of fluoride (or other cariostatic ions) in the oral environment to prevent caries. However, further analyses of LDH compositions, and clinical research investigating any other cariostatic effects, are required."
Tejani et al. (2022)	In vitro study on the effect of layered double hydroxide on fluoride release and recharge from a commercial and an experimental resin varnish	"Evidence of ZnAl-LDH was confirmed by the presence of peaks for zinc and aluminum in EDS spectra. Cumulative fluoride and mean fluoride released between Clinpro, Clinpro + LDH and resin were significantly different (ANOVA, Tukey's HSD post-hoc test, $p < 0.001$) except between the resin and resin + LDH. Mean fluoride concentrations differed significantly after every recharge between Clinpro, Clinpro + LDH and resin, but not between the resin and resin + LDH ($p < 0.01$). The weights and SEMs of the experimental resins +/– LDH, appeared to be stable while the weights of Clinpro samples +/– LDH, fluctuated and fragmented. *Significance:* ClinproXT and experimental resin containing ZnAl-LDH recharged with fluoride did not significantly increase fluoride release compared to the unmodified materials. However, all LDH-F incorporated materials demonstrated fluoride recharging properties which appear beneficial to dentistry and thus further work is required to improve these properties."

(continued)

Table 10.1 (continued)

Authors	Type of study	Authors comments
Glass Ionemer cements Duarte et al. (2022)	In vitro study on enhancing glass ionomer cement features by using the calcium phosphate nanocomposite	"This study showed the synthesis of Glass ionomer cements (GIC) modified with calcium phosphate nanoparticles (nCaP). The nCaP/GIC were submitted to mechanical compression and diametral tensile tests. The biocomposite were characterized by scanning electron microscopy (SEM), energy-dispersive X-ray spectroscopy (EDX), X-ray diffraction (XRD) and Fourier-transform infrared spectroscopy (FTIR). Cytotoxicity and cell viability tests were performed on the human bone marrow mesenchymal stem cells using a 3-(4,5-dimethylthiazol-2yl)2,5-diphenyl-tetrazolium-bromide assay and LIVE/DEAD assays. Statistically significant differences were observed for mechanical properties (Kruskal-Wallis, $p < 0.001$), nCaP/GIC showed higher resistance to compression and diametral traction. The SEM analyses revealed a uniform distribution nCaP in the ionomer matrix. The EDX and XRD results indicated that hydroxyapatite and calcium β-triphosphate phases. The FTIR spectra revealed the asymmetric band of ν3PO43- between 1100–1030 cm-1 and the vibration band associated with ν1PO43- in 963 cm-1 associated with nCaP. The nCaP/GIC presented response to adequate cell viability and non-cytotoxic behavior. Therefore, the new nCaP/GIC composite showed great mechanical properties, non-cytotoxic behavior, and adequate response to cell viability with promising dental applications."
Ghilotti et al. (2023)	Systematic review on the remineralizing ability of resin modified glass ionomers (RMGICs):	"Studies assessing the remineralizing potential of RMGICs on dentin were included in our review. Studies which compared such properties between different RMGICs or with other materials were also eligible. The studies report the remineralizing ability of RMGICs, albeit with differences between different commercial products. RMGICs show a similar ability to conventional GICs to remineralize affected dentin, fulfilling the function for which they are designed. Moreover, the incorporation of additives, such as bioactive glass (BAG) or CCP-ACP, improves their remineralizing potential. The results of this review support the use of RMGICs as restorative materials after selective caries removal."
Grohe & Mittler 2021	Review on advanced non-fluoride approaches to dental enamel remineralization: The next level in enamel repair management	"Synthetic remineralization systems have become indispensable. In addition to fluoride, Some of these systems claim that they are comparable or even superior to fluoride in terms of their ability to remineralize enamel. This article, following an introduction into enamel (re)mineralization and fluoride-assisted remineralization, discusses the requirements for non-fluoride remineralization systems, particularly their mechanisms and challenges, and summarizes the findings that underpin the most promising advances in enamel remineralization therapy."

(continued)

Table 10.1 (continued)

Authors	Type of study	Authors comments
Varnishes Shen et al. (2016)	In vitro study on the effect of calcium phosphate addition to fluoride-containing dental varnishes on enamel demineralization	"All fluoride-containing varnishes significantly inhibited enamel demineralization when compared with the placebo varnish. However, out of the calcium phosphate and fluoride-containing varnishes only MI Varnish, containing fluoride and CPP-ACP was superior to the fluoride alone varnishes. MI Varnish also released the highest levels of calcium, phosphate and fluoride ions. *Conclusions:* MI Varnish containing fluoride and CPP-ACP was superior to the other varnishes in protecting against enamel demineralization."
Godoi et al. (2019)	In vitro study on the remineralizing effect of commercial fluoride varnishes on artificial enamel lesions	"Forty bovine enamel blocks were separated into four groups ($n = 10$): control (no treatment), Enamelast (Ultradent Products), Duraphat (Colgate-Palmolive) and Clinpro White Varnish (3M ESPE). Surface enamel microhardness evaluations were obtained, artificial enamel caries lesions were developed by dynamic pH-cycling, and the varnishes were then applied every 6 days, after which the enamel blocks were submitted to dynamic remineralization by pH cycles. There was a significant decrease in enamel surface microhardness after performing all the treatments ($p < 0.0001$). Enamelast and Duraphat showed significantly higher enamel microhardness values than the control and the Clinpro groups ($p = 0.0002$). Microhardness loss percentage was significantly lower for Enamelast ($p = 0.071$; One-way ANOVA). PLMI showed that subsurface caries lesions were not remineralized with the varnish treatments. No significant differences in the in-depth microhardness levels ($p = 0.7536$; ANOVA) were observed among the treatments. Enamelast presented higher soluble and insoluble fluoride concentrations than the other varnishes ($p < 0.0001$; Kruskal-Wallis and Dunn tests). Enamelast and Duraphat varnishes promoted enamel surface remineralization, but no varnish remineralized the subsurface lesion body. Although insoluble and soluble fluoride concentration values did not correspond to those declared by the manufacturer, Enamelast presented higher fluoride concentration than the others."
Shen et al. (2020)	In vitro study on the remineralization and fluoride uptake of white spot lesions under dental varnishes.	"Both MI and Duraphat varnishes significantly remineralized the covered and uncovered WSLs when compared with the placebo varnish ($P < 0.001$). The WSLs covered with varnish showed greater remineralization than those uncovered. MI varnish produced the highest level of remineralization and significantly greater fluoride uptake (0.44 ± 0.08 wt%) compared with Duraphat (0.24 ± 0.03 wt%) and the placebo varnish (0.06 ± 0.05 wt%). *Conclusion:* Varnish containing fluoride and CPP-ACP was superior to varnish containing fluoride alone in promoting WSL remineralization and fluoride uptake."

(continued)

Table 10.1 (continued)

Authors	Type of study	Authors comments
Manchanda et al. (2022)	Systematic review with network meta-analysis on topical fluoride to prevent early childhood caries:	"Among all the professionally applied topical fluoride interventions reviewed, very low to moderate evidence was found with 0.9% DFS application at 3-monthly intervals, which was ranked highest in prevention of ECC. Among the included studies on self-applied topical fluorides, the evidence was inconclusive due to heterogeneity among studies. *Clinical significance:* The 0.9% DFS varnish applied every 3 months is most effective for preventing early childhood caries. The review recommends that good quality studies be conducted in future, comparing two or more interventions for both self- as well as professionally applied topical fluoride agents with adequate follow-up."
Bioactive glasses (BAG) Al-Eesa et al. (2018)	In vitro study on a fluoride-containing bioactive glass composite for orthodontic adhesives—Apatite formation properties	"The BAG-resin formed apatite on the disk surface, which increased with time, especially in AS4 and AS7. The apatite crystals formed in AS7 were highly orientated and the orientation increased with time. *Significance*: This novel BAG-resin adhesive differs from the currently used adhesives by promoting apatite formation, particularly under acidic conditions. Thus, applied in the clinical situation to bond orthodontic brackets, it may discourage the frequent occurrence of white spot lesion formation around the brackets."
Fernando et al. (2017)	Systematic review	"This review highlights the importance of assessing the mechanical properties of dentin alongside to the newly formed apatite content in order to prove BAGs efficiency to remineralize this tissue. Though studies have confirmed that BAGs stimulate excellent apatite formation in dentin, it should be concluded that there isn't sufficient evidence for bioactive glass to effectively remineralize this tissue as the mechanical properties of the BAG treated dentin haven't been well explored."
Salah et al. (2022)	A randomized controlled trial assessing the efficacy of novel bioactive glass in the treatment of enamel white spot lesion.	"All patients were assessed for change in WSL dimensions using computer assisted analysis based on standardized digital intraoral photographs in addition to laser fluorescence DIAGNOdent assessment before treatment (T0) and at 1 week (T1), 1 month (T2), 3 months (T3), and 6 months (T4) follow-up periods. The combined in-office and home-application of BiominF paste for 4 weeks resulted in greater esthetic improvements of post-orthodontic WSLs compared to Novamin and CPP-ACP. In addition, BiominF showed a significant reduction in fluorescence intensity which indicates potential lesion remineralization."

(continued)

Table 10.1 (continued)

Authors	Type of study	Authors comments
De Caluwé et al. (2017)	In vitro study two types of bioactive glasses (BAG) (45S5F and CF9) are combined with GICs to evaluate the physico-chemical properties and biocompatibility of the BAG-GIC combinations. The effect of the addition of Al^{3+} to the BAG composition and the use of smaller BAG particles on the BAG-GIC properties was also investigated.	"The addition of BAG improves the bioactivity of the GIC, which can be observed by the formation of an apatite (Ap) layer, especially in CF9-containing GICs. More BAG leads to more bioactivity but decreases strength. The addition of Al^{3+} to the BAG composition improves strength but decreases bioactivity. BAGs with smaller particle sizes have no effect on bioactivity and decrease strength. The formation of an Ap layer seems beneficial to the biocompatibility of the BAG-GICs. *Significance:* Bioactive GICs may have several advantages over conventional GICs, such as remineralization of demineralized tissue, adhesion and proliferation of bone- and dental cells, allowing integration in surrounding tissue. CF9 BAG-GIC combinations containing maximum 10 mol% Al^{3+} are most promising, when added in ≤20 wt% to a GIC".
Raszewski et al. (2024)	Bioactive-glass-infused gels for enamel remineralization An in vitro study	"Across the board, the five synthesized gels facilitated the release of calcium, phosphate, and silicon ions, raising the pH from 9.00 ± 0.10 to 9.7 ± 0.0-a range conducive to remineralization. Dissolution in water occurred within 30–50 min post-application. Viscosity readings showed variability, with 45S5 reaching 6337 ± 24 mPa/s and Biomin F at 3269 ± 18 mPa/s after two months. Initial adhesion for the blank gel was measured at 0.27 ± 0.04 Pa, increasing to 0.73 ± 0.06 Pa for the others over time. Gels can release elements upon contact with water (Ca^- Biomin C 104.8 ± 15.7 mg/L; Na^- Biomin F 76.30 ± 11.44 mg/L; P^- Biomin C 2.623 ± 0.393 mg/L; Si^- 45S5-45.15 ± 6.77 mg/L, F^- Biomin F^- 3.256 ± 0.651 mg/L; Cl^- Biomin C 135.5 ± 20.3 mg/L after 45 min). *Conclusions:* These findings highlight the gels' capacity to kickstart the remineralization process by delivering critical ions needed for enamel layer reconstruction. Further exploration in more dynamic, real-world conditions is recommended to fully ascertain their practical utility"
Taha et al. (2017)	Systematic review on the effect of bioactive glasses on enamel remineralization:	"A total of 11 laboratory-based studies were included in this review. The methodological quality was deemed to be high in four, and medium in the remaining studies. Based on the in vitro studies, enamel remineralization improved with bioactive glasses, irrespective of the method of application. Ex vivo signs of remineralization such as increase in enamel hardness, the formation of an enamel-protective layer and reduced intensity of light backscattering were less evident with alternatives including fluoride, and casein phosphopeptide-amorphous calcium phosphate (CPP-ACP). *Conclusions*: Based on in vitro findings only, bioactive glasses may be capable of enhancing enamel remineralization in various formulations, compared with other topical remineralizing materials including fluoride, and CPP-ACP. However, clinical research to confirm their effectiveness is now overdue".

(continued)

Table 10.1 (continued)

Authors	Type of study	Authors comments
Tiskaya et al. (2021)	Critical review on bioactive glass (BAG) in dental composites	"BAGs release C^{a2+}, PO43- and F- ions, raise the pH and form apatite. There are numerous published papers on the bioactivity of BAGs, but the different glass compositions, volume fractions, particle sizes, immersion media, time points, and the characterization techniques used, make comparison difficult. Several papers only use certain characterization techniques that do not provide a full picture of the behavior of the glass. It was noted that in most studies, mechanical properties were measured on dry samples, which does not replicate the conditions in the oral environment. Therefore, it is recommended that samples should be immersed for longer time periods in physiological solutions to mimic clinical environments. *Significance*: BAGs present major benefits in dentistry, especially their capacity to form apatite, which could potentially fill any marginal gaps produced due to polymerization shrinkage."
Selected combination therapies Dionysopoulos et al. (2019)	Effect of CPP-ACPF and Nano-hydroxyapatite preventive treatments on the susceptibility of enamel to erosive challenge	"Eighteen sound bovine incisors were used for this study. Three experimental groups were assigned as follows: Group 1 was the control group; Group 2 specimens received a CPP-ACPF paste treatment; and Group 3 specimens received a treatment with a product containing 1% nano-hydroxyapatite and 455 ppmF-. The specimens were submitted to erosive challenge using a common soft drink (Coca Cola). The erosive activity on the enamel was evaluated by measuring surface microhardness change (Vickers method), surface roughness alterations and surface loss (vertical scanning interferometry (VSI) method). The data were statistically analyzed using one-way analysis of variance (ANOVA) and Tukey's post-hoc test at a level of statistical significance a = 0.05. *Results:* The tested treatments exhibited significantly lower decreases in surface microhardness compared to the control group after the erosive challenge ($p < 0.05$). The tested treatment groups did not show statistically significant lower increases in surface roughness compared to the control group ($p > 0.05$). In addition, the treatment groups exhibited statistically significant lower surface loss than the control group ($p < 0.05$). *Conclusion:* Although the tested treatments reduced erosive activity, none of them provided complete protection against the development of enamel erosion, which means that they should be only used as a part of an individually tailored preventive program."

(continued)

Table 10.1 (continued)

Authors	Type of study	Authors comments
Kamal et al. (2020)	In vitro study on the complementary remineralizing effect of self-assembling peptide (P11-4) with CPP-ACPF or fluoride:	"Six groups: G1-(Control, artificial saliva), G2-(Fluoride varnish), G3-(CPP-ACPF varnish), G4-(Self-assembling peptide), G5-(Self-assembling peptide + fluoride varnish), G6-(Self-assembling peptide+CPP-ACPF varnish). All products were applied according to manufacturer's instructions and specimens were stored in a daily renewed artificial saliva. Surface microhardness (SMH) and scanning electron microscope (SEM) were assessed at baseline, after demineralization, 1 week and 4 weeks storage. SMH values were analyzed using ANOVA and Tukey's post-hoc test. *Results:* The highest statistically significant SMH values were found in G6 followed by G5, G4, G2 and G3 while the lowest values were found in G1. No statistically significant difference was found between G5 and G6. Also, no statistically significant difference was found between G2 and G3. SEM showed that G4, G5, G6 resulted in more pronounced remineralization, reversing the demineralized enamel fish scale pattern compared to G2 and G3 after 1 week and 4 week remineralization. *Conclusions:* Complementary effect was obtained after combining self-assembling peptide with CPP-ACPF or fluoride showing the highest remineralizing potential early after 1 week and even after 4 weeks compared to when each agent used alone. Added benefits can be obtained through combining self-assembling peptide with other remineralzing agents allowing faster and enhanced regeneration of non-cavitated caries lesions"
Xie et al. (2023)	Systematic review and network meta-analysis on a comparison of therapies of white spot lesions	"Forty-two articles were included in the systematic review. Thirty-one of them, with a total of 1906 participants, were included in the network meta-analysis. The studies owned a low and moderate risk of bias. This analysis does not suffer from significant inconsistency. The difference between 4 groups 'self-assembled peptide (SAP) P11-4′, 'P11-4 + Fluoride Varnish (FV)', 'Resin Infiltration (RI)', 'casein phosphor peptides-amorphous calcium fluoride phosphate (CPP-ACFP)' and the 'Control' group was found to be statistically significant. Compared to the 'FV' and 'casein phosphor peptides-amorphous calcium phosphate (CPP-ACP)' groups, the 'P11-4 + FV" group and 'RI" group made a significant difference. The hierarchy was evident in the SUCRA values of 7 therapies. P11-4 + FV and RI were considered effective therapies compared to the control group or the FV group (gold standard group). *Conclusions:* The available evidence suggests that resin infiltration and P11-4 in combination with fluoride varnish had advantages over gold standard (FV). The effect of tricalcium phosphate-based drugs and fluoride is not very noticeable. Overall, drugs based on P11-4 and resin infiltration will be better therapies. Using more than two drugs in combination also would increase efficacy".

(continued)

Table 10.1 (continued)

Authors	Type of study	Authors comments
Kobeissi et al. (2020)	A clinical randomized trial on the effectiveness of self-assembling peptide P_{11}-4 compared to tricalcium phosphate fluoride varnish in remineralization of white spot lesions:	"The result of the current study revealed a significant quantitative and qualitative increase in remineralization of WSLs in both groups and over time intervals. However, the WSL recovery was significantly better in the self-assembling peptide group, reflecting an excellent remineralization potential of the WSLs by the SAP_{11}-4 compared to TCPF varnish. *Conclusion:* Both TCPF and SAP_{11}-4 were effective in treating WSLs. However, the success of guided enamel regeneration by the SAP_{11}-4 through the biomineralization has proven superiority of this material compared to TCPF."
Novel varnishes *Xylitol varnish* Cardoso et al. (2016)	In situ study on the effect of xylitol varnishes on remineralization of artificial enamel caries lesions in situ	"Enamel surface remineralization was significantly increased by Duraphat™, Duofluorid™ and 20% xylitol formulations. Significant subsurface mineral remineralization could also be seen for the experimental and commercial varnishes, except for Duraphat™, when the parameter "lesion depth" was considered. *Conclusions***:** 20% xylitol varnish seem to be a promising alternative to increase surface and subsurface remineralization of artificial caries lesions in situ."

The following products are include in the review (1) Self-assembling peptides, (2) hydroxyapatite toothpastes, (3) Silver diamine fluoride (SDF) Riva star, (4) ACP, (5) Calcium phosphate, (6) Layered double hydroxide (LDH), (7) Glass ionomers, (8) Varnishes, (9) Bioactive glass, fluoride releasing composites, (10) Combination therapies and (11) Novel products

There is no doubt that the development of novel and innovative products is essential in replacing lost dental tissue, this will range from early mineral loss from the enamel surface to replacing existing failing restorations. Several problems may however be apparent with some of these products, for example, (i) will the material release calcium, phosphate, and fluoride ions into the surround tissue, (ii) will the surface layer be able to resist future acid challenges and (iii) will the material successfully fill the cavity (to avoid marginal gaps between the resin/tooth interface and prevent any bacterial infiltration. For example, with the requirements of replacing amalgam restorations following the Minamata Convention on Mercury Treaty (2013) that was a need for a more environmentally friendly material. Currently, some of the products listed in Table 10.1 such as glass ionomer cements are used to replace lost tissue in a cavitated lesion. For larger replacement of tooth mineral loss, dental composites are currently used to replace existing amalgam restorations. There are, however, problems with these materials as outlines in Fig. 10.1.

The question therefore remains is there a suitable material that can resolve the problems with the current dental composites. One possible solution is the introduction of Bioactive Glass Composites (see Table 10.1).

Ongoing studies in the development of novel materials to treat dentine hypersensitivity, demineralization, white spot lesions and replacing dental composites with bioactive glass composites has provided supporting evidence for these products (See Table 10.1 and Figs. 10.2, 10.3, 10.4, 10.5, 10.6, 10.7 and 10.8).

There is evidence that a radio-opaque surface layer is formed with the presence of needle like crystals (Fig. 10.2) It is also possible that an apa-

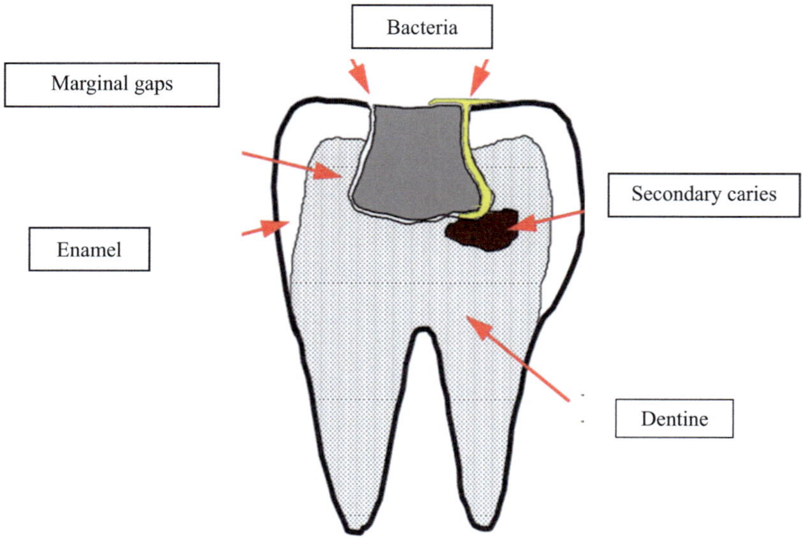

Fig. 10.1 Diagram illustrating the problems with dental composite materials

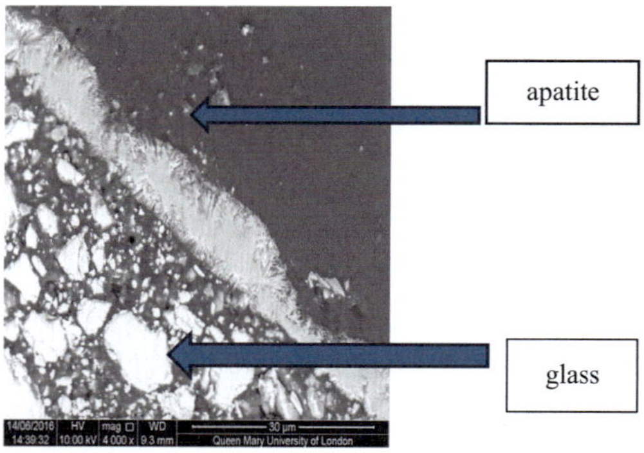

Fig. 10.2 Back Scattered SEM Cross-Section BG Composite ReMin AS pH = 7

tite layer may form in marginal gaps on surface of carious lesions within cracks and voids.

A further study to assess the remineralization potential of a fluoride BAG composite restoration demonstrated the ability to remineralize dental tissue around the restoration. (Figs. 10.3, 10.4 and 10.5).

To summarize Figs. 10.2, 10.3, 10.4, 10.5, 10.6, 10.7 and 10.8, it can be suggested that calcium, phosphate, and fluoride release is possible from a bioactive composite restoration and can result in the remineralization of a carious lesions which could be beneficial in minimally invasive dental procedures such as atraumatic restorative treatment (ART). There is also evidence of the exchange of H^+ for Ca^{2+} resulting in a basic pH particularly in water filled marginal gaps that inhibit acidophilic bacteria as well the presence of apatite formation within the marginal gaps (between the restoration and dentine) resulting in the infill within the gap and potentially stopping bacterial penetration and secondary caries.

A final example of the work ongoing at QMUL is the development of a fluorine containing bioactive glass orthodontic adhesive, see Fig. 10.9.

The ability to prevent demineralisation of teeth during orthodontic treatment is a major advantagem.

10.2 Conclusions

It is evident from reviewing the effectiveness of the available remineralization products that while some of the products appear to be of promise, the consensus from the published reviews such as systematic reviews with/without meta-analysis appears somewhat inclusive. Part of the problem as expressed in several reviews is the lack of standardization of both in vitro and in vivo studies and perhaps this should be addressed in the future.

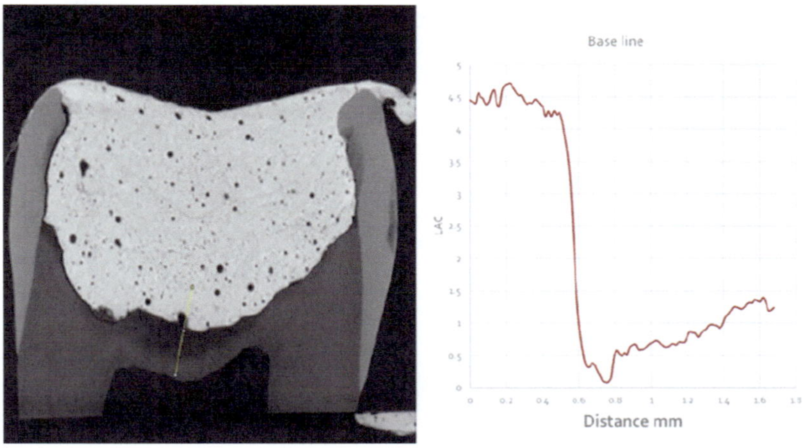

Fig. 10.3 XMT image of Tooth1 immediately (0 time)

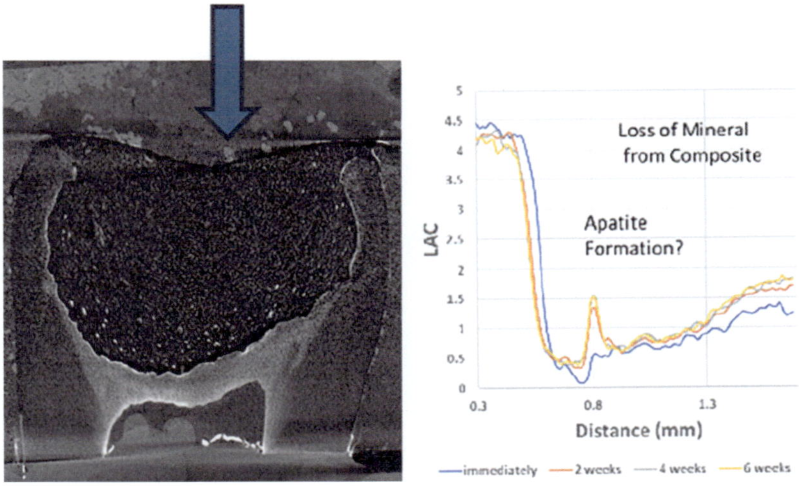

Fig. 10.4 XMT image of Tooth1 difference image at 2 weeks, plus 2-, 4-, and 6-weeks Line Scans). *A* occlusal surface of composite, *B* marginal gap, *C* composite-sound dentine interface, *D* composite carious dentine interface

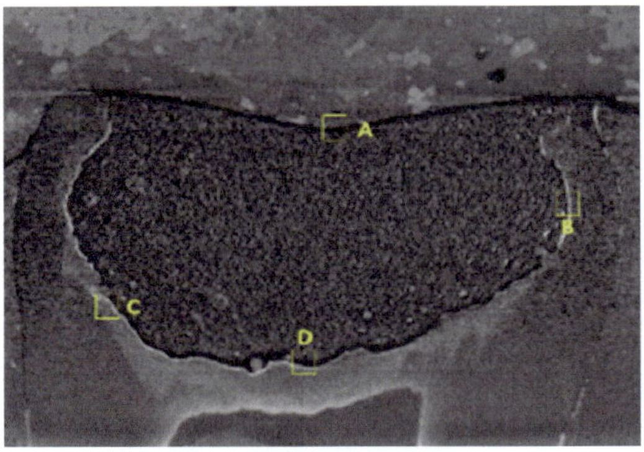

A = Occlusal Surface of Composite. B= Marginal Gap.
C=Composite-Sound Dentine interface
D= Composite Carious Dentine Interface.

Fig. 10.5 After XMT Tooth 1 was cut with a Diamond Saw Polished and Scanning Electron Microscopy carried out the Areas A-D were examined

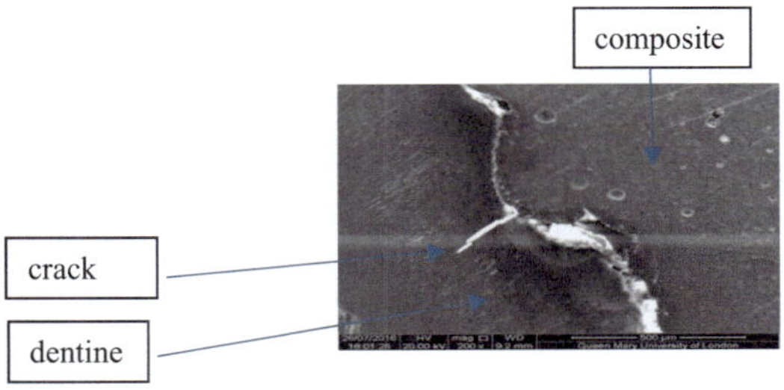

Fig. 10.6 XMT showing apatite forming in the margins and cracks between the dentine and composite

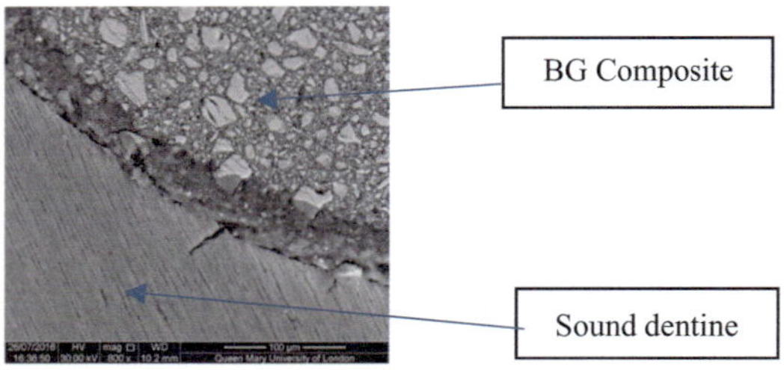

Fig. 10.7 SEM showing sound dentine and the BG composite interface

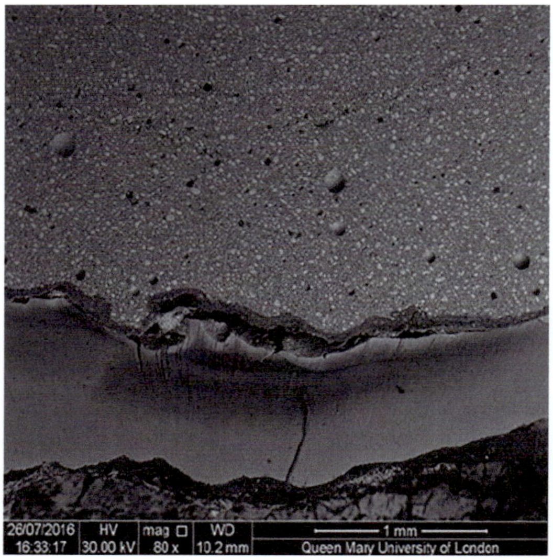

Fig. 10.8 SEM showing the carious dentine BG composite interface

Acknowledgments The authors would like to acknowledge the contributing of our colleagues in the development and evaluation of the novel products currently being developed at QMUL namely: Professor Graham Davis, Professor Mangala Patel, Professor Delia Brauer, Dr. Natalia Karpukhina, Professor Padhraig Fleming, Dr. Saroash Shahid, Dr. Melissa Tiskaya as well as the numerous undergraduate and postgraduate students who have been invaluable in these formative studies.

Future Research

Although the bioactive glasses being developed at QMUL show promise as remineralizing agents, there is a need for further clinical research in well controlled randomized clinical trials.

Disclosure Statement

The authors have one or more patents on the bioactive glass formulations and other oral care products and are currently directors of BioMin Technology Ltd., UK.

References

Al-Eesa NA, Johal A, Hill RG, Wong FSL. Fluoride containing bioactive glass composite for orthodontic adhesives—apatite formation properties. Dent Mater. 2018;34(8):1127–33. https://doi.org/10.1016/j.dental.2018.04.009. Epub 2018 May 17. PMID: 29779628.

Fig. 10.9 In vitro comparison of a leading inert glass orthodontic adhesive (left) with a novel fluorine containing bioactive glass orthodontic adhesive (right). (Premolars with orthodontic brackets after immersion in artificial saliva pH 4)

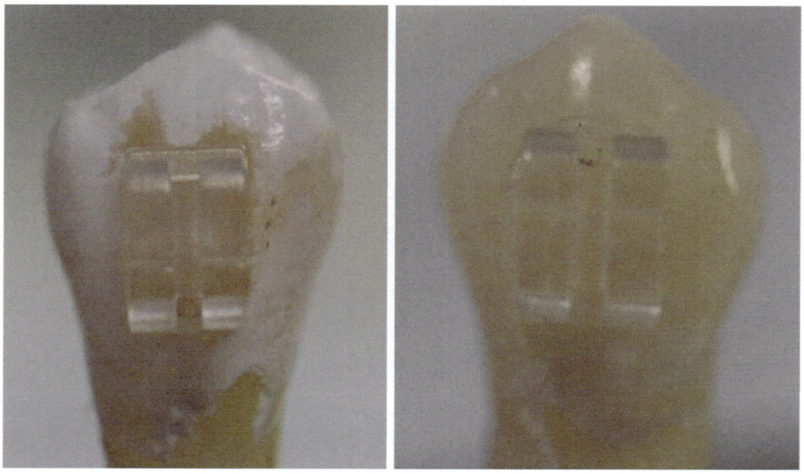

Atteya SM, Amer HA, Saleh SM, Safwat Y. The effect of nano silver fluoride, self-assembling peptide and sodium fluoride varnish on salivary cariogenic bacteria: a randomized controlled clinical trial. Clin Oral Investig. 2024;28(3):167. https://doi.org/10.1007/s00784-024-05562-0. PMID: 38388987; PMCID: PMC10884112.

Bartlett D. The implication of laboratory research on tooth wear and erosion. Oral Dis. 2005;11(1):3–6.

Bossù M, Saccucci M, Salucci A, Di Giorgio G, Bruni E, Uccelletti D, Sarto MS, Familiari G, Relucenti M, Polimeni A. Enamel remineralization and repair results of biomimetic hydroxyapatite toothpaste on deciduous teeth: an effective option to fluoride toothpaste. J Nanobiotechnoly. 2019;17(1):17. https://doi.org/10.1186/s12951-019-0454-6. PMID: 30683113; PMCID: PMC6346538.

Cardoso CA, Cassiano LP, Costa EN, Souza-E-Silva CM, Magalhães AC, Grizzo LT, Caldana ML, Bastos JR, Buzalaf MA. Effect of xylitol varnishes on remineralization of artificial enamel caries lesions in situ. J Dent. 2016;50:74–8. https://doi.org/10.1016/j.jdent.2016.03.011. Epub 2016 Mar 23. PMID: 27032722.

Crystal YO, Niederman R. Evidence-based dentistry update on silver diamine fluoride. Dent Clin N Am. 2019;63(1):45–68. https://doi.org/10.1016/j.cden.2018.08.011. PMID: 30447792; PMCID: PMC6500430.

De Caluwé T, Vercruysse CW, Ladik I, Convents R, Declercq H, Martens LC, Verbeeck RM. Addition of bioactive glass to glass ionomer cements: effect on the physico-chemical properties and biocompatibility. Dent Mater. 2017;33(4):e186–203. https://doi.org/10.1016/j.dental.2017.01.007. Epub 2017 Feb 10. PMID: 28196604.

Dionysopoulos D, Tolidis K, Sfeikos T. Effect of CPP-ACPF and Nano-hydroxyapatite preventive treatments on the susceptibility of enamel to erosive challenge. Oral Health Prev Dent. 2019;17(4):357–64. https://doi.org/10.3290/j.ohpd.a42690. PMID: 31204397.

Duarte ACA, Pereira RDFC, Carvalho SM, Silva AGD, Araújo CTP, Galo R, Dumont VC. Enhancing glass ionomer cement features by using the calcium phosphate nanocomposite. Braz Dent J. 2022;33(3):99–108. https://doi.org/10.1590/0103-6440202204887. PMID: 35766723; PMCID: PMC9645200.

Ekambaram M, Mohd Said SNB, Yiu CKY. A review of enamel remineralisation potential of calcium- and phosphate-based remineralisation systems. Oral Health Prev Dent. 2017;15(5):415–20. https://doi.org/10.3290/j.ohpd.a38779. PMID: 28785750.

Fernando D, Attik N, Pradelle-Plasse N, Jackson P, Grosgogeat B, Colon P. Bioactive glass for dentin remineralization: a systematic review. Mater Sci Eng C Mater Biol Appl. 2017;76:1369–77. https://doi.org/10.1016/j.msec.2017.03.083. Epub 2017 Mar 14. PMID: 28482504.

Ghilotti J, Mayorga P, Sanz JL, Forner L, Llena C. Remineralizing ability of Resin Modified Glass Ionomers (RMGICs): a systematic review. J Funct Biomater. 2023;14(8):421. https://doi.org/10.3390/jfb14080421. PMID: 37623665; PMCID: PMC10455182.

Godoi FA, Carlos NR, Bridi EC, Amaral FLBD, França FMG, Turssi CP, Kantovitz KR, Basting RT. Remineralizing effect of commercial fluoride varnishes on artificial enamel lesions. Braz Oral Res. 2019;33:e044. https://doi.org/10.1590/1807-3107bor-2019.vol33.0044. PMID: 31141037.

Gohar RAAEG, Ibrahim SH, Safwat OM. Evaluation of the remineralizing effect of biomimetic self-assembling peptides in post-orthodontic white spot lesions compared to fluoride-based delivery systems: randomized controlled trial. Clin Oral Investig. 2023;27(2):613–24. https://doi.org/10.1007/s00784-022-04757-7. Epub 2022 Oct 26. PMID: 36287272; PMCID: PMC9889428.

Golzio B, Navarro Cavalcante, Schulze Wenning A, Szabó B, László Márk C, Hegyi P, Borbély J, Németh O, Bartha K, Gerber G, Varga G. Combined casein phosphopeptide-amorphous calcium phosphate and fluoride is not superior to fluoride alone in early carious lesions: a meta-analysis. Caries Res. 2024;58(1):1–16. https://doi.org/10.1159/000533547. Epub 2023 Oct 26. PMID: 37883928.

Grohe B & Mittler S (2021) Advanced non-fluoride approaches to dental enamel remineralization: The next level in enamel repair management Biomater Biosyst 2021 Oct 29:4:100029. https://doi.org/10.1016/j.bbiosy.2021.100029. eCollection 2021 Dec.

Hoxha A, Gillam DG, Bushby AJ, Agha A, Patel MP. Layered double hydroxide fluoride release in dental applications: a systematic review. Dent J (Basel). 2019;7(3):87. https://doi.org/10.3390/dj7030087. PMID: 31480648; PMCID: PMC6784472.

Hoxha A, Gillam DG, Agha A, Karpukhina N, Bushby AJ, Patel MP. Novel fluoride rechargeable dental composites containing MgAl and CaAl layered double hydroxide (LDH). Dent Mater. 2020;36(8):973–86. https://doi.org/10.1016/j.dental.2020.04.011. Epub 2020 Jun 11. PMID: 32536588.

Kamal D, Hassanein H, Elkassas D, Hamza H. Complementary remineralizing effect of self-assembling peptide (P11-4) with CPP-ACPF or fluoride: an *in vitro* study. J Clin Exp Dent. 2020;12(2):e161–8. https://doi.org/10.4317/jced.56295. PMID: 32071698; PMCID: PMC7018478.

Keeper JH, Kibbe LJ, Thakkar-Samtani M, Heaton LJ, Desrosiers C, Vela K, Amaechi BT, Jablonski-Momeni A, Young DA, MacLean J, Weyant RJ, Zandona AF, Sohn W, Pitts N, Frantsve-Hawley J. Systematic review and meta-analysis on the effect of self-assembling peptide P_{11}-4 on arrest, cavitation, and progression of initial caries lesions. J Am Dent Assoc. 2023;154(7):580–591.e11. https://doi.org/10.1016/j.adaj.2023.03.014. Epub 2023 May 26. PMID: 37245138.

Kobeissi R, Badr SB, Osman E. Effectiveness of self-assembling peptide P_{11}-4 compared to tricalcium phosphate fluoride varnish in remineralization of white spot lesions: a clinical randomized trial. Int J Clin Pediatr Dent. 2020;13(5):451–6. https://doi.org/10.5005/jp-journals-10005-1804. PMID: 33623327; PMCID: PMC7887159.

Li J, Xie X, Wang Y, Yin W, Antoun JS, Farella M, Mei L. Long-term remineralizing effect of casein phosphopeptide-amorphous calcium phosphate (CPP-ACP) on early caries lesions in vivo: a systematic review. J Dent. 2014;42(7):769–77. https://doi.org/10.1016/j.jdent.2014.03.015. Epub 2014 Apr 3. PMID: 24705069.

Llena C, Leyda AM, Forner L. CPP-ACP and CPP-ACFP versus fluoride varnish in remineralisation of early caries lesions. A prospective study. Eur J Paediatr Dent. 2015;16(3):181–6. PMID: 26418918.

Manchanda S, Sardana D, Liu P, Lee GH, Li KY, Lo EC, Yiu CK. Topical fluoride to prevent early childhood caries: systematic review with network meta-analysis. J Dent. 2022;116:103885. https://doi.org/10.1016/j.jdent.2021.103885. Epub 2021 Nov 12. PMID: 34780874.

McReynolds D, Duane B. Systematic review finds that silver diamine fluoride is effective for both root caries prevention and arrest in older adults. Evid Based Dent. 2018;19(2):46–7. https://doi.org/10.1038/sj.ebd.6401304.

Minamata Convention on Mercury; 2013. https://minamataconvention.org/en/about. Accessed 7 July 2024.

Muntean A, Mzoughi SM, Pacurar M, Candrea S, Inchingolo AD, Inchingolo AM, Ferrante L, Dipalma G, Inchingolo F, Palermo A, Bordea IR. Silver diamine fluoride in pediatric dentistry: effectiveness in preventing and arresting dental caries-a systematic review. Children (Basel). 2024;11(4):499. https://doi.org/10.3390/children11040499. PMID: 38671716; PMCID: PMC11049537.

Oliveira BH, Rajendra A, Veitz-Keenan A, Niederman R. The effect of silver diamine fluoride in preventing caries in the primary dentition: a systematic review and meta-analysis. Caries Res. 2019;53(1):24–32. https://doi.org/10.1159/000488686. Epub 2018 Jun 6. PMID: 29874642; PMCID: PMC6292783.

Rahmath Meeral P, Doraikannan S, Indiran MA. Efficiency of casein phosphopeptide amorphous calcium phosphate versus topical fluorides on remineralizing early enamel carious lesions—a systematic review and meta-analysis. Saudi Dent J. 2024;36(4):521–7. https://doi.org/10.1016/j.sdentj.2024.01.014. Epub 2024 Feb 6. PMID: 38690375; PMCID: PMC11056415.

Raszewski Z, Chojnacka K, Mikulewicz M. Investigating bioactive-glass-infused gels for enamel remineralization: an in vitro study. J Funct Biomater. 2024;15(5):119. https://doi.org/10.3390/jfb15050119. PMID: 38786631; PMCID: PMC11122500.

Salah R, Afifi RR, Kehela HA, Aly NM, Rashwan M, Hill RG. Efficacy of novel bioactive glass I the treatment of enamel white spot lesions. A randomised controlled trial. J Evid Based Dent Pract. 2022;22:101725.

Sari M, Ramadhanti DM, Amalina R, Chotimah, Ana ID, Yusuf Y. Development of a hydroxyapatite nanoparticle-based gel for enamel remineralization—a physicochemical properties and cell viability assay analysis. Dent Mater J. 2022;41(1):68–77. https://doi.org/10.4012/dmj.2021-102. Epub 2021 Sep 2. PMID: 34471039.

Shen P, Bagheri R, Walker GD, Yuan Y, Stanton DP, Reynolds C, Reynolds EC. Effect of calcium phosphate addition to fluoride containing dental varnishes on enamel demineralization. Aust Dent J. 2016;61(3):357–65. https://doi.org/10.1111/adj.12385. PMID: 26541509.

Shen P, McKeever A, Walker GD, Yuan Y, Reynolds C, Fernando JR, Chen YY, MacRae CM, Schneider P, Reynolds EC. Remineralization and fluoride uptake of white spot lesions under dental varnishes. Aust Dent J. 2020;65(4):278–85. https://doi.org/10.1111/adj.12787. Epub 2020 Aug 5. PMID: 32678914.

Tejani TH, Milosevic A, Patel M, Gillam D. The effect of layered double hydroxide on fluoride release and recharge from a commercial and an experimental resin varnish. Dent Mater. 2022;38(1):e1–9. https://doi.org/10.1016/j.dental.2021.10.002. Epub 2021 Nov 8. PMID: 34763905.

Taha AA, Patel MP, Hill RG, Fleming PS The effect of bioactive glasses on enamel remineralization: A systematic review Journal of Dentistry 2017;67:9–17 https://doi.org/10.1016/j.jdent.2017.09.007.

Tiskaya M, Shahid S, Gillam D, Hill R. The use of bioactive glass (BAG) in dental composites: a critical review. Dent Mater. 2021;37(2):296–310. https://doi.org/10.1016/j.dental.2020.11.015. Epub 2021 Jan 10. PMID: 33441250.

Wei SL, Lin DJ, Yen UJ. Novel dental resin composites containing LiAl-F layered double hydroxide (LDH) filler: fluoride release/recharge, mechanical properties, color change, and cytotoxicity. Dent Mater. 2019;35(5):663–72. https://doi.org/10.1016/j.dental.2019.02.002. Epub 2019 Mar 5. PMID: 30850280.

West NX, Sanz M, Lussi A, Bartlett D, Bouchard P, Bourgeois D. Prevalence of dentine hypersensitivity and study of associated factors: a European population-based cross-sectional study. J Dent. 2013;41(10):841–51.

Wierichs RJ, Carvalho TS, Wolf TG. Efficacy of a self-assembling peptide to remineralize initial caries lesions—a systematic review and meta-analysis. J Dent. 2021;109:103652. https://doi.org/10.1016/j.jdent.2021.103652. Epub 2021 Mar 30. PMID: 33798639.

Wierichs RJ, Wolf TG, Campus G, Carvalho TS. Efficacy of nano-hydroxyapatite on caries prevention-a systematic review and meta-analysis. Clin Oral Investig. 2022;26(4):3373–81. https://doi.org/10.1007/s00784-022-04390-4. Epub 2022 Feb 1. PMID: 35103837; PMCID: PMC8979882.

Xie Z, Yu L, Li S, Li J, Liu Y. Comparison of therapies of white spot lesions: a systematic review and network meta-analysis. BMC Oral Health. 2023;23(1):346. https://doi.org/10.1186/s12903-023-03076-x. PMID: 37264364; PMCID: PMC10233982.

Zero DT, Lussi A. Erosion—chemical and biological factors of importance to the dental practitioner. Int Dent J. 2005;55(4 Suppl 1):285–90.

Closing Remarks Quo Vadis? 11

David G. Gillam

There's no end to the publishing of books, and constant study wears you out so you're no good for anything else. (Ecclesiastes 12:12)

The main purpose of the 2015 book was to provide an overview on DH to both educate and update readers on the latest research results regarding the development of new products and any advances in clinical management strategies and perhaps more importantly for clinicians the implications for everyday clinical practice. However, there has been considerable research undertaken in the last decade since the publication in 2015. There is no doubt, however, that for both the hard-pressed researcher and the busy clinician, the problem of both diagnosing and managing dentine hypersensitivity (DH) continues to challenge both the clinician and the researcher to develop new strategies and new products to treat the condition. As Gottfried Schmalz indicated in the foreword of the book, the topic of DH has attracted considerable interest in recent years as demonstrated by the number of publications listed in the published literature. This observation concurs with the earlier concerns of Emling (1982) who indicted that:

> There may well be no single phenomenon in all of science which has occupied so much attention over so much time and yielded so few results as dentin hypersensitivity. Its causes have remained obscured throughout the existence of mankind (Emling 1982).

D. G. Gillam (✉)
Centre for Oral Bioengineering, Institute of Dentistry, Barts and the London School of Medicine and Dentistry, Queen Mary University of London, London, UK
e-mail: d.g.gillam@qmul.ac.uk

The question may, however, arise, why write another book on DH? Perhaps the reader will have some sympathy with the exhortation expressed by Solomon in the book of Ecclesiastes regarding the need of researchers to constantly study and publish the outcomes of their labours. There is no doubt, however, that previously, as indicated in Chap. 1, there were concerns expressed by both researchers and clinicians regarding the apparent lack of knowledge and understanding of the condition, and in particular, the terminology used to define DH (Emling 1982; Johnson et al. 1982; Dababneh et al. 1997). Nevertheless, as Addy and Gillam indicated in Chap. 1, there have been considerable advances in both the knowledge and understanding regarding DH in recent years and yet as expressed by the various contributors in this book there are still areas of research and clinical practice that need to be addressed. For example, the question of the role of pulpal inflammation in DH is still relatively unclear and somewhat controversial (Dababneh et al. 1997) and there are questions relating to whether the Hydrodynamic Theory can explain all aspects of stimulus transfer to the pulp (see Chap. 5). The role of the odontoblast in DH is also enigmatic, most published texts have consigned its role to the past and yet as Markowitz and Pashley (2008) have indicated that following more recent evidence this require a reappraisal of

D. G. Gillam (ed.), *Dentine Hypersensitivity*, https://doi.org/10.1007/978-3-031-74321-4_11

its role (see Chap. 6). Furthermore, according to Markowitz and Pashley (2008) although there was evidence to suggest that by increasing dentine permeability teeth become more sensitive, however, what is uncertain is the degree to which dentine permeability needs to be reduced to effectively desensitize teeth.

The question as to whether the true prevalence of DH is reported in the published literature has also been addressed (see Chap. 2) and there appears to be confusion with what is exactly being reported. For example, there are a wide range of values from the questionnaire and clinically based studies and where the studies were conducted (e.g., general or private practice, university/hospital, patients with or without periodontal disease, consumer based, etc.). Furthermore, the methodology used when conducting these studies also varies and therefore there appears a need for more consistent and reproducible methodology when reporting the prevalence of DH. One of the problems that has also caused controversy was the redefining of DH and root sensitivity (RS) (Sanz and Addy 2002), although to date there does not appear to be any published studies that have separated the precise prevalence values based on the treatment history of these individuals to distinguishing the two clinical aspects of tooth sensitivity. Perhaps another development in terminology as discussed in Chap. 1 by Marin Addy and David Gillam is the potential confusion when diagnosing clinical conditions that have similar pain features to Dentine Hypersensitivity. Perhaps this is an area that merits further discussion.

Undoubtedly there are several diagnostic challenges facing the busy clinician when examining patients complaining of dental pain in general, and more specifically with DH (Gillam 2013). For example, (1) are clinicians under or overestimating the problem, (2) is the condition being adequately diagnosed and successfully managed by clinicians in daily practice, (3) are clinicians aware of the impact (real or imagined) on the quality of life (QOL) (see also Chap. 3) in patients complaining with DH, and (4) is the condition adequately monitored by clinicians in daily practice. According to Gillam (2013) clinicians do not routinely screen/examine their patients for DH unless the patient prompts them, and this practice therefore needs to be reconsidered.

These questions have, however, been addressed by Ryan Olley and David Bartlett (see Chap. 4) although it should be acknowledged that a thorough clinical examination with a detailed medical and dental history may not only take time but may also challenge the clinician to provide an accurate differential diagnosis of DH within the constraints of a busy dental practice. It may therefore be suggested that consideration should be made to incorporating the various relevant aetiological factors and predisposing features implicated in the initiation and development of DH by recording dietary histories, clinical evidence of tooth wear (e.g., BEWE scores), clinical models (from impressions), and photographs, pain and QOL scores, etc. in the patient's clinical record (see Chaps. 4 and 8).

From the published literature, there are a plethora of recommended products and treatments that have been claimed to be successful for treating DH, nevertheless, there has been inconsistencies in the design and methodology of in vitro, in situ and in vivo models used by researchers. For example, it is very difficult to mimic the oral environment in the laboratory environment and care should therefore be taken not to extrapolate the results from the in vitro studies into the clinical environment.

Nevertheless, as Victor Mosquim and colleagues have indicated in Chap. 7, the in vitro investigation of an experimental desensitizing product may provide evidence of the potential effectiveness in successfully blocking the dentine tubules when the product is applied onto the dentine surface. The question however arises as to whether these in vitro models (including laboratory methodology, e.g., scanning electron microscopy, etc.) are suitable for evaluating all potential desensitizing agents, for example potassium containing toothpastes may not provide evidence of the mechanism of action of potassium in a dentine disk section (see Chap. 7). Furthermore, most if not all the OTC toothpastes require the interaction of saliva to enable the ingredients to be precipitated onto the tooth surface and if saliva is not incorporated into the experimental design, would the precipitated deposit be like that deposited in the oral environment. It should be noted however, that the development of a desensitizing product from concept through to the introduction of the product into the professional or consumer market is a lengthy and well-regulated process and depending on the specific claims made for the product (e.g., medicinal claims) may also involve exacting regulatory oversight (e.g., USA Food and Drug Administration [FDA] and the Medicines and Healthcare Products Regulatory Agency [MHRA], UK) prior to its acceptance as a desensitizing product. The development and evaluation of current, novel and future products designed to treat DH either from an In-Office or over-the-counter perspective has been addressed in Chaps. 7, 9 and 10, and there is no doubt that there is currently more emphasis in developing new biomimetic materials for the remineralizing of both enamel and dentine (Chap. 10). For example, the development of bioactive glass (calcium phospho-silicate or bioactive glass toothpastes), self-assembling peptides, Protease inhibitors, functionalized tricalcium phosphate (f TCP) and polymer-induced liquid-precursors (PILP), etc., for possible dental applications including remineralization, anti-caries, and tubule occlusion (Niu et al. 2014, see Chaps. 7, 9, and 10). However, for the clinician, the availability of the number of these products that are available for treating DH are somewhat overwhelming and to some extent has caused a degree of confusion as to which product was the most appropriate to use. It is also evident that rather than enabling the clinician to be more aware of the appropriate use of these products, the converse may be true in that clinicians have reported a lack of confidence when using these products when treating DH (Cuhna-Cruz et al. 2010). The question that may therefore be considered is whether the clinician's awareness of desensitizing products was (1) based on a commercial or marketing perspective that was driven by the industry literature, (2) based on personal exposure or awareness from colleagues in the practice environment or (3) derived from personal reading of the evidence-based clinical studies published in the literature. In fairness to the busy clinician, it may be unreasonable to expect them to spend hours reading papers or attending lectures without the hands-on experience of using these materials under supervision. The onus therefore may be for both Industry and Academia to provide more appropriate and practical guidelines for treating DH in clinical practice (see Chap. 8).

There are, however, several problems that may, however, be encountered by the clinician when evaluating the efficacy of a desensitizing product in the clinical environment as previously addressed by Curro and Gillam (2015). From a historical perspective (pre-1997), these studies have been criticized for the lack of homogeneity in the methodology used to evaluate DH and in the study design per se (Cummins 2010). Following the recommendations of Holland et al. (1997), it was evident that there were improvements in terms of the controls used as well as in the objective methodology employed in the studies. However, Curro and Gillam (2015) indicated the clinical outcomes from these studies were not person-centred in nature and therefore failed to address the impact of the clinical outcomes from the subject's perspective. More recently there has been a greater emphasis of the impact of DH on the quality of life (QoL) of those individuals who experience pain associated with DH and no doubt these measures will increasingly be included in the study design of clinical trials (Robinson 2014, see also Chap. 3).

The shift of a top-down practitioner-centred model to a person-centred model as indicated in Chaps. 3 and 8 may therefore have implications not only for research but also for the clinical management of the condition. The emphasis in the future evaluation and management of DH should there involve the individual in the development of (1) the clinical trial process and (2) the management and treatment strategies. This undoubtedly will mean a change in the mind set of both the clinician and the individual in the clinical trial and practice environment, for example the clinician should take steps to include the individual in the research and treatment process and the individual needs in return to be fully motivated and compliant (see Chap. 8).

Furthermore, as indicated by Gillam et al. (2013) the management of DH should not be simply providing an In-office prescription/procedure or an OTC product without first removing any aetiological factor associated with DH and providing the necessary advice to minimize any future detrimental effects on the hard and soft tissues (see Chaps. 4 and 8). In other words, one of the most importance aspects in the management of DH is the education of both the clinician and individual under treatment. It is also important to emphasis to the clinician that there is no-one treatment therapy for all the problems associated with DH and that the condition should be monitored depending on the extent and severity of the problem (Orchardson and Gillam 2006; Gillam et al. 2013; Gillam 2017).

There have also been some interesting developments in developing novel and innovative products to treat Dentine Hypersensitivity (as discussed in Chaps. 7, 9 and 10), particularly with the development of bioactive glasses in toothpastes, prophylaxis polishing pastes, air abrasion powders and more recently in dental composite materials. It is evident that as discussed in Chaps. 4 and 9 there is an abundance of both in vitro and in vivo evidence for the effectiveness of these products in treating Dentine Hypersensitivity. The question proposed in Chap. 9 by Robert Hill and David Gillam is what constitutes an ideal desensitizing product. According to these authors, such a product should have (1) the ability to adhere to dental tissues, (2) provide a controlled release of ions such as Ca, P, F to improve protection of the tooth surface, (3) provide smaller particle size (e.g., 5 microns average) to enable penetration into the dentinal tubule, (4) have the capability to dissolve faster at a lower pH to protect the tooth against acid dissolution (dental erosion) and restore the pH balance in the mouth, (5) provide the formation of an acid resistant fluorapatite on the tooth surface. The ideal product should also be n toxic and pleasant to use. It should be noted, however, as discussed by David Gillam and Christoph Ramseier in Chap. 8 that simply providing a treatment (e.g., toothpaste) or procedure without (1) resolving the aetiological features that were responsible for the problem of Dentine Hypersensitivity or (2) putting into place a maintenance programme including dietary advice and control (e.g., reduction of acidic food and drinks) and oral hygiene advice to modify toothbrushing techniques, etc. will not resolve the patient's clinical problem in the long term.

Although most of these products were originally designed to treat Dentine Hypersensitivity, there does appear to be a shift in treating acid erosion and to some extent remineralization of the early caries lesion. The question as to whether dental erosion should be considered the main aetiological and subsequently considered a separate clinical condition from Dentine Hypersensitivity is interesting and may be worthwhile discussing particularly when the aetiological factors are virtually the same for both conditions.

11.1 Summary

There is always the temptation when reviewing the literature to be very selective in one's interpretation in what has been previously described and it is evident that the topic of DH has been thoroughly discussed in numerous publications and journals. The authors of this book have however, not ignored the valuable contributions of those researchers and clinicians who have made a major impact on our understanding of the condition. There have been major improvements in our understanding in both the development of new products as well as improvements in the clinical management of DH although it is important to recognize that as we consider and implement these changes, there are still challenges to be overcome in the future.

Obtundants have been tried by hundreds of dentists and then faded out of the memory of men. Such has been the fate of every obtundant for sensitive dentine, except for a few now on trial, that have come forward during 70 or more years of clinical practice. But the relief of suffering is an ever-present duty and the search for this very desirable thing should continue (Black 1908).

References

Black GV. The pathology of the hard tissues of the teeth. In: A work of operative dentistry in two volumes, vol. 1. Chicago: Chicago Medico-dental publishing Co; 1908. p. 149–50.

Cummins D. Recent advances in dentin hypersensitivity: clinically proven treatments for instant and lasting sensitivity relief. Am J Dent. 2010;23(Spec A):3A–13A.

Cunha-Cruz J, Wataha JC, Zhou L, Manning W, Trantow M, Bettendorf MM, Heaton LJ, Berg J. Treating dentin hypersensitivity: therapeutic choices made by dentists of the northwest PRECEDENT network. J Am Dent Assoc. 2010;141(9):1097–105.

Curro FA, Gillam DG. Chapter 7: Challenging the traditional approach to the conduct of dentine hypersensitivity studies: person-centric studies connecting the patient with their practitioner to optimize the clinical outcome. In: Gillam DG, editor. Dentine hypersensitivity: advances in diagnosis, management, and treatment. Cham: Springer; 2015. p. 85–99. https://doi.org/10.1007/978-3-319-14577-8.

Dababneh RH, Khouri AT, Addy M. Dentine hypersensitivity—an enigma? A review of terminology, mechanisms, aetiology and management. Br Dent J. 1997;187(11):606–11. discussion 603

Emling RC. Historical overview of causes and treatment of dental hypersensitivity. Compend Contin Educ Dent Suppl. 1982;3:92–4.

Gillam D. Current diagnosis of dentin hypersensitivity in the dental office: an overview. Clin Oral Investig. 2013;17(Suppl 1):21–9.

Gillam DG. A New Perspective on Dentine Hypersensitivity – Guidelines for General Dental Practice. Dent Update. 2017;44(1):33–6, 39–42. https://doi.org/10.12968/denu.2017.44.1.33. PMID: 29172308.

Gillam D, Chesters R, Attrill D, Brunton P, Slater M, Strand P, Whelton H, Bartlett D. Dentine hypersensitivity—guidelines for the management of a common oral health problem. Dent Update. 2013;40(7):514–6, 518–20, 523–4.

Holland GR, Narhi MN, Addy M, Gangarosa L, Orchardson R. Guidelines for the design and conduct of clinical trials on dentine hypersensitivity. J Clin Periodontol. 1997;24(11):808–13.

Johnson RH, Zulqar-Nain BJ, Koval JJ. The effectiveness of an electro-ionizing toothbrush in the control of dentinal hypersensitivity. J Periodontol. 1982;53:353–9.

Markowitz, K. and D. H. Pashley. Discovering new treatments for sensitive teeth: the long path from biology to therapy. J Oral Rehabil. 2008;35(4):300–15.

Niu LN, Zhang W, Pashley DH, Breschi L, Mao J, Chen JH, Tay FR. Biomimetic remineralization of dentin. Dent Mater. 2014;30(1):77–96.

Orchardson R, Gillam DG. Managing dentin hypersensitivity. J Am Dent Assoc. 2006;137(7):990–8. quiz 1028-9

Peterson EH. Ecclesiastes 12:12 from THE MESSAGE: The Bible in contemporary language; 2002. © 2002 by Eugene H. Peterson. All rights reserved.

Robinson PG. In: Robinson PG, editor. Dentine hypersensitivity, developing a person-centred approach to Oral health. 1st ed. New York: Academic Press, Elsevier B.V; 2014.

Sanz M, Addy M. Group D summary. J Clin Periodontol. 2002;29(supplement 3):195–6.

MIX
Papier aus verantwortungsvollen Quellen
Paper from responsible sources
FSC® C105338

If you have any concerns about our products,
you can contact us on
ProductSafety@springernature.com

In case Publisher is established outside the EU,
the EU authorized representative is:
Springer Nature Customer Service Center GmbH
Europaplatz 3, 69115 Heidelberg, Germany

Printed by Libri Plureos GmbH
in Hamburg, Germany